Inpatient Behavior Therapy for Children and Adolescents

Inpatient Behavior Therapy for Children and Adolescents

Edited by

VINCENT B. VAN HASSELT

Center for Psychological Studies
Nova University
Fort Lauderdale, Florida

AND

DAVID J. KOLKO

Western Psychiatric Institute and Clinic
University of Pittsburgh School of Medicine
Pittsburgh, Pennsylvania

PLENUM PRESS • NEW YORK AND LONDON

Library of Congress Cataloging-in-Publication Data

Inpatient behavior therapy for children and adolescents / edited by
Vincent B. Van Hasselt and David J. Kolko.
p. cm.
Includes bibliographical references and index.
ISBN 0-306-44079-2
1. Behavior therapy for children. 2. Behavior therapy for
teenagers. 3. Child psychotherapy--Residential treatment.
4. Adolescent psychotherapy--Residential treatment. I. Kolko,
David J. II. Van Hasselt, Vincent B.
[DNLM: 1. Behavior Therapy--in adolescence. 2. Behavior Therapy-
-in infancy & childhood. 3. Behavior Therapy--methods.
4. Institutionalization. WS 350.6 I583]
RJ505.B4I55 1992
618.92'89142--dc20
DNLM/DLC
for Library of Congress 92-14198
CIP

ISBN 0-306-44079-2

A Division of Plenum Publishing Corporation
233 Spring Street, New York, N.Y. 10013

Printed in the United States of America

To the memory of my grandparents—Helen and Rudolph
—VVH

To my grandparents—Esther, Reuben, Ada, and Hyman
—DJK

Contributors

ROWLAND P. BARRETT, Department of Psychiatry and Human Behavior, Brown University School of Medicine, Emma Pendleton Bradley Hospital, East Providence, Rhode Island 02915

CHRIS BRADEN, Department of Psychiatry and Human Behavior, University of California, Irvine Medical Center, Orange, California 92668

OSCAR G. BUKSTEIN, Department of Psychiatry, Western Psychiatric Institute and Clinic, 3811 O'Hara Street, Pittsburgh, Pennsylvania 15213

GABRIELLE A. CARLSON, Department of Psychiatry and Behavioral Science, State University of New York at Stony Brook, Stony Brook, New York 11794-8790

WALTER P. CHRISTIAN, The May Institute, Inc., 100 Sea View Street, Chatham, Massachusetts 02633

JOHN F. CURRY, Department of Psychiatry, Duke University Medical Center, Durham, North Carolina 27710

C. J. DAVIS, Department of Psychology, Louisiana State University, Baton Rouge, Louisiana 70803-5501

MICHAEL J. DOLGIN, Children's Hospital of Los Angeles, and University of Southern California, Los Angeles, California 90089-1061

ERICH G. DUCHMANN, Department of Psychology, Louisiana State University, Baton Rouge, Louisiana 70803-5501

CARL FEINSTEIN, Department of Psychiatry and Human Behavior, Brown University School of Medicine, Emma Pendleton Bradley Hospital, East Providence, Rhode Island 02915

GRETA FRANCIS, Department of Psychiatry and Human Behavior, Brown University School of Medicine, Emma Pendleton Bradley Hospital, East Providence, Rhode Island 02915

JACK FUNDANISH, Attention and Conduct Evaluation Service, Western Psychiatric Institute and Clinic, 3811 O'Hara Street, Pittsburgh, Pennsylvania 15213

KATHLEEN J. HART, Department of Psychology, Xavier University, Cincinnati, Ohio 45207

YIFRAH KAMINER, Center for Alcohol and Addictions Studies, Brown University, and Adolescent Substance Abuse Intervention Center, Emma Pendleton Bradley Hospital, East Providence, Rhode Island 02915

MARGARET KLITZKE, Department of Psychiatry and Human Behavior, Brown University School of Medicine, Emma Pendleton Bradley Hospital, East Providence, Rhode Island 02915

DAVID J. KOLKO, Western Psychiatric Institute and Clinic, University of Pittsburgh School of Medicine, 3811 O'Hara Street, Pittsburgh, Pennsylvania 15213

LINDA L. LOAR, Association for Children and Adults with Learning Disabilities, 4900 Girard Road, Pittsburgh, Pennsylvania 15227

JOHN E. LOCHMAN, Department of Psychiatry, Duke University Medical Center, Durham, North Carolina 27710

STEPHEN C. LUCE, The May Institute, Inc., 100 Sea View Street, Chatham, Massachusetts 02633

JOHN J. McGONIGLE, Department of Psychiatry, Allegheny Neuropsychiatric Institute, 7777 Steubenville Pike, Oakdale, Pennsylvania 15071

ARTHUR F. MERCURIO, Department of Psychiatry and Human Behavior, Brown University School of Medicine, Emma Pendleton Bradley Hospital, East Providence, Rhode Island 02915

CAROLY S. PATAKI, Department of Psychiatry and Behavioral Science, State University of New York at Stony Brook, Stony Brook, New York 11794-8790

MARK D. RAPPORT, Department of Psychology, University of Hawaii, Honolulu, Hawaii 96822

RICHARD R. RUMER, Department of Psychiatry, Duke University Medical Center, Durham, North Carolina 27710

LAWRENCE J. SIEGEL, Ferkauf Graduate School of Psychology, Yeshiva University, Bronx, New York 10416

JOSEPH STRAYHORN, Medical College of Pennsylvania, Allegheny General Hospital, Early Childhood Clinic, Pittsburgh, Pennsylvania 15212

VINCENT B. VAN HASSELT, Center for Psychological Studies, Nova University, Fort Lauderdale, Florida 33314

JAMES W. VARNI, Orthopaedic Hospital, and University of Southern California, Los Angeles, California 90089-1061

GARY A. WALCO, Schneider Children's Hospital of Long Island Jewish Medical Center, and Albert Einstein College of Medicine, New Hyde Park, New York 11042

ANNE S. WALTERS, Department of Psychiatry and Human Behavior, Brown University School of Medicine, Emma Pendleton Bradley Hospital, East Providence, Rhode Island 02915

KAREN J. WHITE, Department of Psychology, University of Notre Dame, St. Joseph, Indiana 46556

DONALD A. WILLIAMSON, Department of Psychology, Louisiana State University, Baton Rouge, Louisiana 70803-5501

Preface

Behavior therapists on child and adolescent psychiatric inpatient units have played an increasing role in the treatment of a wide range of disorders. Indeed, behavioral assessment and treatment strategies in these settings have been applied to a diversity of problems, including depression, mental retardation, autism, conduct disorders, attention-deficit hyperactivity disorder, anorexia, and bulimia. More recently, the heuristic value of behavioral methods with substance abuse, pediatric pain, and child maltreatment has been documented as well. Because of the multifaceted and complex challenges posed by children and adolescents who reach inpatient units, behavioral clinicians have worked closely with other professionals (e.g., psychiatrists, social workers, psychiatric nurses) in an effort to provide broad-spectrum, comprehensive intervention. However, as a burgeoning body of clinical research attests, the significant contribution of behavior therapy to successful treatment outcome is now indisputable.

Yet, surprisingly few texts have been published concerning inpatient treatment of children and adolescents. The few extant efforts in this area have not covered the broad array of issues and diagnostic populations treated, nor have they considered the pragmatic day-to-day difficulties encountered by behaviorally oriented practitioners working in child and adolescent inpatient settings. This text is an attempt to remedy such shortcomings by providing a comprehensive yet practical approach to the functions of behavior therapists on inpatient psychiatric services for children and youth.

The book is divided into four parts, with Part I (General Issues) consisting of a historical overview, an analysis of staff training and consultation, and a description of the medical aspects of care. Parts II and III deal with the treatment of children and adolescents, respectively. Each of the nine chapters in these sections includes a precise clinical description of the disorder, a discussion of how to evaluate it behaviorally and psychiatrically, presentation of behavioral treatments and their frequent integration with psychopharmacologic approaches, case illustrations, and a discussion of specific problem areas. Finally, Part IV (Special Topics) considers the topics of child abuse, academic and educational aspects of inpatient treatment, and the role of social and family work, all of which cut across the disorders covered in the previous two parts.

Many people have contributed their time and effort to the development and production of this volume. We would first like to thank our colleagues who agreed that this book was needed and who willingly contributed chapters. Next, we would like to extend our appreciation to Tracey Eck, Jane A. Null, and Maria Smith for their technical assistance in preparation of the volume. Finally, we thank our friends at Plenum for their willingness to undertake this project and for their assistance and skill in all aspects of production.

Vincent B. Van Hasselt, Ph.D.
Fort Lauderdale, Florida

David J. Kolko, Ph.D.
Pittsburgh, Pennsylvania

Contents

PART I: GENERAL ISSUES

PART II: TREATMENT OF CHILDREN

PART III: TREATMENT OF ADOLESCENTS

I

General Issues

1

Historical Overview

DAVID J. KOLKO

INTRODUCTION

Inpatient psychiatric services for children and adolescents have been in full operation since the 1920s (see American Psychiatric Association, 1957). Following World War I, three facilities opened to provide medical and psychiatric care for children with postencephalitic behavior disorders: the Children's Ward of Bellevue Psychiatric Hospital (New York, New York), the Children's Service at Kings Park State Hospital (Kings Park, New York), and the Franklin School (Philadelphia, Pennsylvania). Soon thereafter, residential programs were established for primarily delinquent populations, notably, the Aichorn Institution in Vienna and the Psychopathic Institute of the Jewish Hospital in Cincinnati. These services attempted to provide an environment in which troubled youth could be cared for and raised, managed, and trained.

The findings and experiences that emerged from this period actually helped to highlight among these youthful populations the potential interferences in their development and personality caused by institutional care and, thus, provided the impetus for psychiatric treatment for children with emotional problems. At that time, the primary reasons for the growth in residential psychiatric treatment centers included the fol-

DAVID J. KOLKO • Western Psychiatric Institute and Clinic, University of Pittsburgh School of Medicine, 3811 O'Hara Street, Pittsburgh, Pennsylvania 15213.

Inpatient Behavior Therapy for Children and Adolescents, edited by Vincent B. Van Hasselt and David J. Kolko. Plenum Press, New York, 1992.

lowing: (1) lack of sufficient impact of outpatient child guidance clinics, (2) parental inability to implement programs at home, (3) the perception that skilled psychotherapists were needed to effect improvements, (4) recognition of the need to provide specialized treatments for children, and (5) the evolution of the concept of milieu therapy and attendant findings which suggested the feasibility of residential treatment. In the 1940s, these developments were associated with the establishment of residential programs with either university or private affiliations across the country. This decade in which an emphasis was placed upon prosocial habit training with primarily delinquent populations gave way to a more balanced appreciation for the mental health needs of children and the nature of their emotional disturbances, before giving rise to the development of the community mental health system (Rivlin & Wolfe, 1985). By the early 1970s, community centers routinely provided inpatient or hospitalization services for children. The number of such programs has increased until the present.

A brief review of selected considerations used by the American Psychiatric Association in 1956 provides a context in which to appreciate the need for inpatient psychiatric treatment programs. For example, the typical profiles of cases seen in four hospitals in 1955 were as follows: chronic brain syndromes, mental deficiency, personality disorders, psychoneurotic disorders, psychotic disorders, and transient situational personality disorders (see American Psychiatric Association, 1957, p. 137). Although some of these disorders may not be as common on today's inpatient units, many of the goals, principles, and practices described in the association's initial "needs assessment," conducted nearly 35 years ago, are clearly contemporary. Six major elements of treatment were identified: parent participation, a therapeutic atmosphere, individual psychotherapy, somatic therapies, education, and medical services. Current programs may differ in their emphasis of specific elements, but the majority generally attempt to incorporate all six elements.

Of course, there are several differences between early and current perspectives on residential and inpatient treatment. As noted by Chelimsky (1985), residential care institutions are less likely today to view corporal punishment as a legitimate therapeutic measure. In addition, current trends suggest a reduction in the number of young children in residential programs, but an increase in voluntary commitments, juvenile court involvement, private sector support, and adoption of a mental health perspective governing the treatment of children. The number of mentally ill or emotionally disturbed children referred for residential psychiatric treatment almost doubled between the years 1966 and 1981 (cf. Chelimsky, 1985, p. 5). The 10 most common problems manifested by children in residential care facilities in 1981 were: family problems, peer problems, delinquency, status offenses, depression, property crimes, history of abuse, learning problems, drugs and alcohol, and violence. Predictors of placement in residential care included a history of criminal behavior or status offenses, prior residential experiences, a history of abuse, violent behavior, and Medicaid eligibility. Such problems clearly underscore the difficulties associated with the individual child and the family system.

The Growth in Inpatient Psychiatric Units

The past few decades have witnessed significant developments in the general field of child psychiatry, including diagnostic instruments, methods of evaluation, and psychopharmacologic intervention (American Academy of Child Psychiatry, 1983). Such improvements have been closely tied to advances in training and research sophistication that address the many unique issues that arise in the inpatient treatment enterprise (Rancurello, 1987). In an effort to integrate some of these developments and issues, I first will briefly review some of the primary reasons for the growth and use of inpatient psychiatric units for children and adolescents.

Inpatient units have paralleled the development of more specialized psychiatric services for child populations in general. Experience suggests that children require different inpatient programs than do adults in light of differences in developmental sophistication, legal status, and family context. There is also greater recognition of the need for specialized care for specific types of child problems. A second reason implicates developments achieved in our understanding of the severity and chronicity of child psychiatric disorders. Aspects of the clinical picture of children with depression, hyperactivity and attentional problems, and conduct problems or antisocial behavior have been examined in empirical studies. Recent research has begun to document the characteristics, correlates, biological underpinnings, and courses of these conditions, suggesting in all three cases a greater continuity across time or chronicity than was previously understood (see Barkley, Fischer, Edelbrock, & Smallish, 1990; Kazdin, 1987; Kovacs, Feinberg, Crouse-Novak, Paulauskas, & Finkelstein, 1984).

A related improvement concerns the identification and evaluation of newer methods of management and treatment. Specialized pharmacological agents and, to some extent, psychosocial interventions, provide a more diverse and balanced approach toward the resolution of severe behavioral and emotional problems during an intensive, albeit brief, hospital stay. The inpatient setting offers multiple opportunities for therapeutic contact, for monitoring of dangerous or disturbing symptomatology, and for decision-making as to follow-up and disposition (Grizenko & Sayegh, 1990). Psychotropic medications, such as lithium and imipramine, can be used efficaciously in the treatment of several serious psychiatric disorders. Accordingly, there may be greater confidence that inpatient treatment has clinical merit. A final consideration involves the growing need to provide specialized programming for psychiatrically disturbed children who are victims of severe family dysfunction, instability, or chaos. Such children, many of whom have been physically and/or sexually abused, or neglected, often require at least short-term intervention and disposition planning (see Gabel & Shindledecker, 1990). Providing for their protection from hostile and damaging family interactions and advocating for their placement out of the home are, unfortunately, becoming part of the routine services provided by hospital staff. Although the tools and tactics have expanded, so too have the personal tragedies that surround a child's admission.

CURRENT FUNCTIONS AND PRACTICES

Historically, the inpatient unit has evolved from a long-term care facility to a clinical environment that is designed to achieve gains in patient adjustment and functioning following brief exposure to an intensive therapeutic regimen. In many instances, the need to bolster parent and family functioning is a notable precipitant of psychiatric hospitalization. Of course, there are several specialized functions that may be fulfilled on the inpatient psychiatric unit (see Jemerin & Philips, 1988; Nurcombe, 1989; Woolston, 1989a). For purposes of illustration, some of these functions are annotated using recent advances and applications in this section.

Specialized Assessment/Evaluation

Standardized Comparisons. Various assessment and diagnostic functions are served during inpatient hospitalization that are otherwise more difficult to perform on an outpatient basis. Methods for more accurately documenting and examining individual problems, in particular, are among the most frequently utilized. Use of the parent-reported Child Behavior Checklist (CBCL, Achenbach & Edelbrock, 1983) has allowed for the accumulation of normative data on the range and severity of general psychopathology exhibited by troubled children and adolescents upon admission (Jones, Latkowski, Kircher, & McMahon, 1988). Jones *et al.*, (1988) found that their inpatient sample scored above the 98th percentile on virtually all of the behavior problem factors, notably, the depressed, hyperactive, aggressive, and delinquent factors. Interestingly, this heightened level of severity was found to be true for both males and females. Apart from permitting comparison with both outpatients and nonreferred children, these normative data should facilitate within-group comparisons following discharge that reflect follow-up adjustment. Indeed, recent evidence suggests a significant reduction in CBCL scores at follow-ups of 6 months (McMahon *et al.*, 1984) and at 1 year (Kazdin, 1989; Kazdin & Bass, 1988). Continued applications of standardized assessment measures will be able to document the correlates and predictors of clinically significant scores on the CBCL (Towle & Schwarz, 1987).

Repeated and Multiple Measures. Measures have been administered to provide ongoing and comprehensive assessment of psychiatric symptoms evinced during hospitalization. Repeated measurement of salient symptoms has been a primary function of inpatient treatment as reflected in an early rating scale described by Jenkins & Shoji (1967). Related assessment tools that have been disseminated recently include the Inpatient Global Rating Scale (IGRS) (Conners, 1985) and the Child Behavior Rating Form (CBRF) (Edelbrock, 1985; Kolko, 1988a). Both measures include factors that appear to tap conduct problems, inattention and hyperactivity, and anxiety. However, the IGRS also includes specific factors reflecting mood (e.g., euphoric-active), cognition (e.g., conceptual dysfunction), and somatic functioning, whereas the CBRF includes factors that assess depression/withdrawal, negative self-image/self-injury, compliance/self-control, and positive/adaptive social. Some evidence suggests the reliability and the concurrent and criterion validity of the CBRF (Kolko, 1988a). Continued refinement of these and other measures is needed to enhance treatment planning and prediction of response to treatment (see Overall & Pfefferbaum, 1982; Rapoport, Conners, & Reatig, 1985).

Problem-Focused Assessment and Validation. Inpatient assessment is also directed toward careful problem-focused assessment and examination of specific characteristics of individual disorders or special populations. Nurcombe (1989) provided a comprehensive and compelling discussion of the general elements inherent in goal-directed treatment planning during brief hospitalization that bear relevance to a broad range of disturbances. Accordingly, a series of specific steps have been articulated to clarify each problem behavior, identify salient correlates, link diagnosis to short-term treatment, and facilitate both evaluation and revision of stated objectives in a given case. The usefulness of this general approach during brief treatment is difficult to overemphasize. Treatment planning along these lines and the generalization of gains may be promoted when parents and teachers are directly involved (Woolston, 1989b).

In terms of instrument development and specific evaluation findings, a measure of the antisocial and delinquent behaviors exhibited by children with conduct disorder (CD) was developed using both in-hospital and self-report data (Kazdin & Esveldt-Dawson, 1986). The result was the Interview for Antisocial Behavior (IAB) which consisted of 30 items that were rated by parents in terms of severity and duration. Scores on the IAB were found to correlate to CBCL scores, scores on a measure of aggression and hostility, performance on a behavioral role-play, and scores on a social skill inventory. In addition, the IAB distinguished CD from non-CD children, because CD children received significantly higher scores on almost all of the individual items in the IAB than did the non-CD children.

Berg, Rapoport, and Flament (1986) obtained interview and behavioral ratings in an effort to validate the Leyton Obsessional Inventory—Child Version (LOI—CV). Scores on this self-report measure were obtained from hospitalized children with obsessive-compulsive disorder and compared with scores on several rating scales. The LOI—CV was found to differentiate patients from nonpatients, to possess adequate test–retest reliability, and to discriminate placebo and drug treatment conditions. However, the instrument did not correlate with observer ratings of obsessive-compulsive behavior and general psychopathology obtained at baseline. A similar blending of parent ratings and in-hospital behavioral frequencies was found helpful in documenting the specific characteristics of inpatient children with a history of sexual abuse (Kolko, Moser, & Weldy, 1988). Both home and hospital behaviors were found to differentiate sexually abused, but not physically abused, children. Interestingly, there was no relationship between ratings of symptoms exhibited at home and in the hospital.

Evaluation of Response to Medication. An additional function on the inpatient setting concerns the evaluation of response to pharmacological and behavioral interventions. Two of the many examples of the application and behavioral assessment of pharmacotherapy are briefly mentioned here. Brown, Jaffe, Silverstein, & Magee (1991) found that methylphenidate had a significant effect on teacher ratings of conduct problems and academic performance in a classroom, but had no effect on impulsivity.

Evaluation of the impact and side effects of other medications used with autistic children is a related inpatient application (Campbell *et al.*, 1988). Campbell *et al.* (1988) employed a parallel group design in order to study the effects of fenfluramine or placebo during a 12-week hospital trial with 28 autistic children. Multiple measures (e.g., discrimination learning) and behavioral ratings (e.g., children's psychiatric rating scale) were obtained along with measures of side effects. Interestingly, fenfluramine did not result in greater symptom reduction overall and, at the same time, it was associated with suppressed discrimination learning. No major side effects on medication were observed, although some children showed weight loss. The integration of standardized measures of medical status, behavior, and learning in the context of placebo-controlled design are among the strengths of this evaluation.

Management: Consistent Exposure to Corrective Contingencies

Many of the children and adolescents referred for inpatient treatment have been exposed to inconsistent, inadequate, or harsh disciplinary measures (cf. Patterson, 1982). One specialized function of the inpatient setting is the provision of structure and consistent expectations through which judicious consequences can be used to motivate children to engage in prosocial behavior and, at the same time, refrain from deviant behavior. Contingency management programs, such as the token economy or point system, provide patients with a clear set of rules and a variety of reinforcing activities that are earned for compliance with these rules (see Chapter 8). Exposure to the consistency of the inpatient environment, in an effort to shape increasingly more responsible behavior by incorporating established behavioral principles, is perhaps one of the major benefits to initiating intervention in this type of setting (see Kazdin, 1977).

Apart from providing all residents with specific guidelines, the token economy embodies several other noteworthy characteristics, such as fairness, comprehensiveness, and predictability. These characteristics are necessary in order to successfully address the diverse behaviors of children who have become accustomed to engaging in undesirable behaviors and in the absence of any contingent consequences, both positive and negative. For example, severely dysfunctional children with attention deficit/hyperactivity disorder (AD/HD), conduct disorder (CD), and major depressive disorder (MDD), or bipolar affective disorder, often exhibit a broad range of troublesome, frequent, and resistive behaviors both as components of their psychiatric disorders (e.g., overactivity, swearing) and their reactions to management or control efforts (defiance, tantrumming). In many instances, severe out-of-control behavior, including assault and serious property destruction, are evinced during the initial period of hospitalization.

Therefore, the focus of contemporary contingent management programs is likely to be diverse, with equal attention being paid to increasing desired behaviors as with decreasing negative behaviors. Unlike the outpatient setting, the need to motivate children to engage in various self-care and mealtime behaviors, small group activities, and recreational or leisure activities is of equal therapeutic importance to that of improving self-control skills. Consequently, such programs target behaviors in all settings and activities from wake-up to bedtime, which requires consistent monitoring, frequent as well as delayed reinforcement, multiple reinforcers, and ongoing supervision and feedback.

Inpatient settings have also examined more critically the specific types of behavioral techniques used to effect change in serious behaviors. Hogan and Johnson (1985) implemented a token economy following a baseline condition with emotionally disturbed adolescents. The token economy consisted of point earnings and costs for engaging in desired and undesired behaviors, respectively. Behavioral goals were expressed in negative terms as behaviors in which the adolescents were not to engage. The final condition involved an elimination of the response cost procedure and a revision of goals into more positive terms. The results indicated that introduction of the token economy was associated with several improvements (e.g., frequency of problem incidents, use of time-out room) and that elimination of response-cost resulted in even further gains along these lines. Plausible explanations for the findings include improvement in client behavior and overall morale, suggesting the utility of examining alternative methods of improving and then maintaining behavioral control.

Despite their widespread application, the use of restraint and seclusion procedures for the control of serious aggression and agitated behavior has been examined more critically in recent years. Both of these procedures have been found to help children gain control of out-of-control behaviors (Gair, Bullard, & Corwin, 1984). Aggression has been found to be a common target for the use of seclusion (Garrison, Ecker, Friedman, Davidoff, Haeberle, & Wagner, 1990). One recent study provided a short-term examination of the use of seclusion on a children's inpatient unit (Joshi, Capozzoli, & Coyle, 1988). Across a 6-week period, the authors found reductions in both the rates and duration of seclusion, with many seclusions being self-imposed. Children with oppositional or attention deficit disorders required the most frequent use of seclusion. Moreover, in one half of the seclusions, the children were able to state the reason for this intervention. Continued evaluation of the benefits of this procedure and its parameters is likely to enhance the overall therapeutic impact of an inpatient program.

Brief Treatment of Psychiatric Disorders

As the number of children referred for serious behavioral (e.g., aggressive, defiant, impulsive) and emotional (e.g., depressive, suicidal) problems has increased, so too has the range of therapeutic interventions designed to address these problems. For example, methods to deal with violent behavior have been refined and integrated, such as verbal and physical crisis control strategies, behavioral procedures for reinforcement and punishment, and pharmacotherapy. Children with severe hyperactivity and attentional problems have likewise been referred so that alternative medications and behavioral programs can be monitored, evaluated, and revised to produce maximum benefit. Procedures for treating other types of externalizing problems are detailed elsewhere (see Chapters 8 and 9).

At the same time, children with disabling depressive symptoms or pain behavior have profitted from close monitoring and intensive treatment during short-term hospitalization (see Chapters 4 and 7). Both social and cognitive methods of behavior change have been implemented on an intensive basis (see Kolko, 1988b). Likewise, several advances in psychopharmacologic treatments have been evaluated during inpatient admission to alleviate depressive symptoms (Puig-Antich, 1984). The inpatient setting also offers a specialized environment for the administration of treatment protocols directed toward other problems (Kolko, 1987, 1989).

Protection and Respite

The decision to hospitalize often involves a consideration of the severity of a child's symptomatology, as well as parental and family dysfunction, among other concerns. In some cases, children who have been the victims of various forms of abuse or harsh management practices are clearly at risk for serious injuries which may prompt social service agencies to seek their admission (Jemerin & Philips, 1988). In many other instances, a short-term hospital stay is significantly influenced by the fact that a child's generally unmanageable behavior appears to be intimately tied to escalating family conflict and tension. The possibility of considerable harm to the child is of equal concern in such cases.

A child's physical and psychological welfare may be threatened because of serious psychiatric disturbances in the parents, including major depression, substance and drug abuse, schizophrenia, and antisocial behavior. Unfortunately, other characteristics of children referred to inpatient facilities that have become increasingly more common include homelessness, severe financial disadvantage, single-parent household status, social and community insularity, and medical complications. It may not be obvious for some time that a given child's referral for treatment is the ultimate consequence of general family breakdown. Accordingly, many children are separated from their parents, if only temporarily, in order to protect the child, impose some stability upon the child's behavior, and carefully examine the sources of the family's toxic interactions, before initiating formal therapeutic interventions.

Disposition and Placement

Difficulties in achieving successful outcomes with respect to all of the aforementioned unit functions may prompt the need to consider changing a child's school or family situation, if not both. Not surprisingly, out-of-home placement is frequently implied, if not requested outright, by an accompanying parent at the time of admission. Yet, with fewer available residential programs or community-based resources, the likelihood of ascertaining a sufficient placement is slim at best. As articulated by Jemerin and Philips (1988), the short-term unit often has to delay discharging a patient until plans for placement have been solidified. In the meantime, utilization review and insurance considerations are raised that compel a discharge that is "sooner than later." It is plausible that advances in both psychosocial and pharmacological treatments will expedite a child's rehabilitation in order to facilitate a prompt return either home or to a less restrictive but appropriate placement site.

CHALLENGES: PRACTICAL AND PROGRAMMATIC CONSIDERATIONS

Staff Training and Consistency

The importance of adequate preparation and training of staff cannot be overemphasized in light of the ever-diminishing complement of staff members and other resources, and concurrent attempts to expand assessment and brief treatment services (see Chapter 2). Examination of previous applications of staff-training procedures has yielded mixed results in terms of actual behavior change with patients (Milne, 1984). Compounding the difficulty in achieving beneficial outcomes within a short time period is the need to familiarize numerous staff members with individual programs and/or train a few staff in the implementation of specific techniques.

The diffusion of both expertise and accountability that occurs when multiple behavior change agents are involved, albeit at different times, often impedes consistency and, ultimately, good outcomes. Lack of adequate communication regarding behavioral programs can similarly limit the impact of even the most simplistic interventions. This is especially pertinent when behavioral frequencies are to be monitored across different shifts in order to determine whether predetermined criteria for improvement have been achieved (e.g., differential reinforcement of other behavior [DRO] or of a low rate of behavior [DRL]). Some recent data highlight the variability in implementation of contingent management procedures on a child inpatient unit and some of the variables that may influence procedural consistency (Kolko, McCanna, & Donaldson, 1989). Specifically, descriptive observational data revealed considerable variability in the rates of staff–patient interactions and the consistency with which specific consequences were administered. Work history and nursing stress variables were predictors of staff behavior. In effect, a staff member whose responsibilities include providing care for several conduct problem children simultaneously during a hectic or disruptive shift may not have time or energy to implement special behavioral programs.

Time Pressures

The transition toward shorter periods of hospitalization provides institutional limitations to the accomplishment of many treatment goals. Quite often, the pressure is reflective of financial rather than therapeutic considerations. Jemerin and Philips (1988) poignantly articulate this concern in the form of a "hello–goodbye" cycle through which patients revolve in rapid succession. This cycle contributes to weakened peer relationships, staff frustration, disappointment, fatigue, more frequent escalations in serious behaviors, and system conflicts about the overall purpose of admission. It is not uncommon for the average length of stay to be in the neighborhood of 2 to 8 weeks. In many cases, assessment or diagnostic work is concluded by the 3rd week, leaving roughly 4 weeks or so for the initiation, evaluation, and revision of various treatments.

Consequently, treatments are abbreviated or, not infrequently, postponed until after discharge. The hectic pace of the inpatient unit has similar implications for training and research (Rancurello, 1987).

Constraints of a Controlled Setting

Sometimes the primary benefit of a controlled setting serves, at the same time, as the primary obstacle to successful intervention. Children referred for various conduct-problem behaviors simply cannot engage in these activities during hospitalization, thus precluding observation and modification of the very acts for which admission was sought. Examples include separation anxiety, school phobia, family interactional conflicts and violence, academic underachievement, and various "covert" antisocial behaviors (e.g., fire-setting, shoplifting, gang activities, running away, truancy, and drug use). In contrast, certain behaviors may receive more complete examination in the hospital, such as depressive mood and irritability, sleep onset latency, eating problems, hyperactivity, inattention, and manic symptoms. Aggression and suicidality, perhaps the most common referral reasons, are more variably exhibited during hospitalization. Difficulties in accurately depicting the severity of a child's actual involvement in problem behaviors may hinder efforts at both diagnosis and intervention.

Additional constraints include the tight structure of the unit's daily schedule and the restricted number of settings or activities to which children are exposed. Finding an appropriate time for conducting behavioral treatments is, on occasion, as difficult as training new staff to implement novel procedures. One is then required to employ considerable creativity in arranging for intervention, as well as in designing methods to measure a child's unique problem behaviors. At the same time, the fact that the children exhibit multiple problem behaviors in different activities provides various opportunities to employ multiple-baseline designs across behaviors or settings.

Concurrent Treatments

The goals of hospitalization are often accomplished by initiating several concurrent intervention programs. Common treatments include medical/nursing health care, contingency management, skills training, social and family work, parent management training, academic rehabilitation, group and/or arts therapy, and psychopharmacology. In some instances, multiple behavioral and psychopharmacological interventions are employed to contain severe agitation, aggression, or suicidality. Not unexpectedly, it is difficult to isolate the cause of change during hospitalization. To withhold recommended treatments or stagger their introduction to avoid multiple treatment interference would be both impractical and inappropriate. Treatment teams hope to strike a balance between implementing critical interventions and determining the relative impact of specific procedures in order to render clinically useful plans for follow-up disposition and treatment.

Multiple Service Agency Involvement

A long history of prior contacts with agencies representing various disciplines and services is common among hospitalized children. In part, this history is a reflection of the diverse service needs of multi-distressed families in the face of ever-shrinking community resources. Prior to inpatient admission, a child may have had contact with Children and Youth Services, an outpatient therapist in a community mental health center, school guidance counselors or other representatives, juvenile court, and/or other social service agencies (e.g., Welfare). Parents may have been involved with their own outpatient therapists, a psychiatric hospital, the courts or justice system, or a family therapist. Cases of child abuse, in particular, are noted for their involvement in numerous clinical, social, and legal agencies. Thus, both children and their parents may share the same dubious status as a chronic patient.

Although involvement in these services is, unfortunately, a necessity for many children, it is not without its drawbacks and costs. The families are frequently required to "re-tell their stories" to yet another compassionate diagnostician and to complete the administrative paperwork that documents their financial, psychiatric, social, and personal disadvantages. Moreover, with continued specialization, it becomes more improbable that the family's diverse needs can be served by one or just a few service providers. As noted by Jemerin and Philips (1988), this fragmentation of the service delivery process may subvert the maintenance of prior treatment gains and hinder a child's ability to establish attachments. Although difficult to ascertain, the adverse impact of multiple agency involvement may be experienced in the form of diminished family motivation for change and heightened confusion about being pulled in different therapeutic directions.

SUGGESTIONS AND FUTURE DIRECTIONS

Recent reviews of advances in inpatient child psychiatric services provide several worthwhile recommendations to enhance the administrative, organizational, fiscal, clinical, and therapeutic integrity of a comprehensive child inpatient unit (Jemerin & Philips, 1988; Nurcombe, 1989; Woolston, 1989b). The following suggestions are designed to support and extend these developments and needed directions. One of the more basic recommendations concerns the process of identifying realistic goals for short-term hospitalization. Specific guidelines for developing focused treatment plans and procedures for use during brief inpatient (Nurcombe, 1989; Woolston, 1989b) and long-term residential treatment (Barker, 1988) are pertinent in this context. These recommendations include the use of clearly defined goals, specific desired outcomes, operational criteria, the inclusion of positive terms, a designated time frame, and circumstances under which changes are expected. Nurcombe (1989) provided an excellent discussion of specific examples and applications of problem-oriented treatment plans that nicely extends details commonly obtained via a comprehensive functional analysis. Progress achieved toward these specific goals could be supplemented with other objective data and standardized assessment measures obtained just prior to admission. Potential measures include parent ratings (e.g., Child Behavior Checklist), diagnostic interviews (Kiddie-SADS), parent daily reports of problem behaviors at home and at school (Parent Daily Report), nurses' ratings and observations, weekly clinician interviews, and records of critical hospital incidents. These measures are likely to facilitate clinical decision-making, treatment selection, and research (see Chapter 8).

There is also a greater need to evaluate the follow-up outcomes of hospitalization. For example, Pfeiffer (1989) and Pfeiffer and Strzelecki (1990) have suggested that greater attention be paid to improvements in conceptualization, clinical-description, and methodology. The improvements include greater description of the salient dimensions of treatment (e.g., scope, content), definitions of follow-up improvement (e.g., positive and negative symptoms, community adjustment), use of rigorous statistical methods and designs (e.g., multivariate analyses), and expansion of predictors (e.g., treatment regimen, family involvement). The examination of diverse program outcomes may be examined as a function of different demographics, populations, and settings. Further, follow-up intervals have varied both within and across studies, ranging from 2 months to 20 years (Davids & Salvatore, 1976; Lampen & Neill, 1985; Parham, Reid, & Hamer, 1987; Wergeland, 1980), with most studies reporting one- to two-year outcomes. Programs that conduct formal follow-ups may be in a better position to both document the benefit of hospitalization and to identify targets or conditions worthy of modification. Few inpatient programs, for example, have evaluated many of their services (e.g., intake, assessment, feedback, discharge planning), though such information would clearly enhance program development efforts (Charlop, Parrish, Fenton, & Cataldo, 1987; Harper, 1989). Various types of program outcome data highlight the benefit of inpatient treatment (Kazdin, 1989; Orchard & MacLeod, 1990) and both the correlates and predictors of limited, short-term improvement at follow-up (Kolko, in press).

An integrated, interdisciplinary data base in which all relevant issues are summarized is likely to facilitate rapid understanding of the child's and the family's history so that the "next step" in the therapeutic enterprise can be designated (Rancurello, 1987). For some children, this may merely involve the decision to initiate a specific behavioral program or medication, whereas for others this will entail a revision in diagnostic formulation and treatment direction. The need for a comprehensive evaluation is especially warranted in light of the multiple problems evinced by the children (e.g., medical, psychiatric, psychological, cognitive, social/behavioral, academic) and their families (e.g., parental psychopathology, poverty, social insularity). Staff members can be encouraged to acquire specialized expertise in a given area in order to serve as designated unit "resource staff" for particular types of disorders (e.g., anxiety) or treatments (e.g., bell-and-pad).

There is a need for greater reliance upon training or instructional methods that teach specific cognitive or behavioral skills. To achieve greater success during hospitalization, staff members should be trained in crisis intervention procedures to diffuse rapidly escalating sequences and functional analysis principles that emphasize the incorporation of specific antecedent or precipitating variables in the form of preventive methods (see Katz, 1988). Although contingent consequences for various behaviors remain the backbone of most unit management programs, the overall utility of behavioral treatment may be enhanced by paying greater attention to situational or interpersonal influences on behavior.

A related direction involves the integration of psychosocial and pharmacological approaches to intervention. Combined interventions that address complementary foci may better promote short- and long-term improvement than single-modality interventions. Evidence has accumulated to support the use of each approach in the treatment of aggression, hyperactivity, depression, anxiety, and pain, among other problems. This requires greater collaboration between psychologists and psychiatrists, as well as other treatment team collaborators (see Hersen, 1986).

The establishment and maintenance of family involvement in treatment is one of the understated obstacles encountered during hospitalization. Apart from conducting preadmission interviews and tours, it is important to make various arrangements (e.g., phone calls, compliance contingencies) to motivate the parents to attend family sessions and support the child's treatment plan. A salient component of this overall plan may involve parent referral for evaluation and treatment, the initiation of marital counseling, and/or child management skills training. A specific family plan is likely to be needed not only to clarify the expectations of all parties involved, but also for use in corroborating subsequent clinical and legal decisions about the child's care and welfare. The methods and modalities of contemporary family work require considerable flexibility in order to accommodate variations in life-styles, family constellation, and ethnic and cultural background, single-parent households, and parents with limited intellectual and personal resources.

As the impact of these and other family circumstances is felt, the importance of disposition planning and out-of-home placement will most likely increase. It is therefore necessary to be familiar with the child's history of placement, state laws governing child welfare and dependency status, and the hierarchy of available placement options that address the child's unique characteristics and circumstances (e.g., child's age, parent's capacity for rehabilitation, prior efforts at treatment, chronicity of problems, parent motivation/investment). Permanency planning may be abetted to the extent that the following are employed: specific time frames, case reviews/contracting, active collaboration with community agencies, continued parental involvement, and attention to relevant legal requirements (see Maluccio, 1988).

Administration of the aforementioned services and operations is likely to be maximized in a therapeutic institution that provides a continuum of care. The development of more centralized services for children (Jemerin & Philips, 1988) would expedite a child's referral for an appropriate level of care and for as many coordinated programs as would be deemed necessary. Inpatient settings that are more closely tied to outpatient clinics or to day treatment programs may promote more efficient and painless transfer between programs. The provision of coordinated services is likely to reduce involvement in often related, and sometimes redundant, agencies, and to promote more continued involvement in the treatment of psychiatric disorders whose chronicity is now well documented (e.g., conduct disorder, attention deficit disorder, major depressive disorder). Accordingly, generalization of treatment gains from the hospital to the natural environment and across time would be maximized. To the extent that these general objectives are fostered, the management, treatment, and ultimate rehabilitation of psychiatrically hospitalized children will be more fully realized.

REFERENCES

Achenbach, T. M., & Edelbrock, C. S. (1983). *Manual for the Child Behavior Checklist and Revised Child Behavior Profile*. Burlington, VT: University Associates in Psychiatry.

American Academy of Child Psychiatry. (1983). *Child psychiatry: A plan for the coming decades*. Washington, DC: Author.

American Psychiatric Association. (1957). *Psychiatric inpatient treatment of children*. Baltimore, MD: Lord Baltimore Press.

Barker, P. (1988). The future of residential treatment. In C. E. Schaefer and A. J. Swanson (Eds.), *Children in residential care: Critical issues in treatment* (pp. 1–16). New York: Van Nostrand Reinhold.

Barkley, R. A., Fischer, M., Edelbrock, C. S., & Smallish, L. (1990). The adolescent outcome of hyperactive children diagnosed by research criteria: I. An 8-year prospective follow-up study. *Journal of the American Academy of Child and Adolescent Psychiatry, 29*, 546–557.

Berg, C. J., Rapoport, J. L., & Flament, M. (1986). The Leyton Obsessional Inventory—Child Version. *Journal of the American Academy of Child and Adolescent Psychiatry, 25*, 84–91.

Brown, R. T., Jaffe, S. L., Silverstein, J., & Magee, H. (1991). Methylphenidate and adolescents hospitalized with conduct disorder: Dose effects on classroom behavior, academic performance, and impulsivity. *Journal of Clinical Child Psychology, 3*, 282–292.

Campbell, M., Adams, P., Small, A. M., Curren, E. L., Overall, J. E., Anderson, L. T., Lunch, N., & Perry, R. (1988). Efficacy and safety of fenfluramine in autistic children. *Journal of the American Academy of Child and Adolescent Psychiatry, 27*, 434–439.

Charlop, M. H., Parrish, J. M., Fenton, L. R., & Cataldo, M. F. (1987). Evaluation of hospital-based outpatient pediatric psychology services. *Journal of Pediatric Psychology, 12*, 485–503.

Chelimsky, E. (1985). *Residential care: Patterns of child placement in three states*. Gaithersburg, MD: U.S. General Accounting Office.

Conners, C. K. (1985). Inpatient global rating scale. *Psychopharmacology Bulletin, 21*, 832–834.

Davids, A., & Salvatore, P. D. (1976). Residential treatment of disturbed children and adequacy of their subsequent adjustment. *American Journal of Orthopsychiatry, 46*, 62–73.

Edelbrock, C. S. (1985). Child behavior rating form. *Psychopharmacology Bulletin, 21*, 835–837.

Gabel, S., & Shindledecker, R. (1990). Parental substance abuse and suspected child abuse/maltreatment predict outcome in children's inpatient treatment. *Journal of the American Academy of Child and Adolescent Psychiatry, 29*, 919–924.

Gair, D. S., Bullard, D. M., Jr., & Corwin, J. M. (1984). Guidelines for children and adolescents. In K. Tardiff (Ed.), *The psychiatric uses of seclusion and restraint* (pp. 69–85). Washington, DC: American Psychiatric Press.

Garrison, W. T., Ecker, B., Friedman, M., Davidoff, R., Haeberle, K., & Wagner, M. (1990). Aggression and counteraggression during child psychiatric hospitalization. *Journal of the American Academy of Child and Adolescent Psychiatry, 29*, 242–250.

Grizenko, M., & Sayegh, L. (1990). Evaluation of the effectiveness of a psychodynamically oriented day treatment program for children with behaviour problems: A pilot study. *Canadian Journal of Psychiatry, 35*, 519–525.

Harper, G. (1989). Focal inpatient treatment planning. *Journal of the American Academy of Child and Adolescent Psychiatry, 28*, 31–37.
Hersen, M. (Ed.). (1986). *Pharmacological and behavioral treatment: An integrative approach*. New York: John Wiley.
Hogan, W. A., & Johnson, D. P. (1985). Elimination of response cost in a token economy program and improvement in behavior of emotionally disturbed youth. *Behavior Therapy, 16*, 87–98.
Jemerin, J. M., & Philips, I. (1988). Changes in inpatient child psychiatry: Consequences and recommendations. *Journal of the American Academy of Child and Adolescent Psychiatry, 27*, 397–403.
Jenkins, R. L., & Shoji, T. (1967). Charting disturbed children's behavior. *Hospital and Community Psychiatry, 24*, 230–233.
Jones, R. N., Latkowski, M. E., Kircher, J. C., & McMahon, W. M. (1988). The Child Behavior Checklist: Normative information for inpatients. *Journal of the American Academy of Child and Adolescent Psychiatry, 27*, 632–635.
Joshi, P. T., Capozzoli, J. A., & Coyle, J. T. (1988). Use of a quiet room on an inpatient unit. *Journal of the American Academy of Child and Adolescent Psychiatry, 27*, 642–644.
Katz, M. (1988). Crisis intervention in residential care. In *Children in residential care: Critical issues in treatment* (pp. 30–49). New York: Van Nostrand Reinhold.
Kazdin, A. E. (1977). *The token economy: A review and evaluation*. New York: Plenum Press.
Kazdin, A. E. (1987). *Conduct disorders in childhood and adolescence*. Beverly Hills, CA: Sage Publications.
Kazdin, A. E. (1989). Hospitalization of antisocial children: Clinical course, follow-up status, and predictors of outcome. *Advances in Behaviour Research and Therapy, 11*, 1–67.
Kazdin, A. E., & Bass, D. (1988). Parent, teacher, and hospital staff evaluations of severely disturbed children. *American Journal of Orthopsychiatry, 58*, 512–523.
Kazdin, A. E., & Esveldt-Dawson, K. (1986). The Interview for Antisocial Behavior: Concurrent validity with child psychiatric inpatients. *Journal of Psychopathology and Behavioral Assessment, 8*, 289–303.
Kolko, D. J. (1987). Simplified inpatient treatment of nocturnal enuresis in psychiatrically disturbed children. *Behavior Therapy, 2*, 99–112.
Kolko, D. J. (1988a). Daily ratings on a child psychiatric unit. *Journal of the American Academy of Child and Adolescent Psychiatry, 27*, 126–132.
Kolko, D. J. (1988b). Depression. In M. Hersen & V. B. Van Hasselt (Eds.), *Behavior therapy with children and adolescents* (pp. 137–183). New York: Wiley.
Kolko, D. J. (1989). Inpatient intervention for chronic functional encopresis in psychiatrically disturbed children. *Behavioral Residential Treatment, 4*, 232–252.
Kolko, D. J. (in press). Short-term follow-up of child psychiatric hospitalization: Clinical description, predictors, and correlates. *Journal of the American Academy of Child and Adolescent Psychiatry.*
Kolko, D. J., Moser, J. T., & Weldy, S. R. (1988). Behavioral/emotional indicators of sexual abuse among child psychiatric inpatients: A comparison with physical abuse. *Child Abuse & Neglect, 12*, 529–541.
Kolko, D. J., McCanna, M., & Donaldson, L. (1989). Sequential assessment of staff administration of contingency management procedures on a child psychiatric unit. *Behavior Modification, 13*, 216–244.
Kovacs, M., Feinberg, T. L., Crouse-Novak, M. A., Paulauskas, S. L., & Finkelstein, R. (1984). Depressive disorders in childhood: I. A longitudinal prospective study of characteristics and recovery. *Archives of General Psychiatry, 41*, 229–237.

Lampen, J., & Neill, T. (1985). "A bucket of cold water:" A follow-up study of a residential special school. *Journal of Adolescence, 8*, 271–287.

Maluccio, A. N. (1988). Promoting permanency planning. In *Children in residential care: Critical issues in treatment* (pp. 175–190). New York: Van Nostrand Reinhold.

McMahon, W. M., King, K., Harris, F. N., Latkowski, M., Ferre, R., & Jenson, W. R. (1984, October). *Inpatient follow-up: Use of the Child Behavior Checklist.* Paper presented at the 31st annual meeting of the American Academy of Child Psychiatry, Toronto.

Milne, D. (1984). The development and evaluation of a structured learning format introduction to behavior therapy for psychiatric nurses. *British Journal of Clinical Psychology, 23*, 120–131.

Nurcombe, B. (1989). Goal-directed treatment planning and the principles of brief hospitalization. *Journal of the American Academy of Child and Adolescent Psychiatry, 28*, 26–30.

Orchard, J. M., & MacLeod, R. J. (1990). Adolescent day program: A two year retrospective review. *Canadian Journal of Psychiatry, 35*, 554–556.

Overall, J. E., & Pfefferbaum, B. (1982). The brief psychiatric rating scale for children. *Psychopharmacology Bulletin, 18*, 10–16.

Parham, C., Reid, S., & Hamer, R. M. (1987). A long-range follow-up study of former inpatients at a children's psychiatric hospital. *Child Psychiatry and Human Development, 17*, 199–209.

Patterson, G. R. (1982). *Coercive family process.* Eugene, OR: Castalia Publishing.

Pfeiffer, S. I. (1989). Follow-up of children and adolescents treated in psychiatric facilities. *Psychiatric Hospital, 20*, 15–20.

Pfeiffer, S. I., & Strzelecki, S. C. (1990). Inpatient psychiatric treatment of children and adolescents: a review of outcome studies. *Journal of the American Academy of Child and Adolescent Psychiatry, 29*, 847–853.

Puig-Antich, J. (1984). Psychobiology in prepubertal major depression. In E. B. Welle & R. A. Weller (Eds.), *Current perspectives on major depressive disorders in children.* (pp. 78–90). Washington, DC: American Psychiatric Association.

Rancurello, M. (1987). Special aspects of the care of the severely disturbed child and use of psychiatric inpatient services. In R. L. Cohen & M. K. Dulcan (Eds.), *Basic handbook of training in child and adolescent psychiatry* (pp. 105–116). Springfield, IL: Charles C. Thomas.

Rapoport, J., Conners, C. K., & Reatig, N. (Guest Eds.). (1985). Rating scales and assessment instruments for use in pediatric psychopharmacology research. *Psychopharmacology Bulletin, 21*, 713–1125.

Rivlin, L. G., & Wolfe, M. (1985). *Institutional settings in children's lives.* New York: Wiley.

Towle, P. O., & Schwarz, J. C. (1987). The Child Behavior Checklist as applied to archival data: Factor structure and external correlates. *Journal of Clinical Child Psychology, 16*, 69–79.

Wergeland, H. (1980). A follow-up investigation of 39 antisocial children 4–20 years after discharge from hospital. *Acta Paedopsychiatria, 46*, 39–55.

Woolston, J. L. (1989a). Issues in child and adolescent psychiatric hospitalization. *Journal of the American Academy of Child and Adolescent Psychiatry, 28*, 20.

Woolston, J. L. (1989b). Transactional risk model for short and intermediate term psychiatric inpatient treatment of children. *Journal of the American Academy of Child and Adolescent Psychiatry, 28*, 38–41.

2

Staff Training and Community Consultation

JOHN J. MCGONIGLE

INTRODUCTION

Continuity of care refers to a planned coordination of the movement of a patient along the various components of a care delivery system (Perris, Radhe, Palm, Hellgren, Lilja, & Soderman, 1985). The issue of continuity of care has long been a concern of health care professionals for the simple fact that much of the time and effort involved in the treatment of patients in psychiatric inpatient units is literally wasted because of a breakdown in the care system. Fragmented services, poor case management, appropriate living arrangements post discharge, as well as the lack of capable and knowledgeable individuals to deliver the care are issues of concern. It truly takes a coordination of services both in the hospital and following the patient's discharge from the hospital to maintain symptoms or problems at minimal rates. In many instances, the patients who are discharged from inpatient psychiatric hospitals return to the community with little, if any, follow-up or aftercare. The patient may be discharged back to a setting which may exacerbate the problem and require the patient to be readmitted to the hospital.

JOHN J. MCGONIGLE • Department of Psychiatry, Allegheny Neuropsychiatric Institute, 7777 Steubenville Pike, Oakdale, Pennsylvania 15071.

Inpatient Behavior Therapy for Children and Adolescents, edited by Vincent B. Van Hasselt and David J. Kolko. Plenum Press, New York, 1992.

A review of the literature on continuation of patient care reveals little mention of the continuity of care and service delivery within the hospital setting and even less attention to the transition from inpatient hospitalization to the community. Automatic assumptions are made that there are minimal problems with the continuity of care for patients being treated in an inpatient hospital ward or unit. The assumption is that patients' problems are well controlled because they are followed by a treatment team 24 hours a day. Another assumption is that there is a high degree of consistency in the implementation and monitoring of patients' treatment. This chapter will explore some of the issues regarding staff training, continuity of care of patients within the hospital setting, and the role of the consultant in facilitating the patient's transition back to the community.

THE SOCIAL ENVIRONMENT OF AN INPATIENT PSYCHIATRIC FACILITY

Landesman-Dwyer and Knowles (1987) wrote about the social environment of the residential facility in the community. Just as every residential facility has an ambience of its own, the same can be said for an inpatient hospital program. The social environment of a psychiatric inpatient unit is an extension of the composition of the workers on the unit. Psychiatric aides or child care workers, milieu therapists, nurses, teachers, psychologists (behavior specialists), social workers, psychiatrists, and special therapists (speech therapists, physical therapists, occupational therapists) combine to make up the social environment of the unit or ward. The knowledge, expertise, and interaction of this group not only affects the behavior of individual staff members but also affects the patients that are being treated (Landesman-Dwyer & Knowles, 1987). These individuals comprise both professional and nonprofessional staff. Thinking in terms of continuity of care and staff training within the hospital setting, it is essential to understand that in order to provide quality care to the inpatient, the entire milieu staff must formulate and carry out a consistent treatment plan. The above statement and the theory supporting this treatment process sound easy, but when team members are extremely diverse in their knowledge and approach to treating the patient (i.e., developmental vs. humanistic vs. behavioral), it can lead to many problems with consistency. Consistent treatment and management of the inpatient by the staff is a major variable in successful treatment outcomes. Consistency not only helps the patient learn and understand about his or her individual problems, but it also assists in the maintenance and generalization of treatment gains following discharge.

Staff training and consultation are an essential part of any successful hospital program. Of course, even the inpatient staff needs to have some understanding of the patient beyond the confines of the hospital milieu. Such considerations as the circumstances around the admission of the patient, the current needs of the patient, and what happens to the patient following discharge should be known. When evaluating a patient in this perspective, it is clear that there is much more to be aware of than simply providing interim treatment for a short time period and then discharging the patient back to the home environment.

For example, consider the standard design for a child or adolescent who is receiving evaluation and treatment in a psychiatric inpatient program. Following the patient's arrival to the hospital, a baseline period lasting from 1 to 2 weeks goes into effect. The baseline is usually followed by a 2- to 4-week treatment period (i.e., medication, behavioral intervention). Following the treatment or intervention phase, the patient is then discharged to the community. Oftentimes, there is minimal or no training or aftercare provided.

Inpatient programs must look at the patient on a much broader scope (the patient outside of the hospital) when determining the individual needs of the patient. A more inclusive course of treatment would extend beyond the inpatient hospital setting. Using this design, the patient is evaluated in the home setting and receives follow-up or aftercare services. With the shortening of patient hospital stays, it has become more difficult to provide an evaluation, develop an effective treatment plan, and implement the prescribed treatment. The development and the maintenance of consistent patient care require that the inpatient staff receive the proper training and consultation in the management of individuals with psychiatric diagnoses.

STAFF-TRAINING PROCEDURES IN INPATIENT SETTINGS

In this chapter, I will define and summarize staff-training techniques that have been utilized to effect behavior change in patients who are receiving treatment in inpatient psychiatric hospitals. Methods employed to train staff range from group inservice training (Delamater, Connors, & Wells, 1984) to providing token reinforcement for staff to public posting (Welsch, Ludwig, Radiker, & Krapil, 1973). Research on staff training and patient outcomes have evaluated ways to suppress aberrant behaviors (Peed, Roberts, & Forehand, 1977), to increase prosocial responding (Kissel, Whitman, & Reid, 1983), and to eliminate maladaptive behaviors (Jones & Eimers, 1975).

A common element underlying many of the limited outcomes of a patient who frequently returns to the hospital is that there is inadequate preparation for the patient's return home. An inadequately prepared staff can be one of the reasons a patient may fail both in and out of the hospital. Staff training is one of the ways to improve the success rates of patients who leave the hospital setting. The descriptions that follow are some of the many ways that inpatient psychiatric hospital programs attempt to train and provide consultation for staff.

Group Inservice Training

One of the most frequently employed ways to train staff in inpatient settings is by way of large and small group instruction. Although inservice staff training by itself is one of the most frequently used methods to develop the skills of the inpatient staff, it is the least likely to affect behavior change in the patients. Results of previous research (Delamater *et al.*, 1984; Gardner, 1972; McKeown, Adams, & Forehand, 1975; Quilitch, 1975) have noted that inservice staff training is a very good way to develop knowledge, vocabulary, and theory about specific patient problems or symptomatology; however, without the combination of verbal feedback, behavior rehearsal, modeling, or role-playing sessions, the training has little effect on staff behaviors and ultimately on behavior change in the patient. Delamater *et al.* (1984) compared three staff-training procedures on a child psychiatric inpatient setting: (1) inservice training, using Brown and Presbie's (1974) Behavior Management Skills; (2) direct feedback of actual staff performance; aand (3) role-playing, involving instruction, modeling, behavior rehearsal, feedback, and reinforcement. The phases of the 21-week study included: inservice training, inservice training plus direct feedback, and role-playing. Results of the study indicated that (1) inservice training had little effect on staff behavior; (2) direct feedback in some cases resulted in increased frequency of staff responding including greater use of positive reinforcement; and (3) the greatest gains in the staff behavior occurred as a result of role-playing. The results of this study concur with previous research in showing that inservice training is limited to providing staff with a knowledge base but is minimally effective in changing the staff's behavior.

Inservice training involves explaining or demonstrating to the staff specific ways to manage client or patient behaviors. These instructions are given to increase the likelihood that the staff will intervene in appropriate ways and at the appropriate times. Martin and Pear (1983) stated that instructions are most effective when they are within the understanding of the targeted individual, specify the behavior to be displayed, are comprised of systematic steps, are delivered courteously, and are sequenced from easy to difficult.

Verbal and Written Instruction/Direct Feedback

The use of verbal and written instruction in staff training is clearly more specific and related to the individual needs of the patient. The training assists the staff in acquiring knowledge and understanding of specific target symptoms or problem behaviors. Instructions providing both written, verbal, or direct feedback involve telling or showing staff members how to behave with or to teach patients. Instructions are most effective when they are within the understanding of the targeted individual, specify the behavior to be displayed, are comprised of systematic steps, and are sequenced from easy to difficult (Martin & Pear, 1983).

The use of verbal and written instruction to affect behavior change in patients and staff has been reported with varying degrees of success. Fielding, Erickson, and Bettin (1971) investigated the use of instruction to reduce staff's use of physical coercion to move a resident in a 24-hour care facility. Initially, the staff received inservice training (verbal instructions) in the application of behavior modification techniques to move residents with severe handicaps from one area to another. Although staff responded to the verbal instruction during the training session, the inservice training was ineffective in changing staff behavior in the work setting.

A poster was presented to the staff which likened physical coercion of the residents to placing them on a flatbed "tow truck." Staff responded by correctly escorting residents throughout the ward. Experimental control of the independent variable was not demonstrated; however, the authors' impressions noted that instructional manipulations consisting of the poster in conjunction with an inservice training workshop were successful in changing staff performance. Another drawback to this study was that the authors did not report on resident behavior.

A comparison of staff-training procedures by Delameter *et al.* (1984) evaluated the effects of direct feedback in addition to inservice training to increase appropriate interactions of staff and children on a ward in an inpatient psychiatric care facility. The direct feedback condition was implemented following an inservice training program and began in weeks

9 and 10 of the study. For a 2-week time period, the staff received feedback concerning their interactions with the children. The feedback was given to the staff at predetermined time periods and consisted of factual presentation of percentages of time the staff member engaged in a variety of behaviors that were being observed. Reinforcement for appropriate staff interaction was also provided. The feedback session occurred in a one-to-one session. A review of the data suggests that the first significant change in staff behavior occurred as a result of the implementation of the feedback condition. This increase in appropriate staff/child interaction was not observed in all staff members, and these acquired behaviors did not consistently maintain over time. The results of the study demonstrated that the feedback condition in conjunction with inservice training was effective in producing behavior changes with some staff members but not with others. It was the authors' impression that the differences in staff response were related to the staff's perception of the feedback. Some staff may have viewed the feedback as positive and an opportunity to better interact with the children on the ward. Yet other staff members perceived the feedback to be negative and a criticism of their performance.

This reactivity issue is most noteworthy when using verbal and written instruction/direct feedback to train staff members. Hagen, Craighead, and Paul (1975) reported that in order for feedback to be effective, a good, open, nondefensive working relationship is required. Another issue that has been reported concerning the use of feedback relates to the position or role of the person who administers the feedback. In the Delameter *et al.* (1984) study, a research assistant with much less authority provided the performance feedback and may have been associated with the unresponsiveness of a few staff members. The authors suggested that the effects of feedback may vary with the perceived valence or weight attributed to the person giving the feedback.

In conclusion, verbal and written instruction and direct feedback have been reported with varying degrees of success. Feedback appears to be more successful in improving staff/patient or client interaction and is more effective than inservice training. Issues of concern when using this method of staff training include the role of authority in the individual who is providing the feedback, the positive nature of the feedback, and the staffs' understanding of the role and use of the feedback procedure.

Figure 1 is an example of a behavior modification program which was designed to treat the aggressive and self-injurious behavior of a hospitalized adolescent boy. The program is designed as a staff-training tool that can provide written and verbal feedback with regard to con-

BEHAVIOR MODIFICATION PROGRAM

Name: Frequency of target behaviors ____

Date: No. of times program was implemented ____

Goals: To reduce self-injurious behavior and aggressive behavior to zero rates

Target Behaviors: Hand biting; raising hand to hit

Setting: ICF/MR Program

Method: Differential reinforcement of other behaviors

Program Restrictions: There are no program restrictions. This is a positive reinforcement program.

Program Outline

Differential reinforcement of other behaviors (DRO)

	YES	NO
An audio tape cueing the staff to reinforce patient every 10 minutes is supplied and is intended to be used during all program hours.		
1) Whenever the cue sounds, staff assigned to patient should attend to him.	____	____
a) If patient is engaged in an appropriate behavior (i.e., following directions and all behaviors except for hand biting, threatening others), he should be reinforced with verbal praise.	____	____
b) If patient is displaying undesirable behaviors (above-mentioned behaviors), he should <u>not</u> be reinforced.	____	____
2) For every third interval (30 minutes) patient will receive primary reinforcers (edibles) paired with social praise.	____	____
3) Edibles should always be accompanied with social touching (pat on back) and verbal praise.	____	____
4) <u>Reinforcer List</u>	____	____

1)
2)
3)
4)
5)

Figure 1. A behavior modification program designed in a step-by-step description. The evaluation procedures for the behavior modification are intended to reduce self-injurious behaviors in community settings.

Example: Treatment Course

Baseline in hospital Symptom Problems	Treatment/ Interventions	Discharge
One week	Two weeks	
1-2 weeks	2-4 weeks	

Treatment Course in and out of the Hospital

Baseline in the home	Treatment/ Intervention	Parent/Agency Training	Discharge Follow-up School Home
	2-4 weeks	2 weeks	As needed basis

Figure 1. (Continued)

sistency in program implementation and staff performance related to the treatment of the patient's specific referred or targeted behaviors. In order for this program to be carried out and consistently implemented, the staff must first know the specific target behaviors and the method or means by which the behavior is being treated, and must understand all the steps in the program. The staff-training procedures that can be utilized with this format include the written instructions in having the staff fill in the specific target behaviors for the patient and the verbal feedback and praise to the staff for implementation of the program according to the stepwise procedures listed in numerical order. Staff members can also self-assess by filling out the checkmark section in the right-hand column (see Figure 3) following treatment sessions.

Role-playing has been used as a training technique in a variety of clinical and applied settings. For example, individual and group psychotherapy sessions and social skills groups are frequently practiced by nurse clinicians, therapists, psychologists, and developmental therapists (teachers), prior to independently conducting therapy sessions. Delamater *et al.* (1984) compared role-playing, inservice training, and feedback on increasing rates of staff performance and staff/patient interactions. The results of the study noted that (1) inservice training alone had little effect on behavior change in staff-to-patient interaction, (2) the feedback condition was effective in producing behavioral changes in some staff but not in others, and (3) the most dramatic improvements in staff responding occurred as a result of role-playing.

Gardner (1972) compared the effectiveness of two instructional methods—role-playing and lectures—in evaluating the effectiveness of teaching behavior modification to institutional attendants. Staff dependent measures for outcome variables were (1) knowledge of behavior modification principles and (2) ratings of ability to apply behavior modification techniques. The psychiatric attendants were matched according to social economic status, knowledge of the retarded population, and knowledge of nursing skills. The attendants were randomly assigned to one of two groups: role-playing or lecture. The Behavior Modification Test, which is a true/false test that measures knowledge of behavior principles, was administered as a pretest. Following the pretest, the subjects entered into one of two training phases: role-playing or lectures. Role-playing consisted of six 1-hour sessions in which various behavior modification techniques were demonstrated. Emphasis was placed on methods of administering reinforcers and shaping behavior. Psychiatric attendants worked in pairs, each alternately assuming the role of the resident or trainer. The pairs were supervised by experienced behavior modification technicians.

The lecture series consisted of eight 1-hour sessions designed to present behavior modification principles in everyday language. The lectures covered three major areas: (1) reinforcement, (2) shaping techniques, and (3) stimulus control. The results indicated that role-playing was more effective in teaching behavior modification skills whereas the lectures were more effective in teaching principles of behavior modification.

A study conducted by Jones and Eimers (1975) evaluated role-playing to train elementary teachers to reduce disruptive behavior in two third-grade classrooms. Both child and teacher behaviors were observed and recorded. A multiple-baseline design was employed using the two teachers as multiple subjects. A training program utilized a role-playing procedure in which teachers were trained in the effective use of a classroom management "skills package." Child measures included: talking aloud, out-of-seat, inappropriate talking (i.e., name calling, laughing, etc.).

The results of the study demonstrated that all classroom disruptive behavior was significantly decreased when teacher-training methods using role-playing were implemented. Out-of-seat behavior and inappropriate talking were immediately affected in the teacher-training phase of the study. Experimental control over the role-playing session was achieved by employing the role-playing procedure across teachers and settings.

Case Observation/Video Tape Sessions

An effective teaching and training tool noted in the literature (Dowrick & Johns, 1976; Gary, 1974) is the use of direct observation. The training in most reported cases involves the therapist's observing the patient through a one-way observation mirror or in the milieu. The therapist is required to write a short observation or log of the patient's target symptoms and behaviors. The staff person is then asked to present the observation to the trainer and then give feedback. Videotaping in conjunction with direct observation is a tool that has also been used frequently in the training of staff in inpatient psychiatric programs.

The videotape method of staff training has been utilized in classrooms (Hall, Panvan, Rabon, & Broden, 1968), counseling sessions (Waltz & Johnston, 1963), and psychiatric residential facilities (Gary, 1974). Dowrick and Johns (1976) and Gray (1974) have documented the use of videotaping as feedback. The training involves the use of videotaping for feedback purposes. Gary (1974) evaluated the effectiveness of video feedback plus positive reinforcement delivered to the therapist to increase on-task attending of children in a day treatment program in a psychiatric hospital. During the group treatment session, a video recording was made of the whole group. Immediately following the sessions, the therapist was shown the recording, and the supervisors made comments and delivered verbal praise when the therapist reinforced the children for on-task attending. The intervention was assessed systematically by way of withdrawal of treatment design. Data were presented on the therapist's attending to on-task behavior using videotapes as compared to baseline and no feedback. The results of the study indicated that the therapist's skills (attending to on-task behavior) were at lower rates without feedback. With a reintroduction of videotapes and praise, the therapist had maximized both attending and on-task activity and ignored off-task. Generally, the approach that is taken is that the therapist/clinician is observed conducting a session, and the videotape is then viewed at a later time period. The advantage that a videotape session has over a case observation is that the tape is a permanent product that can be scored or reviewed at a later date.

Hands-on Training

Another frequently employed staff-training technique is hands-on training. Many inpatient programs do not have the luxury of videotapes or time to spend with staff members in individual training sessions. For this reason, many staff members working on inpatient psychiatric units are oriented to the unit/ward with the patients under the direct supervision of an experienced staff trainer. In many cases, this is a "learn-as-you-go" or "baptism-by-fire" approach. The staff person being trained is directly supervised at all times until a specific level of criteria is achieved. The trainee is observed by the trainer, who follows the implementation of the specific behavior programs and then provides the trainee with immediate feedback. Once the trainee has achieved criteria for success (determined by the trainer), the trainer then makes periodic checks on the systematic implementation of the prescribed program.

A review of the literature revealed that no study employed hands-on training alone. This approach was always reported in combination with other training methods (e.g., inservice training, verbal feedback, or videotaping). Although the hands-on approach is not well documented, it would appear to be a very efficient and effective way for training staff. With the direct observation and continuous feedback desired staff behaviors can be shaped and maintained.

METHODS OF EVALUATION

All the studies reviewed for staff-training techniques utilized various types of evaluations, such as pre-post testing (Gardner, 1972; Peed, *et al.*, 1977), multiple-baseline designs (Jones and Eimers, 1975; Quilitch, 1975; Realon, Lewallen, & Wheeler, 1983; Sanders & Glynn, 1981), and withdrawal of treatment (Delamater *et al.*, 1984; Hollander & Plutchik, 1972). Foremost among the reasons for assessment is that evaluation generally determines the gains made by both staff and clinicians who work with the patients. The following are two examples of ways to evaluate the effectiveness of a staff-training program.

In using an anecdotal record, the trainer observes and literally describes (in a written log) the implementation of the treatment program for a given patient. This initial observational note is then followed by a training package that is designed to meet specific deficit areas of the staff. Comparisons can then be made between pre- and postobservations. Clearly, the problems inherent in this method are that it is subjective and there is no reliability. It is solely based on clinical impressions.

A more popular method involves the use of a single-case design, such as an "A-B" design with extended follow-up, or multiple-baseline designs (Hersen & Barlow, 1976). In the A-B extended follow-up format, the staff is given an assessment (pretest) to determine the individual skill level that each staff brings to the training session. Following this pretest, the staff is then involved in a formal or informal training program. The program can include any or all of the previously mentioned training methods. Following this training session, the trainees are administered a posttest. Comparisons are made between pre- and posttests and a level of criteria is established. Staff persons who do not reach this level of criteria are required to retrain to acceptable levels. Those staff members who have demonstrated success are assigned individual cases. Follow-up measures are periodically conducted through written, verbal, and direct observation assessments and completed in order to maintain the skill level acquired during staff-training sessions. The objective for any training program is the maintenance and generalization of the skills acquired by staff as a result of the staff training (i.e., taking the skills learned in the individual training session and applying them across all other settings). The hands-on method of training is very well suited for the maintenance and generalization of skills. With a hands-on approach and direct supervision, the trainer is able to program for generalization by training staff in a variety of settings (i.e., learning center, lunch room, outings) and under a variety of conditions.

Follow-up measures on the staff's acquired skills can be achieved in most cases by using a procedure reliability checklist. Figure 1 also is an example of the use of a designed behavior program as an evaluation tool to evaluate the degree of consistency in the implementation of a specific behavior program. The program is outlined in a stepwise fashion to ensure consistency and to assist in preventing the freelance implementation of programs or drift from the program's purpose. The right-hand column of the assessment form has categories, such as the number of times target behavior occurred, number of times procedure was implemented, and a yes/no column that is adjacent to each of the steps in the program. The procedure check is simply achieved by the trainer or evaluator's observing the staff member during program hours. Such items as the patient's target behaviors, the reaction of staff (number of times the patient displays a target behavior), and staff consistencies in the implementation of each step in the program are noted. Following the observation, feedback and supervision are given. This procedural check can also be coupled with a videotape session so that the staff member can self-record. Self-recording and supervision programs have been noted to be a successful way to increase interaction between staff and patients (Burg, Reid, & Lattimore, 1979).

STAFF/PARENT TRAINING AND CONSULTATION/LIAISON IN THE COMMUNITY

Inpatient psychiatric care facilities seek to accomplish a great deal of work in a very short time period. Inpatient programs must conduct a comprehensive assessment, develop and implement a treatment plan, and provide for disposition planning within a 20- to 30-day time period. Psychiatric hospitalization can range from a diagnostic or evaluation period of a few days to 4 to 6 weeks, depending upon the course of treatment and the patient's symptoms or disability. With a trend toward reduced hospital stays, much of the focus of treatment involves follow-up and aftercare services. Consequently, outpatient and aftercare services have expanded and are basically doing much of the work (e.g., individual/group therapy, pharmacotherapy, and behavior therapy) that traditionally has been accomplished in inpatient programs. Aftercare and follow-up services are necessary for the maintenance and generalization of hospital gains (Rosenfield, Caton, Nachumi, & Robbins, 1986). In far too many cases, the patient is admitted to an inpatient program, receives treatment for a number of weeks, and then is discharged back to the community without follow-up. Within a relatively short period of time, the patient regresses (i.e., patient does not take medications, caregivers do not know how to deal with the patient, or patient has no support group), and is readmitted to the hospital (Horn, 1986). This is particularly true for the mentally retarded and developmentally delayed individuals with psychiatric concerns (Marcos, Gil, Vazquez, 1986). Patients who have multiple needs and severely and profoundly mentally retarded individuals who were admitted to inpatient psychiatric care facilities have a more difficult time in maintaining and generalizing treatment gains than individuals who are within the borderline or normal range of intellectual functioning and who have psychiatric diagnoses. With this trend toward shorter inpatient stays and expanded services following the patient's discharge, staff training and community consultation/liaison are becoming a very important part of the patient's overall treatment package. As was previously noted, developing a consistent patient care plan within the hospital setting is necessary for the continuation of the patient's treatment plan after discharge and is ultimately a major factor in successful patient outcomes. Management of the patient following discharge provides the opportunity for the individual to maintain hospital gains and, in turn, reduces the opportunity for the patient to regress to the point whereby hospitalization is again necessary. Providing proper training to the patient's caregivers, school personnel, and community agencies goes hand in hand with the patient's total treatment package. The days of inpatient programs with caregivers working independently and in isolated settings are rapidly changing. Good inpatient care should be accompanied by good aftercare. Because of many sophisticated assessment (i.e., video, EEG, MRI, neuropsychiatric and psychological testing) and specialized services (i.e., communications, behavior therapy, expressive arts, etc.), it is very difficult for the average local community mental health system to have enough individuals on staff to provide expertise in all of these service areas. It is therefore extremely important that inpatient hospital programs share this information through training and consultation to ensure good quality care.

Training for both the parents of patients and staff of referring agencies is similar in many ways to that of inpatient staff training, except that the training is geared for the natural or home setting. The environment of most inpatient programs is highly structured, provides 24-hour programming if necessary, and controls the variables that may influence the patient's target symptoms or behaviors. Thus, it becomes important that the course of treatment, treatment plan, and program be adapted for a variety of settings, including the home setting. All too often treatments that have been effective during the patient's inpatient hospital stay are unable to be adapted so that the programs can be implemented in the home setting. An example of this scenario follows.

An adolescent suffering from depression was admitted to an inpatient hospital program. The patient had a history of lying, stealing, running away, and suicidal ideation. During the course of hospitalization, the patient responded to pharmacotherapy (antidepressant medication) and a dual contingency token system (earning and losing tokens). The token system provided opportunities for the patient to earn privileges and rewards for the absence of the target symptoms. The program also included fines whenever the patient displayed any of the undesirable target behaviors (response cost). The combination of pharmacotherapy and behavior therapy was effective in eliminating the problem behavior. The inpatient staff was required to monitor, evaluate, and give tokens periodically throughout the day. Medications were also given and monitored by staff on a daily basis. The family situation is such that the adolescent lives at home with his mother who needs to work at night because she provides the only means of support for the family. The patient, for the most part, is often home alone, and the mother does not have time to consistently implement the token system. Given what is known about the child and the family situation, the likelihood of consistent implementation of the program is minimal.

What typically will happen is that the patient will be discharged and the successful token program and possibly the medication will not be implemented on a consistent basis, such that the patient again may need assistance. The above-mentioned scenario would have ended the same way even though the mother may have been involved in countless hours of training in the hospital. Part of the problem is that the programs that were established could not be generalized across settings. Program planning for treatment and generalization could have been accomplished by adapting the specific program to the family or home situation. Timely staff training and consultation in many cases may avert regression and a return of a patient to the hospital. Staff training and consultation for those outside of the hospital and community agencies have also been achieved in a variety of ways, the most common of which are group inservice training, role-playing, case observation, and hands-on training/feedback.

Group Inservice Training

Group training is provided in most cases without the presence of the patient or client. Generally, the staff is called together during the day while the client is participating in his or her day or school program. All permanent and part-time staff are scheduled for training. Many of the community agency staff have other daytime jobs, so it has been helpful to videotape the training session or offer the inservice a second time. This training is provided both in the hospital and in the natural environment.

Role-Playing

Training staff in community settings by role-playing is another technique that is probably used more frequently than large group staff training. Staff members who work in the community are less concerned about the patient's diagnosis but are more interested in knowing "If the patient displays a problem and we're out shopping, what do I do?" This is where role-playing becomes a very effective teaching tool. The trainer or consultant can train the staff by having each member take the role of the patient as well as the role of a staff member. Generally, this type of training answers most of the if/what questions (e.g., "If the client destroys property, what then do I do?").

Case Observation

The training of community staff and parents by using case observation is identical to the training of inpatient staff. The training usually takes place in the hospital setting. Community staff members observe through one-way mirrors the way in which the patient is managed and the intervention that is implemented. Then the staff asks questions regarding specific program steps and their application or adaptation in the home setting.

Hands-on Training

Because of the limited financial resources of community agencies and the availability of staff, hands-on training is probably the most frequently employed method to train staff in the management of the patient. The hands-on training typically follows the case observation in which the community staff or parent observes the inpatient staff working with the patient on the unit or ward. The community staff will then work under a consultant or trainer. The trainee is supervised at all times during the session and feedback is given along the way. The trainer or consultant must also take into account the application of the intervention in the home setting. The environment and contexts of the sessions can be modified to simulate those that the patient will experience following discharge. After the patient has been discharged, the trainer/consultant provides hands-on training in the home or school environment.

STAFF TRAINING AND CONSULTATION ACROSS SETTINGS: AN ILLUSTRATION

Lisa, a 17-year-old autistic and severely mentally retarded girl who resided in a community residential facility (CRF) with two other females, was referred to an inpatient unit for treatment of pica behavior. According to the DSM-III, *pica* refers to the persistent eating of nonnutritive substances (American Psychiatric Association, 1980). Pica is a severe and occasionally life-threatening behavior which may be associated with intestinal obstruction and gastrointestinal parasites. Lisa was admitted to an acute inpatient psychiatric care facility because she was ingesting tacks and paper clips. Prior to her hospitalization, various medications and behavioral interventions had been tried, but with a very limited degree of success.

The psychiatric team determined with the input of Lisa's parents and CRF staff that her behavior was life threatening and thus warranted restrictive behavioral interventions. A survey was completed by the patient's community program (see Figure 4) to determine the kinds of interventions that could be implemented within the community setting. This information is extremely important to obtain because the inpatient hospital program may identify a very successful program but because of the restrictive nature of the program, the referring agency may be unable to implement the program. Understandably, the philosophy of the agency and the social palatability of the program (how the community views the intervention) are important factors to consider when transporting interventions.

The community survey revealed that the referring agency was able to implement a wide variety of restrictive programs. A literature search for articles regarding the treatment of pica behavior was then completed. A systematic evaluation was made on deceleration or reduction techniques. It was found that both contingent water mist (Dorsey, Iwata, Ong, & McSwean, 1980; Peterson & Peterson, 1977) and aromatic ammonia (Baumeister & Baumeister, 1975; Tanner & Zeiler, 1975) had been reported to be effective interventions for eliminating pica behavior. Therefore, these two procedures were implemented using an alternating treatments design. Figure 2 shows the phases of the controlled study that evaluated treatment effectiveness for pica behavior (see Rojahn, McGonigle, Curico, & Dixon, 1989). The study consisted of three conditions—two active treatments and one no treatment. Each of the three conditions was assessed daily and implemented in a counterbalanced fashion. Phase 1 was an initial baseline followed by alternating treatments that evaluated the effects of water mist, aromatic ammonia, and no treatment control condition on the reduction of pica behavior.

The results of Phase 2, the alternating treatments phase, indicated that both of the active treatments (water mist and aromatic ammonia) were successful in eliminating pica behaviors following eight treatment sessions. Phase 3 of the study involved choosing between the two successful interventions. Based on information from the community program, water mist was chosen simply because the community perceived this intervention to be more socially acceptable when compared to aromatic ammonia. The third phase of the study (see Figure 2) discontinued the aromatic ammonia and implemented the water mist program as the

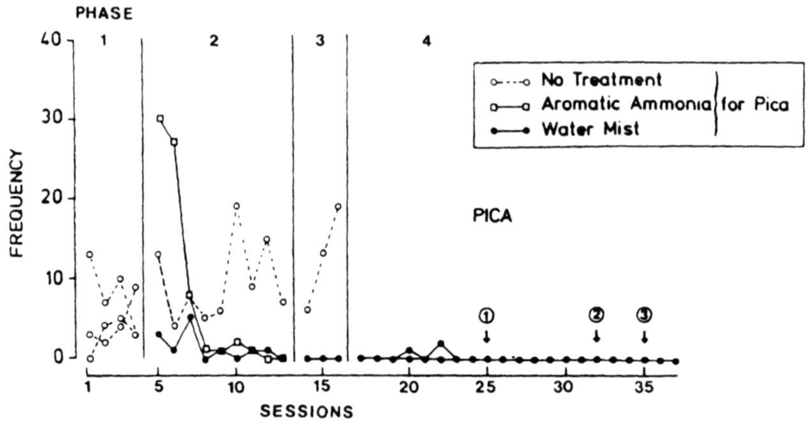

Figure 2. Frequency or occurrence of pica behavior across baseline, treatment, and staff-training sessions. From "Suppression of Pica by Water Mist and Aromatic Ammonia: A Comparative Analysis" by J. Rojahn, J. R. McGonigle, C. Curico, and M. J. Dixon, 1989, *Behavior Modification,* 11, pp. 65–74. Copyright 1989 by the Sage Publications, Inc. Reprinted by permission.

treatment of choice. The final phase of the study included systematic fading of the water mist bottle and training of the CRF staff as therapists. Because of the specialized nature of the intervention, the community staff members completed a verbal and written assessment regarding program implementation. The staff members were also involved in hands-on training by the therapist within individual treatment sessions. When it appeared that the community staff members clearly understood the procedures in the program, the patient was discharged back to her previous residence. Follow-up data collected in the home 3 months postdischarge reflected zero rates of pica. Through participation in an intense inpatient psychiatric program followed by successful staff training and consultation to the community agency, the patient's successful response to her program was well maintained long after discharge. Though the intervention described above was very exclusive, staff training still played an integral role in promoting the overall success of the patient, independent of the restrictive or complicated nature of the intervention. One of the main purposes for any inpatient hospital program is to treat patients whose symptoms or problems cannot be managed or cared for in the community. The individual is in need of 24-hour care. The job of an inpatient program is to evaluate and determine the motivation for the patient's problems and design and implement interventions to alleviate or reduce the symptoms. After this is achieved, the most important task of the inpatient staff is that of helping those around the patient to know and understand the problems at hand. This is accomplished by utilizing staff training through community consultation and liaison.

FACILITATING THE TRANSITION FROM THE HOSPITAL TO OTHER SETTINGS

Facilitating a transition from the hospital setting to the community is no small task. Depending on the severity of the patient's problems and the willingness of those involved with the patient, the trip home can be a disaster. Therefore, it is very important that the consultant have as much information about the patient and the settings as is possible. The types and varieties of settings that the patient is discharged to following the inpatient program are as wide and varied as the patients themselves. The settings are set up on a continuum ranging from a least restrictive to a more restrictive setting. The setting to which the patient is discharged depends greatly on the interventions or programs that it would take to maintain the patient in a particular setting. The settings to which patients are discharged following inpatient psychiatric care are diverse. The facilities listed below range from most restrictive to least restrictive:

1. *State Institution/State Facility.* Most restrictive of all settings. State facilities are long-term and have maximum security with locked wards and 24-hour supervision. Patients discharged to these settings are not yet ready for living in a community.
2. *Acute Psychiatric Care.* Short-term hospitalization on inpatient floor. Generally, 20- to 30-day evaluation period. Maximum security with 24-hour supervision. Patients are discharged to long-term care facilities as well as to a variety of community settings.
3. *Large and Small Intermediate Care Facilities (ICF).* Small programs generally have 4 to 8 beds. The larger facilities range from 50 to 100 beds. These facilities in all cases attempt to meet the needs of medically involved, mentally retarded individuals. Dually diagnosed patients (mentally retarded with psychiatric diagnoses) at times are discharged to these settings. The ICF/MR settings provide 24-hour supervision with a treatment team available on an as-needed basis. Depending on treatment gains, both short- and long-term stays are offered.
4. *Community Residential Facilities (CRF)/Group Homes.* Group homes are residential facilities in most cases with 3:1 or 3:2 staff ratio

depending on the needs of the patient. Minimum to maximum supervision is provided. Patients access the community for day and evening activities.

5. *Living at Home or Foster Placement*. The least restrictive setting for discharged patients. The patient is discharged back to the home setting or a home setting with foster parents. Least amount of supervision.

The consultation/liaison specialist provides the training across all settings and must have some understanding of community programs and the ability of community staff members to provide consistent quality care. Community agencies vary in their ability to implement behavioral techniques. Clinicians in acute short-term psychiatric care facilities have come to learn that cognitive and behavior therapy approaches are a must in the treatment of child and adolescent aberrant behavior. Many of the children discharged from the inpatient hospital setting take with them very specific and detailed behavior modification programs. However, the patient's chances for failure are high if the parents or community agencies have not been trained in the implementation of the program, or the programs are so restrictive or time consuming that they cannot be generalized or adapted to other settings.

The consultant must also have knowledge and understanding of some of the major risk factors that jeopardize community placements. These risk factors are behaviors or symptoms that are mainly referral concerns of the patient for treatment in a psychiatric care facility: (1) violent and destructive behavior, (2) fire setting, (3) sex offenses, (4) self-injurious behavior, (5) elopement, and (6) eating disorders (pica and food refusal). Psychiatric patients who have a discharge diagnosis of any of these will have a difficult time getting accepted into community placements. There are two reasons for the difficulty in placement. First and foremost are the liability issues for the receiving agency. Community agencies do not want to be responsible for a patient who will do harm to himself or herself or to others. Obviously, the community placement is responsible for the child or adolescent and the risk of lawsuits is a consideration. The second reason is that the receiving agencies are concerned with the kind and type of behavior programs that are necessary to be employed in order to keep the individual at home or in the community. Treatment both in and out of the hospital depends on the individual and the topography of the problem behavior. The prescribed and effective treatments range from positive reinforcement to punishment procedures which can vary in degree and intensity. The consultant needs to know the continuum of behavior interventions and the use of least to more restrictive approaches and the social palatability of the recommended program.

"First line" interventions are generally positive reinforcement programs (i.e., shaping, token programs, etc.). If such least restrictive interventions are unsuccessful and the patient continues to display problem behaviors, the next step in the continuum is the use of differential reinforcement programs. These response suppression techniques include differential reinforcement of other behaviors (DRO) (Repp, Deitz, & Speir, 1974) and differential reinforcement of incompatible behaviors (Weiher & Harman, 1975). These reinforcement programs represent positive ways to reduce behaviors. Most community programs have the ability to implement positive reinforcement programs; however, when patients are unresponsive to positive approaches or exhibit life-threatening behavior (i.e., pica, severe head banging, or eye gouging) or aggressive/destructive behavior, more restrictive or intrusive programs may be justified. A few popular behavior reduction techniques that have been employed for reducing and eliminating self-injury and aggressive destructive behaviors include: time out from positive reinforcement (Pendergass, 1972), overcorrection (Foxx & Azrin, 1973), and visual screening (McGonigle, Duncan, Cordisco, & Barrett, 1982).

A recently completed survey by McGonigle and Confer (1988) reviewed the types of behavior modification techniques employed in community residential facilities in the western region of Pennsylvania. Thirty-seven agencies in a 23 county area, with a combined total of 378 homes that cared for approximately 1,200 clients were given the survey. A checklist and a short description of each of the interventions was sent to the agencies with a questionnaire (see Figure 3). The ages of the clients being served in these agencies ranged from 1 year to 86 years of age. Reliability was conducted by random calls to the agencies and in-person visits to randomly selected agencies to again complete the survey.

Results of the survey indicated that all the interventions described were used in community settings (i.e., positive reinforcement, DRO, time out, water mist, etc.). Some agencies used more restrictive techniques (i.e., ammonia, visual screening), whereas others used positive reinforcement programs only (i.e., praise/attention, DRO, tokens, etc.). The prevalence of the techniques employed favored positive and less restrictive techniques than punishment or more restrictive techniques. Ninety-eight percent of the community agencies surveyed employed positive reinforcement.

The information gathered from the survey and the use of the checklist can be very helpful for inpatient staff for providing acceptable inter-

Date: ____________________

Client's Name: ____________________ DOB: ____________

Name of Agency/School: ____________________

Informant's Name: ____________________

Please indicate the programs that can be implemented within your facility.

Yes = Y No = N Not Sure = NS

_____ Differential Reinforcement of Other Behavior
_____ Differential Reinforcement of Appropriate Behavior
_____ Differential Reinforcement of Incompatible Behavior
_____ Nonexclusionary Time Out
_____ Extinction
_____ Planned Ignoring
_____ Systematic Attention
_____ Visual Screening
_____ Reprimands/Simple Correction
_____ Satiation
_____ Sensory Extinction
_____ Response Cost
_____ Response Interruption
_____ Compliance Training
_____ Water Mist
_____ Overcorrection
_____ Positive Practice
_____ Negative Practice
_____ Contingent Exercise
_____ Response Requirement
_____ Exclusionary Time Out
_____ Physical Restraint
_____ Mechanical Restraint
_____ Bitter Substances (lemon juice)
_____ Seclusion (isolation)
_____ Aromatic Ammonia

Figure 3. Intervention Questionnaire.

ventions for parents and for agency providers. If the inpatient treatment team had knowledge of the kinds of programming that can be effectively used in the community, it would help the clinicians to choose more selectively an intervention that increases the likelihood that the programs will be carried out following discharge. Oftentimes inpatient clinicians have labored in many intensive hours of individual behavior therapy sessions and many hours of staff training only to find out that the recommended program will not or cannot be implemented following a patient's discharge. This can be a frustrating situation, one that happens all too often. With the survey list of interventions, the treatment team can quickly choose the kinds of programs the referring parent or agencies are willing to use. This, in turn, will save the inpatient clinician's time and energy in evaluating programs that will be terminated when the patient walks out of the doors of the hospital, which ultimately increases the chances of readmission.

Thirty-five percent to fifty percent of chronic mentally ill patients are readmitted within 1 year of being discharged from the hospital (Anthony, Chen, & Vitalo, 1978; Lamb, 1980). This high rate of recidivism has been blamed on several factors. The two major factors appear to be functional and practical intervention strategies in staff and parent training. With sufficient staff training and community consultation, the patient leaving the hospital has a much greater chance in maintaining and generalizing treatment gains.

The necessary components for a successful treatment outcome for an individual who is receiving treatment in an inpatient hospital program include baseline assessment in the home setting, baseline assessment in the hospital, intervention, parent/staff training, home/school visits, and postdischarge follow-up. The role of staff training and consultation permeates most of the patient's hospital stay. In many cases, the need for training and consultation begins before the patient is even admitted to the hospital. The consultant goes to the community to provide consultation and gathers baseline information on the referral concerns prior to the patient's admission to the hospital. Shortly after the patient's admission, baseline measures are taken within the first 72 hours. Following the initial baseline in the hospital treatment evaluations along with staff and parent training will be the majority of the patient's stay. Once the treatment and the training have been completed, disposition planning includes movement from inpatient hospital settings back to the community.

Needs Assessment

Proper planning by way of a patient's needs assessment and both parent and staff training can be instrumental in making the transition successful from inpatient hospitalization back to the community. The long-term benefit is that the patient maintains treatment gains and reduces the likelihood of reentering the hospital (Perris *et al.*, 1985). One of the most effective ways to ensure continuity of care is to complete an individual needs assessment for each patient. The needs assessment serves two purposes: It will give the inpatient treatment team and clinicians much needed information about what is necessary to maintain the patient in the community. It will also provide information to assist in the development of the patient's treatment plan. The consultation/liaison specialist is the individual who is responsible for completing the patient needs assessment and informs the inpatient treatment team prior to the patient's discharge. The needs assessment is individualized and addresses two areas of major emphasis; namely, patient variables and setting variables. *Variables related to the patient* are the symptoms or problem behaviors that are being treated (i.e., aggression, self-injury, drug/alcohol abuse, etc.). *Variables related to the setting* include (1) the staff's and the parent's knowledge and understanding of the presenting problems, (2) the willingness to implement the prescribed behavioral/pharmacological interventions, and (3) the old versus the new setting. Is the patient returning to the same home prior to admission or is it a new home or community placement?

The patient's needs assessment should be completed shortly after admission to the inpatient program. Figure 4 is an example of a patient's needs assessment. As was previously mentioned, each needs assessment is individually based and the items on the assessment may vary according to the patient's needs. The general use of the assessment is to visit the setting and gather information by observation of the setting as well as to talk to the staff or parents of the patient. The information that needs to be obtained is: What does the patient need in order to be maintained in the community? The consultation/liaison specialist requires information, such as staffing ratio or how the patient is monitored. Does the community setting implement behavior programs? The patient needs to take care of the property of others or safety issues while in the community. Also, how are medications monitored? Following the needs assessment in the community, the liaison specialist then has to determine the current status of the patient in the hospital. This is accomplished by directly observing the patient while in treatment, reviewing the course of treatment via the patient's chart, and participation in the treatment team meeting. The patient's needs can be determined by making a comparison between where the patient needs to be in order to be effectively managed in the community and the current status of the patient. If there are major gaps between where the patient needs to be and the patient's current status, then the likelihood of the maintenance and generalization of hospital gains is significantly lowered.

INDIVIDUAL NEEDS ASSESSMENT

Name: Agency: ____________ Type of Placement: Group Home

Where he is:	Where he needs to be:	YES	NO
Dress: Undress independently	Independent dress	____	____
Eats meals independently	Eats independently	____	____
Takes bath; showers	Independent bathing	____	____
Takes care of toileting needs independently	Independent toileting skills	____	____
Some difficulty in ascending and descending stairs	Able to go up and down steps	____	____
Four-to-one staff ratio waking hours; sleeps through night	Two-to-one staff ratio waking hours; no awake night staff	____	____
Aggressive two times per month	Aggressive two times per month	____	____
Two persons to physically manage	Two-to-one ratio	____	____
Appropriate while out in public	Appropriate use of community	____	____
Behavior programs	Behavior programs employed	____	____
Stays with group	Stays with group	____	____

Figure 4. Sample of items in the patient's individual needs assessment.

Case Histories

Using Figure 4 as a format, the needs assessments for two patients (Sam and Dave), who were discharged from an acute psychiatric inpatient program, are now reviewed. Both patients were 17-years-old, male, moderately retarded, with histories of aggressive and destructive behavior. Disposition for both patients was discharge to a community residential facility (CRF). The only major difference between the two patients was that Dave also had mild cerebral palsy. Following the completed needs assessment and based on the discrepancies between where the patients needed to be and their current status, it was quite clear that Sam was definitely going to have more difficulty following discharge than Dave. As reflected in the individual needs assessment, Sam presents with eight areas that seem to have discrepancies between where he is and where he needed to be. Most of the difficulties appear to be in the behavioral areas (i.e., running away, aggression, destruction of property). Dave, on the other hand, has few discrepancies. The group home staff was well trained, the home uses behavioral techniques, and the staffing ratio can handle episodes of aggression. In light of these differences prior to discharge, it was projected that Sam would not maintain his treatment gains and would eventually return for inpatient treatment, and that Dave would have little difficulty fitting into his new home.

The patients were discharged within 2 weeks of one another, with Dave following Sam 2 weeks later. The second day after his discharge, Sam's group home staff called and said they were having difficulty with his aggression and wanted to know how to manage these difficult behaviors. Consultation was then provided at the group home. Three weeks following discharge, Sam was admitted to the emergency room for aggression, destruction of property, and running away. Subsequently, he was readmitted to the inpatient unit. Dave's situation turned out to be much more positive. Following his discharge, one consultation visit was made to the group home for clarification of behavior programs, and that was all that was needed. Dave made the transition very well and continues to be maintained in the community.

The success and failure of these two cases primarily rested on staff training and consultation. The group home that accepted Sam was not interested in implementing behavior programs or following recommendations about changing the environment to meet his needs. Consequently, the staff rarely observed him while he was an inpatient. The agency that accepted Dave was totally involved in his overall treatment. The group home staff for Dave participated in inservice training in the hospital, observed individual behavior therapy sessions, and were involved in hands-on training. The group home also made adjustments in the home environment. By comparing the needs assessments on the two discharged patients, it was fairly evident that the patient with the most gaps would have a more difficult time when returning to the community.

SUMMARY

Staff training and consultation have been implemented in a variety of ways across the continuum of service delivery systems, and from inpatient hospital settings to programs in the community. This chapter clearly shows that staff training and consultation are essential components for successful patient outcomes. Not only does staff training provide consistent programming, but it can also provide much needed assistance for patients in the transition from the hospital to the community. Many inpatient programs have very little knowledge about the home settings selected for patients. Treatment programs are often developed without the input of those individuals who will be working with patients following their discharge. With the length of hospital stays getting shorter and much of the unfinished work being completed after discharge, inpatient programs can no longer afford to operate in a vacuum. It has become quite clear that inpatient programs must work more closely with community agencies through the judicious use of staff training and consultation in an effort to maximize long-term adjustment.

REFERENCES

American Psychiatric Association. (1980). *Diagnostic and statistical manual of mental disorders* (3rd ed.). Washington, DC: Author.

Andrasik, F., & McNamara, J. R. (1977). Optimizing staff performance in an institutional behavior change system. *Behavior Modification, 1,* 235–248.

Anthony, W. A., Cohen, M. R., & Vitalo, R. (1978). The measurement of rehabilitation outcome. *Schizophrenia Bulletin, 4,*365–383.

Baumeister, A. A., & Baumeister, A. A. (1978). Suppression of repetitive self-injurious behavior by contingent inhalation of aromatic ammonia. *Journal of Autism and Childhood Schizophrenia, 8,* 71–77.

Brown, P. L., & Presbie, R. J. (1974). *Behavior Modification Skills.* Hicksville, NY: Research Media.

Burg, M. M., Reid, D. H., & Lattimore, J. (1979). Use of self recording and supervision program to change institutional staff behavior. *Journal of Applied Behavior Analysis, 12,* 363–375.

Delamater, A. M., Connors, C. K., & Wells, K. C. (1984). A comparison of staff training procedures. Behavioral applications in the child psychiatric inpatient setting. *Behavior Modification, 8,* 39–58.

Dorsey, M. F., Iwata, B. A., Ong. P., & McSween, T. E. (1980). Treatment of self-injurious behavior using a water mist: Initial response suppression and generalization. *Journal of Applied Behavior Analysis, 13,* 324–333.

Dowrick, P. W., & Johns, E. M. (1976). Video feedback effects on therapist attention to on-task behaviors of disturbed children. *Journal of Behavior Therapy and Experimental Psychiatry, 1,* 255–257.

Fielding, L. T., Errickson, E., & Bettin, B. (1971). Modification of staff behavior: A brief note. *Behavioral Therapy, 2,* 550–553.

Foxx, R. M., & Azrin, N. W. (1973). The elimination of autistic self-stimulatory behavior by overcorrection. *Journal of Applied Behavior Analysis, 6,* 1–14.

Gardner, J. M. (1972). Teaching behavior modification to non-professionals. *Journal of Applied Behavior Analysis, 5,* 517–521.

Gary, J. J. (1974). Methods of training psychiatric residents in individual behavior therapy. *Journal of Behavior Therapy and Experimental Psychiatry, 5,* 19–25.

Hagen, R. L., Craighead, W. E., & Paul, G. L. (1975). Staff reactivity to evaluative behavioral observations. *Behavior Therapy, 6,* 201–205.

Hall, R. V., Panvan, M., Rabon, D., & Broden, M. (1968). Instructing beginning teachers in reinforcement procedures which improve classroom control. *Journal of Applied Behavior Analysis, 1,* 315–322.

Hersen, M., & Barlow, D. H. (1976). *Single case experimental designs: Strategies for studying behavior change.* New York: Pergamon Press.

Hollander, M. A., & Plutchik, R. (1972). A reinforcement program for psychiatric attendants. *Journal of Behavior Therapy and Experimental Psychiatry, 3,* 297–300.

Horn, G. H., (1984). Aftercare and readmission: A Dutch psychiatric case register study. *Social Psychiatry, 19,* 111–116.

Jones, F. H., & Eimers, R. C. (1975). Role playing to train elementary teachers to use a classroom management "skills package." *Journal of Applied Behavior Analysis, 8,* 421–433.

Kissel, R. C., Whitman, T. L., & Reid, D. H. (1983). An institutional and staff training and self-management program for developing multiple self-care skills in severely/profoundly retarded individuals. *Journal of Applied Behavior Analysis, 16,* 395–415.

Lamb, H. R. (1982). *Treating the long-term mentally ill.* San Francisco Jossey-Bass.

Landesman-Dwyer, S., & Knowles, M. (1987). Ecological analysis of staff training in residential settings. In J. Hogg & P. Mittler (Eds.), *Staff training in mental handicap.* Cambridge, MA: Brookline Books.

Horn, Len G. H. M. M. (1984). Aftercare and readmission. *Social Psychiatry, 19,* 111–116.

Marcos, L. R., Gil, R. M., & Vazquez, K. M. (1986). Case report. *Hospital and Community Psychiatry, 37,* 171–174.

Martin, G., & Pear, J. (1983). Behavior Modification: What is and how to do it (2nd ed.). Englewood Cliffs: Prentice-Hall.

McGonigle, J. J., & Confer, S. J. (1988, November). *The prevalence and types of behavior modification techniques employed in community living arrangements in the Western Region of Pennsylvania.* Paper presented at the Council for Exceptional Children Pennsylvania Chapter, Harrisburg.

McGonigle, J. J., Duncan, D., Cordisco, L., & Barrett, R. P. (1982). Visual screening: An alternative method for reducing stereotypic behaviors. *Journal of Applied Behavior Analysis, 15,* 461–467.

McKeown, D., Adams, H. E., & Forehand, R. (1975). Generalization to the classroom of principles of behavior modification taught to teachers. *Behaviour Research and Therapy, 13,* 85–92.

Peed, S., Roberts. M., & Forehand, R. (1977). Evaluation of the effectiveness of a standardized parent training program in altering the interaction of mothers and their noncompliant child. *Behavior Modification, 1,* 323–350.

Pendergass, V. E. (1972). Time out from positive reinforcement following persistent high rate behavior in retardates. *Journal of Applied Behavior Analysis, 5,* 85–90.

Perris, C., Radhe, A., Palm, R., Hellgren, S., Lilja, C., & Soderman, H. (1985). Fully integrated in-and-out patient services in a psychiatric sector: Implementation of a new model for the care of psychiatric patients, favoring continuity of care. *Social Psychiatry, 20,* 60–69.

Peterson, R. F., & Peterson, L. R. (1968). The use of positive reinforcement in the control of self-destructive behavior in a retarded boy. *Journal of Experimental Child Psychology, 6,* 351–360.

Quilitch, H. R. (1975). A comparison of three staff-management procedures. *Journal of Applied Behavior Analysis, 8,* 59–66.

Realon, R. E., Lewallen, J. D., & Wheeler, A. J. (1983). Verbal feedback vs. verbal feedback plus praise: The effects on direct care staff's training behaviors. *Mental Retardation, 5,* 209–212.

Repp, A., Deitz, S., & Speir, N. (1974). Reducing stereotypic responding of retarded persons by the differential reinforcement of other behavior. *American Journal of Mental Deficiency, 78,* 279–284.

Rojahn, J., McGonigle, J. R., Curico, C., & Dixon, M. J. (1989). Suppression of pica by water mist and aromatic ammonia: A comparative analysis. *Behavior Modification, 11,* 65–74.

Rosenfield, S., Caton, C., Nachumi, G., & Robbins, E. (1986). Closing the gaps: The effectiveness of linking programs connecting chronic mental patients from the hospital to the community. *Journal of Applied Behavioral Science, 227,* 411–423.

Sanders, M. R., & Glynn, T. (1981). Training parents in behavioral self-management: An analysis of generalization and maintenance. *Journal of Applied Behavior Analysis, 14,* 223–237.

Tanner, B. A., & Zeiler, M. D. (1975). Punishment of self-injurious behavior using aromatic ammonia as aversive stimulus. *Journal of Applied Behavior Analysis, 8,* 53–57.

Waltz, G. R., & Johnston, J. A. (1963). Counselors look at themselves on video tape. *Journal of Counseling Psychology, 10,* 232–236.

Weiher, R. G., & Harman, R. E. (1975). The use of omission training to reduce self injurious behavior in a retarded child. *Behavior Therapy, 7,* 261–268.

Welsch, C. J., Ludwig, C., Radiker, J. E., & Krapil, J. E. (1973). Effects of feedback on daily completion of behavior modification projects. *Mental Retardation, 11,* 24–27.

3

Medical Aspects of Psychiatric Treatment of Children

JOSEPH STRAYHORN

THE NATURE OF MEDICAL DECISION MAKING

There was once an era in which "medical model" thinking and learning theory were seen as opposed and mutually exclusive, as if mental health practitioners could handle only one major conceptual model. Inclusion of this chapter in a book on behavior therapy represents the growing consensus that human behavior is complex enough to require more than one conceptual approach; even as we focus on the one, it is important to remind ourselves of the other. We wish to avoid adopting behavioral methods as our main treatment for brain tumors, just as we wish to avoid drugging children who have learned to get their way through tantrums.

The medical model is most useful when efficacy of treatment is maximized by consideration of diagnoses rather than of individual symptoms or complaints. The diagnostic thinker collects a data base of information, makes hypotheses about diagnoses, then collects more information to confirm or refute these hypotheses, and finally applies treatment accordingly. The data base includes the history, or the infor-

JOSEPH STRAYHORN • Medical College of Pennsylvania, Allegheny General Hospital, Early Childhood Clinic, Pittsburgh, Pennsylvania 15212.

Inpatient Behavior Therapy for Children and Adolescents, edited by Vincent B. Van Hasselt and David J. Kolko. Plenum Press, New York, 1992.

mation the person gives; the physical examination, or the information obtained from looking at, listening to, touching, and tapping on the patient; and the laboratory tests.

One possible way of making diagnoses would be simply to gather all possible information from each of these three sources, to examine the patterns of findings, and to compare them to the patterns produced by various disorders. In practice, however, a more interesting and economical thought process is used, in which initial information generates hypotheses that guide the collection of further information. The patient has a concrete complaint, for example, fatigue and loss of energy. The clinician then generates a list of possible disorders that could cause the symptom—a differential diagnosis. In the case of fatigue and energy loss, this list would include depression, hypothyroidism, mononucleosis, anemia, and many others. The disorders in the differential diagnosis constitute hypotheses to be checked out, one by one. The next step is to check these hypotheses by searching for the other features also likely to be present in each of the disorders. For example, with depression we are likely to find sad mood, difficulty staying asleep, appetite loss, reduced pleasure in activities, and so forth; with hypothyroidism we are likely to find intolerance of cold, constipation, dry skin, slowed heart rate, slowed muscle-stretch reflexes, and abnormal findings on laboratory assays of thyroid hormones. We can proceed most efficiently when there is some feature invariably present with a certain disorder, such that the absence of this feature "rules out" the disorder. In testing one of the hypotheses on the differential diagnosis, we gather first the information obtained inexpensively, that is, from the history and physical examination, and employ more expensive laboratory tests if our hypothesis has not been ruled out by less expensive methods. Each abnormal finding that we accumulate has its own differential diagnosis, and each disorder on that list has its own set of abnormal findings. Diagnosis involves constant reference to these two types of lists; this chapter, accordingly, will be unabashedly full of lists.

I will quickly review the findings consistent with three types of disorders: psychiatric syndromes, side effects of psychotropic drug treatment, and medical disorders that can masquerade as psychiatric symptoms. I will review the significance of frequently obtained laboratory results. Finally, although violent behavior is a symptom, not a diagnosis, I will examine some of the literature on treating it pharmacologically, since it so often is a focus of treatment on inpatient units. In order to condense into one chapter a topic broad enough for several shelves of books, I will select primarily the disorders where treatment seems to make the most difference.

DIAGNOSIS OF PSYCHIATRIC SYNDROMES

In an era in which the American Psychiatric Association's diagnostic and statistical manuals, most recently the DSM-III-R (American Psychiatric Association, 1987), have been given such great emphasis, it is hardly necessary to emphasize the diagnosis of psychiatric syndromes. Nonetheless, in gathering a data base from a child and the family, it is good to have these lists so readily available that when a symptom or two raises a hypothesis of a syndrome, the clinician is able to check out the hypothesis by asking all the remaining questions on the list. Table 1 provides a highly condensed version of the DSM-III-R, which may be an aid to memory in the process of history taking. I exclude most of the personality disorders, which, in my opinion, usually benefit less from syndromal diagnosis than from identification of psychological skills most in need of improvement; I exclude the organic disorders, which usually benefit less from a syndromal diagnosis than from one based on the specific cause of the illness.

The job of the clinician should include looking for treatable psychiatric syndromes in the child's parents. The behavioral clinician who undertakes parent training, for example, will have better results with a severely depressed parent if that parent is first, or simultaneously, treated for depression.

One of the ways in which syndromal diagnosis is helpful is in planning drug treatment. To summarize: psychosis that is due to schizophrenia, mania, or severe depression is usually helped by the antipsychotic or neuroleptic drugs; depression by the antidepressants or lithium or monoamine oxidase inhibitors; bipolar affective disorder by lithium; panic disorder by tricyclic antidepressants or monoamine oxidase inhibitors; alcohol withdrawal by sedatives, such as the benzodiazepines, and attention deficit hyperactivity disorder by the stimulants. The sedative drugs, including the benzodiazepines, often help anxiety symptoms, but sometimes add an addiction problem to the anxiety problem.

DRUG SIDE EFFECTS

The price of a set of drugs efficacious for psychiatric syndromes is a set of side effects that clinicians sometimes confuse with hypochondriasis or primary psychiatric illness or independently occurring medical illness. Before giving a drug, it is a good idea to see whether the patient

Table 1. Criteria for Some Psychiatric Syndromes in Children and Their Relatives

Attention deficit disorder: Fidgety; trouble staying seated; easily distracted; trouble awaiting turns; blurts out answers before questions are completed; trouble following instructions; trouble sustaining attention to tasks; shifts from one uncompleted activity to another; trouble playing quietly; talks excessively; interrupts and intrudes; does not listen to what is being said; loses things.

Oppositional defiant disorder: Loses temper; argues with adults; actively refuses requests; deliberately annoys people; blames others for own mistakes; easily annoyed by others; resentful, vindictive, and swears.

Conduct disorder: Stealing with or without confrontation of victim; running away; lying; deliberate fire setting; truancy; breaking and entering; destroying property; cruelty to animals; forcing of sexual activity; using weapon in fights; initiates fights; physical cruelty to people.

Antisocial personality disorder: Before age 15: was truant; ran away from home; started fights; used weapon in fight; forced sexual activity; was physically cruel to animals; was physically cruel to people; destroyed property deliberately; set fires; lied often, and stole. After age 15: unable to sustain work behavior; repeated unlawful behavior; repeated physical fights or assaults; did not honor financial obligations; did not plan ahead; lied; was reckless about safety; neglected children's needs; squandered money; could not sustain monogamous relationship; and lacked remorse.

Borderline personality disorder: Unstable and intense interpersonal relations characterized by overidealization and devaluation; impulsiveness in potentially self-damaging way; great and rapid shifts in mood; inappropriately intense anger; recurrent suicidal or self-mutilating behavior; uncertainty about self-image, sexual orientation, goals, friends, or values; long-lasting feelings of emptiness or boredom; frantic efforts to avoid real or imagined abandonment.

Separation anxiety disorder: Unrealistic worry about attachment figures' being harmed or leaving; worry about calamitous events that would separate child from attachment figure; refusal or reluctance to go to school; refusal or reluctance to go to sleep without attachment figure present; avoidance of being alone by following attachment figures around; nightmares about separation; physical sumptoms when separation is imminent; great distress when anticipating separation; great distress when separated.

Avoidant disorder: Great shyness despite wish to have friends.

Overanxious disorder: Worries about the future, one's own past behavior, competence, and somatic complaints; self-consciousness; need for reassurance; inability to relax.

Generalized anxiety disorder: Unrealistic worry or apprehension about two or more life circumstances, not related to another disorder if present; trembling, twitching, feeling shaky; muscle tension, aches, or soreness; restlessness; easy fatigability; shortness of breath or smothering sensations; rapid heart rate; sweaty hands; dry mouth; dizziness or lightheadedness; nausea, diarrhea, or other abdominal distress; hot flashes or chills; frequent urination; trouble swallowing or lump in throat; feeling keyed up or on edge; exaggerated startle response; difficulty concentrating or mind going blank because of anxiety; trouble falling or staying asleep; irritability.

(*continued*)

Table 1. (Continued)

Sleep terror disorder: Episodes of abrupt awakening for 1–10 minutes, usually in first third of major sleep period, usually beginning with panicky scream; rapid heart rate; rapid breathing; sweating; no detailed dream recalled; unresponsiveness to efforts of others to comfort; confusion; perseverative motor movements, such as picking at a pillow.

Panic disorder: Discrete episodes of intense fear and discomfort that are unexpected and are not due to being the focus of others' attention. During the attacks, shortness of breath or smothering sensations; dizziness or faintness; rapid heart rate; trembling; sweating; choking; abdominal distress; feeling not oneself or that things are not real; numbness; hot flashes or chills; chest discomfort; fear of dying; and fear of going crazy or doing something uncontrolled.

Panic disorder with agoraphobia: The panic disorders listed above, plus fears and avoidance of places where escape might be difficult or embarrassing in case of a panic attack (e.g., being outside the home alone, being in a crowd, standing in a line, being on a bridge, or traveling in a bus, train, or a car).

Obsessive-compulsive disorder: Recurrent or persistent thoughts experienced as intrusive and senseless, despite attempt to ignore or suppress these thoughts; thoughts realized as product of one's own mind; thoughts not related in content to another disorder the person has. Recurrent intentional behaviors, designed to prevent or neutralize discomfort, behavior excessive or not realistic; person usually realizes behavior is unreasonable. Thoughts and behaviors are distressing and time consuming or interfere with role functioning.

Autistic disorder: Marked lack of awareness of the feelings of others; no or abnormal seeking of comfort in times of distress; no or impaired imitation; no or abnormal social play; gross inability to make peer friendships; impairment of communication; abnormal nonverbal communication; absence of imaginative activity; marked abnormalities in speech volume, pitch, rate, stress, or rhythm; echolalia or pronoun reversal or idiosyncratic phrases; impairment in ability to sustain a conversation; stereotyped movements; preoccupation with the parts of objects or attachment to unusual objects; distress over trivial changes in the environment; unreasonable insistence on following routines in precise detail; preoccupation with one narrow interest or restricted range of interests.

Psychosis secondary to schizophrenia: Delusions, hallucinations, and incoherence or loosening of associations; catatonic behavior (consisting of markedly abnormal movement: (e.g., excited purposeless movement, resistance to being moved, assuming a bizarre posture); flat affect or grossly inappropriate affect; and functioning below the expected level.

Prodromal or residual symptoms of schizophrenia: Social isolation; impairment in role functioning; very peculiar behavior; impairment in hygiene or grooming; blunted or inappropriate affect; disorganized speech; odd beliefs; unusual perceptual experiences; and lack of initiative.

Tourette's disorder: Multiple motor tics, and one or more vocal tics (such as grunts, barks, yelps, words, obscene words, sniffs, or coughs).

(continued)

Table 1. (Continued)

Depression: Depressed or irritable mood; loss of pleasure from activities; increase or decreased appetite with weight gain or loss; insomnia or hypersomnia; agitated movement or slowed movement; fatigue and loss of energy; feelings of worthlessness or inappropriate guilt; trouble concentrating or making decisions; thoughts of death or suicidal ideation.

Mania: Abnormally elevated, expansive, or irritable mood; grandiosity; decreased need for sleep; increased talkativeness; racing thoughts; distractibility; increased activity level; excessive involvement in pleasurable activities with danger of painful consequences; impairment of social or occupational functioning.

Anorexia nervosa: Refusal to maintain body weight greater than 15% less than expected for age and height; fear of getting fat though underweight; perceiving oneself as fat though underweight; absence of three consecutive menstrual cycles in females.

Bulimia nervosa: Recurrent eating binges; feeling of lack of control of eating behavior during binges; self-induced vomiting; use of laxatives, fasting, or vigorous exercise to prevent weight gain; persistent overconcern with body shape and weight.

Alcohol withdrawal symptoms: Cessation or reduction of alcohol consumption within a week; nausea or vomiting; malaise or weakness; rapid heart rate; sweating; elevated blood pressure; anxiety; depressed mood or irritability; transient hallucinations or illusions; headache, insomnia, or delirium.

Psychoactive substance dependence: Taking substance in larger amounts than intended; unsuccessful efforts to cut down on use; large time spent getting substance or recovering from its use; frequent intoxication or withdrawal symptoms that interfere with fulfilling role expectations; important activities reduced or given up because of substance use; continued use despite knowledge of harm; marked tolerance; withdrawal symptoms; and use of the substance to avoid withdrawal symptoms.

already has any of the symptoms in the list of those the drug may produce, in order to prevent confusion of drug side effects with symptoms from other causes. When the drug is prescribed, any symptoms that arise should be monitored; serious side effects prompt a discontinuation of the drug. Table 2 lists the most common side effects of common psychotropic drugs; see also Hyman and Arana (1987).

Medical Problems That Can Masquerade as Psychiatric Symptoms

Differential Diagnosis

The differential diagnosis of behavioral and emotional symptoms is without a doubt the largest and most complex one in all of medicine.

Table 2. Side Effects of Commonly Used Psychotropic Drugs

Stimulants: Loss of appetite, insomnia, depressed mood, toxic psychosis, mild increase in heart rate and blood pressure, headaches, and abdominal pain. Significant but small reduction in growth.

Lithium: Nausea, vomiting, appetite loss, diarrhea, and abdominal pain. Increased urination, with resultant increased thirst and drinking of liquids. Tremor, fatigue, and weakness. Muscle twitching, unsteadiness when walking, lack of coordination, slurred speech, confusion, and memory difficulties. Dulling of affects; "graying" of emotional life. Thyroid goiter; hypothyroidism. Alteration of heart rhythm. Acne, psoriasis. Increased white blood cell count, without impairing function. Birth defects when given to pregnant women.

Antidepressants: Fall in blood pressure, and faintness when standing up. Worsening of certain heart rhythm disturbances. Increased likelihood of seizures in epileptic patients. Anticholinergic side affects: dry mouth, constipation, trouble in starting urinating, more rapid heart rate, blurred vision of close objects, worsening of narrow-angle glaucoma. Anticholinergic toxic effects (usually seen only when dose is too high or when other anticholinergic drugs are also given): warm dry skin, fever, dilated pupils, retention of urine, confusion, disturbance of recent memory, restlessness, slurred speech, hallucinations, delirium, and seizures.

Antipsychotic or neuroleptic drugs: Dystonias (substained involuntary contraction of a muscle or muscle group); akasthisia (an unpleasant continuous need to move); Parkinsonian symptoms (reduced animation in facial expressions, stiffness of muscles, slow movement, tremor, stooped posture, and drooling). Neuroleptic malignant syndrome: rigidity, fever, wide variation in blood pressure and heart rate, and encephalopathy. Tardive dyskinesia: a long-term side effect, consisting of repetitive quick involuntary movements of muscles, which, in the early stages of the disorder, are usually in the tongue, cheeks, lips, or face.

Too much of the hormone prolactin, which can result in lactation in females and impotence in males.

The "low potency" antipsychotics, such as chlorpromazine, have the same anticholinergic effects and the same type of cardiac effects as do the antidepressants, including low blood pressure when the patient stands up, sensitivity to sunburn, and, rarely, liver disease or the shutdown of production of blood cells.

Carbamazepine: Dizziness, unsteady gait, clumsiness, sedation, slurred speech, double vision, nausea, and mild reversible lowered white blood cell count. Less commonly: tremor, memory problems, confusion, and heart rhythm problems. Rarely: rash, opaque bodies in lens of eye, inflammation of liver, shutdown of blood cell production.

Beta-adrenergic blockers (e.g., propranolol): Low blood pressure, slowed heart rate, dizziness, and complications in patients with preexisting heart disease. Worsening of asthma. Worsened low blood sugar reactions in diabetics. Nausea, diarrhea, and abdominal pain. Impotence. Fatigue, energy loss, depression, insomnia, and nightmares.

(*continued*)

Table 2. (Continued)

Benzodiazepines: Fatigue, drowsiness, reduced coordination, impairment of memory and cognition, susceptibility to auto accidents, and disinhibition leading to violence. Seizures and other features similar to alcohol withdrawal syndrome can result during withdrawal.

Monoamine oxidase inhibitors: Low blood pressure on standing up, insomnia, agitation, sexual dysfunction, less severe anticholinergic effects than with tricyclics, weight gain, and swelling of ankles. In response to ingestion of foods containing tyramine, including certain cheeses, certain wines, and other foods, or when given along with sympathomimetic drugs, such as amphetamines or L-dopa, severe high blood pressure may result. When given along with meperidine, fever, delirium, or alteration of blood pressure. Adverse interactions also seen with oral antidiabetes drugs and with tricyclic antidepressants.

Table 3 will present an extensive list of organic illnesses that can be confused with learned maladaptive patterns. The disorders are organized into groups according to the cause: toxic, traumatic, infectious, idiopathic, neoplastic, nutritional, congenital, collagen vascular, endocrine, vascular, metabolic, multiple causes, and degenerative. We will examine some of the most common and/or treatable disorders on the list. For a more extended discussion of these disorders, see Strayhorn (1987).

Toxic: Lead Toxicity

Lead toxicity, especially that of less severe form, is common, is likely to present with behavioral symptoms, and has a much better outcome if treated early; accordingly, it is a problem that behavioral clinicians should be familiar with.

A child with early lead toxicity could have a totally normal physical examination, and only such symptoms as increased irritability, decreased appetite, and decreased play activity. Although paint chips from older houses are a well-known source of lead, the history of eating paint chips is not required for a suspicion of lead toxicity. It is a frightening fact that dirt is often found to have high lead concentrations—sometimes approaching half the concentration in paint chips (Chisolm, 1983; Graef, 1983). Rutter (1983) cited five studies to the effect that children's blood lead levels are related to soil concentrations in their neighborhoods; further evidence (Russell Jones & Stephens, 1983) supports the conclusion that the major source of such lead is that released by the burning of leaded gasoline. Elevated lead levels (over 30 μg/dL) were

Table 3. Differential Diagnosis of Organically Caused Behavioral Symptoms in Children and Adolescents

Toxic

Alcohol and other sedatives: Acute alcohol intoxication; intoxication with other sedatives; alcohol withdrawal syndrome; and withdrawal syndrome from other sedatives.

Over-the-counter drugs: Bromide poisoning; scopolamine poisoning; salicylate poisoning; vitamin A poisoning; vitamin D poisoning; caffeinism; and monosodium glutamate syndrome.

Prescription drugs: Reaction to steroids; isoniazid; digitalis; reserpine; antihistamines; methylphenidate and other stimulants; insulin; propranolol; methyldopa; barbiturates (e.g. phenobarbital); other sedatives; other anticonvulsants; theophylline; lithium; procaine penicillin; narcotics; birth control pills; ergotamine; and catecholamines.

"Recreational" drugs: LSD, phencyclidine, marijuana, mescaline, psilocybin, cocaine, and others.

Heavy metals: Lead, mercury, arsenic, calcium, and manganese.

Fumes and gases: Carbon monoxide, benzene, carbon tetrachloride, gasoline, glue, insecticides, and carbon disulfide.

Idiosyncratic reactions to foods and food additives.

Traumatic

Blow to the head resulting in concussion; contusion; laceration; subdural or epidural bleeding; cerebral edema; postconcussive symptoms; punch-drunk syndrome; and electrical injury. Subdural effusion.

Infectious

Bacterial meningitis; brain abscess; syphilis; viral encephalitis (including, among others, herpes simplex, herpes zoster, rabies, infectious hepatitis, infectious mononucleosis, and mumps). Lyme disease; AIDS; tuberculous meningitis; fungal infections (cryptococcosis, coccidiomycosis, histoplasmosis); rickettsial diseases (including Rocky Mountain spotted fever); parasitic illnesses (including trichinosis, echinococcosis, cysticercosis [tapeworm], toxoplasmosis); brucellosis; Sydenham's chorea; kuru; Creutzfeldt-Jakob disease; and subacute sclerosing panencephalitis.

Idiopathic

Narcolepsy, sleep apnea syndromes, Reyes syndrome.

(*continued*)

Table 3. (Continued)

Neoplastic

Brain tumors, metastatic tumors, remote effects of other tumors.

Nutritional

Folate deficiency, vitamin B_{12} deficiency, scurvy, protein-calorie malnutrition, thiamine deficiency, pellagra (nicotinic acid deficiency), and vitamin A deficiency.

Collagen Vascular, Autoimmune, and Allergic

Systemic lupus erythematosus, periarteritis nodosa, temporal arteritis.

Multiple sclerosis.

Allergies.

Congenital and Hereditary

Hepatolenticular degeneration (Wilson's disease); Huntington's chorea; tuberous sclerosis; Friedreich's ataxia; muscular dystrophies; neurofibromatosis; galactosemia; Gilles de la Tourette's disease.

Aminoacidurias, including phenylketonuria and Hartnup disease.

Acute intermittent porphyria; other porphyrias.

Central nervous system lipidoses, including Gaucher's disease, Niemann-Pick disease, and cerebromacular degeneration.

Leukodystrophies, including adrenoleukodystrophy and metachromatic leukodystrophy.

Mucopolysaccharidoses, including San Filippo's syndrome.

Chromosomal abnormalities, including Down's syndrome, fragile X syndrome, Turner's syndrome, and Klinefelter's syndrome.

Endocrine

Hyperthyroidism, hypothyroidism, Cushing's syndrome, Addison's disease, pheochromocytoma, hypopituitarism, hyperparathyroidism, hypoparathyroidism, diabetes mellitus, insulinoma, hypoglycemia, carcinoid, inappropriate ADH syndrome.

Vascular

Subdural hematoma, epidural hematoma, subarachnoid hemorrhage, hypertensive encephalopathy, migraine, and large unruptured cerebral aneurysms.

(continued)

Table 3. (Continued)

Metabolic
Cerebral hypoxia, uremia, hepatic encephalopathy, dehydration, water intoxication, hyponatremia, sodium depletion, potassium depletion, potassium excess, hypercalcemia, hypermagnesemia, hypomagnesemia, alkalosis, acidosis, hypercapnia, hyperthermia.
Multiple Causes
Vision problems, hearing problems. Epilepsy: petit mal; postconvulsive confusion following grand mal; psychomotor (i.e., complex partial or temporal lobe). Constipation as a cause of encopresis. Anemias. Sleep Apneas.

found in 4.5% of a sample of preschool children screened in 1980 (Graef, 1983). (This figure is down from 8% in 1975; the decrease is thought to be partly due to a decreased use of lead in gasoline.) Increased exposure to lead, without overt clinical toxicity, has been found correlated with greater distractibility from schoolwork, less organization, greater impulsivity, reduced ability to follow directions, and lowered overall classroom functioning; these correlations remained after statistical control for age, sex, and more than 30 demographic and socioeconomic variables (Needleman *et al.*, 1979).

How should the clinician carrying out a behavioral assessment avoid missing lead toxicity? It has been argued that free erythrocyte protoporphyrin levels, and/or blood lead levels, should be candidates for routine laboratory tests performed on children presenting with behavioral symptoms. Aside from routine screening, however, what factors in the clinical history should increase the clinician's suspicion of lead toxicity?

Children with a history of pica, that is, the eating of any nonfood substances, are at higher risk, as are children who live in older housing with crumbling paint. (The use of lead additives in residential paint decreased from the 1950s to the 1970s; in 1977, the use of lead additives in residential paints was banned in the United States (Chisholm, 1983)). Children who are less closely supervised by adults seem to be at higher risk. Exposure to lead in cooking vessels or water pipes, swallowing of lead shot, swallowing of camera or watch batteries, exposure to the fumes from fires where storage batteries have been burned, and exposure to the dust from sanding the walls of old houses should raise the suspicion if these exposures are reported. The report that a child gets a lot of dirt on his mouth should also raise the suspicion of lead toxicity. Abdominal pain, loss of appetite, vomiting, constipation, and anemia accompany the more severe levels of lead intoxication; it is hoped the toxicity will be detected before these symptoms occur. More severe toxicity results in confusion, staggering, persistent vomiting, seizures, and coma; by this time, the child should be hospitalized and the illness should be clearly under the bailiwick of a medical specialist.

Toxic: Toxicity from "Recreational" Drugs

In adolescents, the toxic effects of alcohol, marijuana, cocaine, hallucinogens, and other drugs constitute probably the most frequent biologic cause of behavioral difficulties. I will not discuss here the individual effects of each drug, but simply note that the key to diagnosis is the history of drug ingestion. This may sometimes be obtained from significant others when it is not obtained from the patient. Another clue that might raise the hypothesis of drug toxicity as a cause of altered behavior is the gradual spontaneous remission of symptoms after several days of hospital admission. Urine or blood testing for drugs may be useful, but when carrying out such tests, it is important to recall the half-life of the particular drug in the body and to make sure the sample is taken before the drug has been fully metabolized. Cocaine and morphine, for example, have half-lives of 1 hour and 2½ to 3 hours, respectively (Gilman, Goodman, Rall, & Murad, 1985). Alcohol is metabolized by the body at about 1 ounce per 3 hours (Gilman *et al.*, 1985). The inactive metabolites of marijuana have a half-life of about 30 hours (Gilman *et al.*, 1985).

Toxic: Side Effects of Prescribed Drugs

When assessing a child's behavioral problems, it is important to find out if the child is on any medications, since a variety of prescription drugs produce psychological side effects. I will mention only a few of the most common drug reactions resulting in psychological symptoms.

Theophylline is a drug used in the treatment of asthma. Irritability, insomnia, and tremor have occurred even at therapeutic doses of this drug. The restlessness that can be a side effect of this drug can be mistaken for attention deficit disorder (Bukowskyj, Nakatsu, & Munt, 1984; Weinberger & Hendeles, 1980).

Corticosteroid drugs, such as *cortisone* and *prednisone*, are used in the treatment of asthma, rheumatoid arthritis, inflammatory bowel diseases, and a variety of other illnesses. Emotional lability, depression, mania, and psychosis have been noted with substantial doses of these drugs.

Antihistamine drugs, which are often given for allergies, may produce either excitation or sedation in children; at other times these drugs have been known to cause a decrease in mental alertness resulting in school difficulties.

Phenobarbital, which is often used to control epileptic seizures, has been found to produce symptoms mimicking attention deficit disorder: trouble concentrating, restlessness, hyperactivity, and reduced impulse control. When children have taken psychometric tests with and without phenobarbital, performance has been worse on drug; these results correspond to complaints of impaired school performance (Stores, 1975).

Phenytoin, another drug for epileptic seizures, also can impair concentration, especially when the levels of this drug become too high. The classic picture of toxicity with this drug is staggering, lethargy, slurred speech, and jerky movements of the eyes (Stores, 1975).

Any of the stimulant medications used for attention deficit disorder, such as *methylphenidate, dextroamphetamine,* or *pemoline,* can produce psychiatric symptoms if the dose becomes too high. Such symptoms as agitation, confusion, hallucinations, and highly inappropriate behavior may occur.

When diabetic children who take insulin are found to be confused, "not with it," irritable, irrational, or not their usual selves, one possibility is that the glucose in their bloodstreams may be too low because of too much insulin relative to how much they have eaten. Since the brain requires a constant supply of energy in the form of glucose to function properly, a variety of psychological symptoms can occur with moderately low blood sugar. If the glucose gets even lower, the child can become unconscious, have his brain permanently injured, or die. The other symptoms that accompany low blood glucose are trembling, sweating, pounding of the heart, and a feeling of hunger. If a child with diabetes acts strange or has any of the other symptoms, low blood glucose should be suspected. If the child says that he feels that his sugar is low, he should be taken seriously. He should immediately be allowed to eat or drink whatever is available wiith the highest carbohydrate content.

Vitamins A and D, when taken in too large doses, can cause behavioral toxicity. For vitamin A, symptoms of appetite loss and irritability may be accompanied by itching, limited motion of joints, and tender swelling of bones. For vitamin D, symptoms of appetite loss and irritability may be accompanied by constipation, floppy and loose muscle tone, much urination and drinking of liquids, and pallor (Barness, 1983).

Traumatic: Subdural Effusions

The phrase *subdural effusion* refers to a collection of fluid between the brain and the skull. The subdural space is the space under the dura, which is one of the coverings of the brain. The fluid forms a mass that presses on the brain underneath it, resulting in symptoms that depend upon what brain regions are affected. What symptoms are produced also depends upon how rapidly the fluid collects.

The origin of subdural effusions is bleeding into the subdural space caused by a blow to the head. If the resulting bleeding is very fast, the symptoms are more obviously neurological: the child's head hurts, he vomits, he might have weakness or numbness on one side of the body, and he has other symptoms that effectively route him to a neurosurgeon. The more slowly progressing situation is called a *chronic subdural effusion.* The child can get knocked out from a blow on the head and seemingly recovers totally from the injury. But sometimes blood has escaped from one of the veins over the brain, and the clot that forms in the subdural space liquifies, after which water is drawn into the space around it to maintain osmotic equilibrium. As a result, a gradually bigger and bigger mass begins to push on the brain. The size of the mass and the intensity of the symptoms can increase over the course of days or sometimes weeks. The first symptoms can be behavioral symptoms of any sort. The history of the blow on the head is the main tip-off to suspect a chronic subdural; the appearance of headache, vomiting, or neurological symptoms (e.g., weakness, numbness, seizures, clumsiness, staggering, newly occurring visual problems) should raise the suspicion even further. Since child abuse is one way in which children sustain blows to the head, a suspicion of child abuse should also raise the possibility of a subdural effusion.

Infectious: Rocky Mountain Spotted Fever

Rocky Mountain spotted fever is an infection caused by a microorganism that is bigger than a virus but smaller than a bacterium, and possessing some of the characteristics of each. The infection is introduced into the human body by the bite of an infected tick. (These ticks seem to be most common not in the Rocky Mountains but in the Southeastern United States: North Carolina, South Carolina, Virginia, Tennessee, and their neighboring states.) After the infection has entered the body, it can incubate to 8 days, after which a progression of symptoms begins. Early symptoms may sometimes consist of changed personality or bizarre behavior or restlessness or other psychological symptoms. Headache, fever, and loss of appetite are also frequent early symptoms. As the disease progresses, more obvious medical symptoms rapidly appear, such as a rash that starts on the ankles and legs, muscle pain, intense "sick feeling," and other symptoms. Early treatment is very helpful, because there are antibiotics that can successfully cure this illness if diagnosis is correctly and promptly made.

Infectious: Brain Abscess

An *abscess* is a collection of pus surrounded by infected tissue. In some children with brain abscesses, the disease evolves over a course of several weeks (Till, 1975). Sometimes the first symptom can be irritability. Headache and vomiting can occur, especially if the abscess is big enough or at the right place to cause an obstruction of flow of the cerebrospinal fluid and an increase in the pressure inside the brain. If obvious neurologic signs appear (such as weakness, numbness, trouble with eye movements, trouble with vision, seizures, staggering, newly appearing incoordination, or loss of consciousness), the diagnosis is more readily made. Also, if the child has fever, the diagnostician is clued to search for infections. But all these clues can be absent in the child with a brain abscess. Sometimes the tip-off is the history of an infection elsewhere that could have been spread to the brain: infection of the ear, sinus, scalp, gum, or blood. Children with certain types of congenital heart diseases, such as those where blood can go directly from the right side of the heart to the left, are more likely to get brain abscesses (Till, 1975).

Infectious/Toxic: Reye Syndrome

The exact process causing *Reye syndrome* is unknown. It is not an infection in the usual sense but seems to occur more likely just after recovery from a viral infection (most often an upper respiratory tract infection, or, second, most often after chickenpox). It also is more likely to occur when the child has received aspirin (Hurwitz *et al.*, 1987; Starko, Ray, Dominguez, Stromberg, & Woodall, 1980). It affects the cells of various organs, especially the liver and the brain. Like bacterial meningitis, Rocky Mountain spotted fever, and several other rapidly progressing brain illnesses, Reye syndrome is obviously a medical illness once it gets to its full-blown form; in its early stages it has been known to be confused with psychiatric illness. But time is of the essence with such diseases, because the progression from early to later stages can take place over the course of hours. The illness can start out with manifestations of bizarre behavior, confusion, restlessness, irritability, combativeness, or other behavioral symptoms. More frequently, however, the patient develops severe nausea and vomiting at the beginning of the course. As the disease progresses, the child can become stuporous, have seizures, go into coma, or die. The disease is usually ended within a matter of a few days, either by recovery or by death. Although there is not a specific treatment for it, there are ways of reducing the most dangerous feature of the illness, namely the swelling of the brain. This reduction of swelling is accomplished primarily by intravenous infusion of mannitol, a carbohydrate that absorbs some of the water in the brain. This and other "supportive measures" substantially reduce the chance of dying from Reye syndrome (Riela & Roach, 1983).

Neoplastic: Brain Tumors

Fortunately, *brain tumors* cannot be said to be common in children; the incidence of nervous system tumors in children under 15 is somewhere in the region of 25 per million children per year (Till, 1975). However, tumors are second only to accidents as a cause of death in children, and nervous system tumors are the second most frequent type of tumors in children (Till, 1975).

The symptoms of brain tumors are determined mainly by where in the brain they are located, and how big they have gotten. If the tumor produces an obvious neurologic symptom, such as localized weakness, numbness, impaired movement of the eyes, reduced field of vision in one or both eyes, staggering, newly appearing incoordination, or a seizure, it is likely to be discovered quickly. However, in children, more often than not, tumors develop in "silent" areas that do not produce localized symptoms quickly. Often symptoms develop slowly, insidiously, and nonspecifically. The child may have irritability, poor concentration, and diminished school achievement. Physical symptoms, such as clumsiness of gait, headaches, or slowed growth rate, may be the tip-offs that prompt a search for brain tumor. In children, tension headaches are not nearly so common as they are in adults; thus, persistent headaches should be seriously investigated (Till, 1975). As the tumor progresses, the flow of cerebrospinal fluid in the brain may be obstructed and pressure inside the head may increase; vomiting is a prominent symptom of such a condition.

Hereditary: Wilson's Disease

Wilson's disease is genetic, transmitted by a recessive gene that is autosomal (i.e., not on a sex chromosome). Like all other illnesses caused by recessive genes, it is more common in children whose parents are blood relatives of each other. The primary defect is in the liver, which becomes incapable of properly excreting the copper that is present in small degrees in the normal diet. As copper accumulates in the body, it damages the liver, brain, kidneys, and corneas. In the early stages of the illness, the effects on the brain may mimic psychiatric symptoms; in from 10% to 25% of symptomatic patients, the first clinical manifestation of Wilson's disease is psychiatric (Scheinberg & Sternlieb, 1984). Impaired intellectual performance, irritability, impulsivity, unexplained personality change, emotional lability, or other nonspecific psychological symptoms may occur. As the disease progresses undiagnosed, slurred speech, tremors, muscle rigidity, involuntary twitches, and/or an immobile open-mouthed grinning facial expression may develop. Psychiatric symptoms may progress to manic or schizophrenic symptoms, neurotic symptoms, or bizarre behavior, sometimes including criminal behavior. Almost every patient with clinically manifest Wilson's disease suffers psychiatric symptoms of some sort (Scheinberg & Sternlieb, 1984). For the school child, school academic performance would be expected to deteriorate over the course of the illness. Kayser-Fleisher rings begin to develop around the outer rim of the corneas: these are grayish, start as an arc, and gradually encircle the cornea. Because psychiatric symptoms can be the only manifestations of this treatable illness in its early stages, at least one major psychiatric center runs a laboratory screening test for Wilson's disease on nearly every inpatient. The reason this is not done more frequently is because of the rarity of the illness. Its worldwide incidence is estimated at 3 cases per million new patient visits (Scheinberg & Sternlieb, 1984). Sheinberg and Sternlieb recommend ordering the serum ceruloplasmin, which is a laboratory test for Wilson's disease, in psychiatric patients if there is a family history of the disorder, if there is a history of unexplained liver disease, if the psychiatric illness is less responsive to treatment than expected, or if neurologic signs and symptoms supervene. Early treatment with penicillamine, a drug that binds copper, can abort the progression of the damage.

Hereditary: Tourette's Disease

Little is known of the causation of *Tourette's disease;* however, it does appear to run in families, and most researchers think that it has a genetic contribution (Kidd & Pauls, 1982). It begins in childhood between the ages of 2 and 15 years. The symptoms are interesting: there are several types of involuntary jerky muscle movements; for example, jerks of the shoulders of the arms, jerks of the neck, or twitches of the face. In addition, there are "vocal tics": involuntary grunts, barks, clicks, snorts, mutterings, or other noises. The most bizarre symptom is known as *coprolalia:* irresistable utterings of "obscene words." This symptom occurs in a little over half of the children with Tourette's disorder (Nuwer, 1982). As may be imagined, the syndrome causes social problems for patients that may be quite severe. The prevalence is about one hundredth to five hundredths of a percentage of the population (American Psychiatric Association, 1987). It is somewhat responsive to drug therapy: haloperidol and clonidine are most frequently used. Stimulant medication often worsens the symptoms of Tourette's disorder; this fact is unfortunate since many children with Tourette's disorder have attention deficit symptoms.

Endocrine: Hypothyroidism, Hyperthyroidism

If we compare the body to a motor, thyroid hormone's role seems to be to turn up the idling speed. *Hyperthyroidism* results in greater expenditure of energy, increased heart rate, weight loss despite increased eating, quicker muscle stretch reflexes, increased activity level, faster thought processes, diarrhea, feeling too hot in regions where other people are comfortable, and increased sweating. *Hypothyroidism* results in the opposite: lower expenditure of energy, decreased heart rate, weight gain, slower reflexes, reduced activity level, slowed thought processes, constipation, feeling too cold in temperatures where others feel comfortable, and dryness of the skin.

The increased activity level, reduced ability to concentrate, greater irritability, and greater tendency to cry characteristic of hyperthyroidism may resemble attention deficit disorder. Tip-offs that hyperthyroidism is the culprit may include any of the symptoms or signs listed above. In addition, other symptoms can be clues. A goiter or swollen thyroid gland (located in the lower part of the front of the neck) was reported present in all of one series of patients with juvenile hyperthyroidism (Fisher, 1978). Other frequently appearing signs and symptoms included prominence or bulging of the eyes, rapid heartbeat, nervousness, increased perspiration, and increased appetite with weight loss. Deteriorated school work, emotional disturbance, breathlessness, and diarrhea were also often present in this series (Fisher, 1978).

The apathy, sluggishness, reduced energy level, poor appetite, deteriorated school performance, and constipation characteristic of hypothyroidism may be confused with a depressive syndrome. Any of the symptoms listed earlier might be the tip-off for hypothyroidism. In addition, the complaint or finding that the child's rate of growth has been slower than expected, the finding of coarse, brittle hair, the presence of a sallow complexion, or the presence of the enlarged thyroid gland (or goiter) characteristic of certain causes of hypothyroidism may also be clues that laboratory investigation is warranted.

These conditions rate high on the treatability scale and on the scale of possible confusion with psychiatric syndromes, and fairly low on the scale of frequency.

Endocrine: Diabetes

Diabetes is caused by a shortage of insulin, the hormone that causes glucose to be moved from the bloodstream into the muscles and other tissues where it can be used. (The brain, however, can take glucose into itself without the help of insulin.) When there is too little insulin, and the muscles cannot get glucose, a variety of metabolic changes ensue, resulting in higher and higher blood glucose and eventually in a state known as *diabetic ketoacidosis*. The progression to this state can start with personality change and can move to confusion and bizarre behavior and then to stupor, coma, and to death. In children, the onset often follows a viral illness. The early symptoms are increased frequency and total volume of urine output, increased drinking of liquids, fatigue, and sometimes bedwetting in a child who previously had been dry. Diabetes is a common illness, very treatable, and one that in the early stages can be confused with behavioral problems. Even more likely are psychiatric symptoms occurring once the child is already diagnosed as having diabetes: maladaptive behavior of almost any sort may be the result of either too much or too little insulin, resulting in a blood glucose that is either too low or too high.

Other Endocrine Illnesses

Other endocrine illnesses can sometimes be confused with psychiatric illness: *Cushing's disease* (too much secretion from the adrenal cortex), *Addison's disease* (too little secretion from the adrenal cortex), *pheochromocytoma* (too much secretion, at times, of adrenalin or noradrenalin, the hormones secreted by the adrenal medulla), an *insulinoma* (a tumor of the pancreas that secretes insulin and causes symptoms of low blood glucose), and *hypoparathyroidism* and *hyperparathyroidism* (i.e., shortage or excess of a hormone regulating calcium metabolism). These illnesses are rare enough that I will not go into the symptoms they produce.

Multiple Causes: Epileptic Seizures, Especially Complex Partial

Epileptic seizures of any sort are caused by the repetitive firing of groups of neurons in the brain. In tonic-clonic seizures, such activity spreads widely through the brain and results in the classic fits of falling, shaking, tongue-biting, wetting oneself, becoming unconscious, and being confused after regaining consciousness. These symptoms are almost always clearly recognized as medical problems and the patient is quickly routed to a neurologist.

Complex partial seizures, which have also been referred to as *psychomotor* or *temporal lobe seizures,* usually involve the repetitive firing of neurons in a restricted portion of the brain, almost always a temporal lobe or both temporal lobes. These discharges occur at unpredictable times and can apparently be activated by emotional stress. This fact makes the differentiation of their effects from purely psychological phenomena often difficult.

The temporal lobes connect extensively with other brain regions and serve a variety of functions; therefore, the discharges from these regions can produce a wide variety of symptoms. The psychological symptoms may include hallucinations of sight, sound, smell, or taste. Feelings of depersonalization or unreality of things around one can be produced; feelings of déjà vu (the feeling that the present event has been experienced before), jamais vu (the feeling that familiar things are new and unfamiliar), states of high emotion for which there is no appropriate cause, and the utterance of commonplace or jumbled phrases can also be phenomena of these seizures. The child may experience vertigo. The child may run to the mother in fear, or may reject the mother during the attack and run to her for consolation afterward. Sometimes, but not always, amnesia for the events of the attack and the events just before it occurs; sometimes the child is too embarrassed to talk about the events without a great deal of encouragement. Pallor or flushing can occur during the seizures (Brett, 1983).

The movements carried out during a complex partial seizure can vary greatly from case to case. Sometimes there is no movement but just a blank stare. At other times, there is repetitive fumbling with buttons or clothing, rubbing or patting the body, running, picking up objects and dropping them, smacking the lips, chewing, and swallowing. However, more seemingly purposive or antisocial actions have been reported to occur. Throughout such activities the child appears "out of it" and usually is not responsive to conversation except to a limited degree. The particular pattern of activity during the seizure varies less from episode to episode in one child than among a group of children; therefore, a stereotyped pattern that a given child repeats raises the suspicion more than episodes of widely varying strange behavior.

A seizure usually lasts on the order of a few seconds, but "complex partial status epilepticus," in which the seizure activity has lasted for hours, has occasionally been reported (Brett, 1983).

The diagnosis of complex partial seizures is usually established by the electroencephalogram (EEG). False negatives exist, though; in other words a normal EEG does not rule out complex partial seizures. The ideal diagnostic method is to obtain simultaneous EEG recording and videotape recording of behavior at the times of seizures as contrasted to times of normal behavior. As one might expect, such fortuitous recording of what can be an infrequently occurring event is more easily said than done. Usually, the disorder is at least somewhat responsive to treatment, with anticonvulsant drug therapy or with surgery or other treatment of the underlying cerebral disorder.

The other form of seizure that sometimes may be confused with psychological problems is the *absence seizure*, also called *petit mal seizure*. This seizure involves a different pattern of neuronal firing than does the complex partial seizure. The absence attack is characterized by a blank stare lasting on the order of 5 or 10 seconds, accompanied by unawareness and amnesia and sometimes by flickering eyelids or turned-up eyes. Mild shaking of a limb or drooping or sinking in posture can also accompany these seizures. As is apparent from the above description, these sorts of symptoms are also possible to be produced by complex partial seizures; in fact, blank staring spells are more frequently caused by complex partial seizures than by absence seizures. The distinction, which is confirmed by EEG, is relevant to drug treatment and prognosis. Absence seizures respond to different drugs and tend to go away of their own accord when the child grows up (Brett, 1983).

Multiple Causes: Hearing Problems

Herskowitz and Rosman (1982) reported a typical case in which a 5-year-old child presented with hyperactivity and inattention. His mother complained that the child could "tune her out," and that the child got along poorly with other children. It turned out that this child had a 30 to 40 decibel hearing deficit in both ears, apparently because of collections of fluid in the middle ears. When these were treated, the child's behavioral symptoms improved to the extent that drug treatment for attention deficit problems was not necessary.

Undetected hearing loss can be the cause of a variety of problems with speech and language, with schoolwork, or with relations with people. And these problems can, in turn, create a variety of secondary effects, from fights and disobedience and other conduct problems to somatic complaints or social withdrawal.

The approach to detecting hearing loss might include questioning parents regarding risk factors, such as a history of many ear infections, maternal history of rubella or cytomegalovirus or exposure to these during pregnancy; treatment of the child with aminoglycoside antibiotics, such as streptomycin, kanamycin, or gentamycin, or a family history of deafness or hearing loss. Problems with articulation in the speech of young children should also raise the question of hearing deficit. However, the easiest approach to this problem is a quick gross test of the child's hearing. The examiner asks the child if he or she has had any trouble hearing what people say. Then the examiner explains that he will briefly test the child's hearing, and asks the child to repeat the words that the examiner says. The examiner covers his mouth with his hand (to preclude lip-reading) and softly whispers familiar words. If the child can repeat these words, hearing problems as a cause of psychiatric difficulties are essentially ruled out.

Multiple Causes: Vision Problems

Anything that interferes with a child's performance in school can contribute to behavioral problems. Some school-aged children who are handicapped by uncorrected poor vision essentially diagnose themselves by complaining that they cannot see the blackboard or make out the letters in books. The mental health professional can perhaps pick up some children with visual difficulties simply by asking them if they ever have trouble seeing and recognizing the letters on the blackboard or in books. Charts for screening vision are available at low expense for the professional who would like to include this in the assessment.

Multiple Causes: Anemias

Anemia is a shortage of the red blood cells, whose job is to carry oxygen to the tissues. The anemic child may be irritable, fatigue easily, suffer a decrement in school performance, and have difficulty concentrating. The most prevalent cause of anemia in children is iron deficiency. Apparently, iron deficiency may have an effect on behavior over and above that of the anemia it causes (Pearson, 1983). A history of a diet poor in iron is a clue.

Multiple Causes: Sleep Apnea Syndromes

In *sleep apnea* syndromes, the patient periodically stops breathing during sleep for one of two reasons: either the brain does not send signals to the breathing muscles (*central apnea*), or there is an obstruction produced by closure of the throat that blocks breathing (*obstructive apnea*). People with sleep apneas do not sleep well, as might be imagined; sometimes partially or fullly waking up is the body's mechanism for restarting of breathing. As a result, the patient may complain of excessive sleepiness in the daytime, or troubled sleeping; in addition, personality change or deterioration in intellectual functioning may be noted (Strohl, Sullivan, & Saunders, 1984). Snoring may be noted in patients with obstructive apneas. Diagnosis is made by having the child sleep in a sleep laboratory where the patient's respiration can be continuously monitored throughout the night. When there is snoring that may or may not contain apneic episodes, and the clinician is not certain whether it warrants a referral to a sleep laboratory, taking an hour-long cassette recording of the child's snoring and monitoring it for silent periods of 10 seconds or more will sometimes settle the question of whether or not to refer. Research on these syndromes is at too early a stage to tell how frequently they cause behavioral difficulties in children.

Multiple Causes: Constipation as a Cause of Encopresis

Paradoxically, children who soil their undergarments with feces are very often constipated. Feces may "leak around" a reservoir of retained feces in the rectum. The wall of the rectum responds to distension by sending signals to the body that it is time to defecate. If the wall of the rectum is distended with feces over several weeks or months, the system of signaling in response to distension is disrupted. Tip-offs that fecal incontinence is due to constipation include a pattern of very frequent small accidents causing staining or smearing in the underwear, occasional large bowel movements that may even clog the toilet, and the palpation on physical examination of a large mass of stool in the lower left abdomen.

Constipation has a differential diagnosis that will not be fully explored here. It may be nutritional in origin, that is, not enough fiber in the diet, or it may be due to the child's efforts to hold back defecation, which may, in turn, be due to dirty or nonprivate conditions in school restrooms. Constitutional predispositions may also be a factor. Encopresis can sometimes be successfully treated by the combination of medical and behavioral methods: agents that soften stool and promote its evacuation, combined with great social reward for defecating in the toilet.

Degenerative: Multiple Sclerosis

Multiple sclerosis (MS) is a disease involving the breakdown of myelin, the material lining the axons of neurons. Some evidence implicates the immune system and viral infectioons, but the definitive cause is unknown. Thus, we use the rather unsatisfying term *degenerative* to classify it. MS has been confused with conversion disorder, since it involves neurologic symptoms, such as dizziness and staggering, weakness, blind spots, and double vision, all of which may come and go, and which, at first, may not be accompanied by definitive findings on a neurologic examination. Lumbar puncture and examination of the spinal fluid are useful in making the diagnosis of this illness, but even this examination can be normal in the early stages. MS is, to some extent, treatable with adrenocorticotropic hormone (ACTH), the hormone that causes release of corticosteroids from the outer part of the adrenal gland (Huttenlocher, 1987).

THE REVIEW OF SYSTEMS

When the clinician hears of symptoms that are not clearly recognized as fitting the pattern of a certain syndrome, the best course of action is to get as complete a data base as possible, especially from inexpensively obtained sources, such as asking questions of the patient. Going through a checklist of physical symptoms is called performing a "review of systems." Table 4 (cf. DeGowin, 1987) provides a checklist of physical symptoms to ask about when a physical illness or drug side effect is suspected.

INTERPRETATION OF FREQUENTLY USED LABORATORY TESTS

On inpatient units "routine" laboratory tests are frequently given. What is to be inferred from normal or abnormal values on the most

Table 4. Review of Systems

General: Feel sick or well? Feel feverish? Nature of diet? Fatigue?

Skin, hair, and nails: Change in color of skin, pigmentation, moisture, bumps, itching, scaling, bruising, bleeding. Change in color, texture, or distribution of hair; hair loss, unexpected hair growth. Changes in color of nails, brittleness, ridging, pitting, curvature.

Lymph nodes: Any enlargement of the "glands" that can be felt near the jaw, in the neck, in the armpits, in the groin? Any pain, drainage of pus?

Bones, joints, muscles: Injuries, such as breaks, sprains, and dislocations. Pain in joints or muscles; swelling; stiffness; movement of pain or stiffness from one joint to another; weakness; a muscle getting smaller; cramps.

Blood system: Has an anemia been identified? Has there been unexplained bleeding?

Endocrine system: History of growth, shape of body, and weight. Changes in size of hands, feet, and head. Hair distribution; pigmentation of skin. Weakness. Swelling in front and bottom of neck, where thyroid gland is. Bulging of the eyes; dryness of skin and hair; intolerance to heat or cold; tremor of hands. Increase in drinking of liquids; urination. Have signs of puberty come early, late?

Immune system, allergies: Reddened, painful, itchy, blistery skin (dermatitis); short-lived pale itchy ridges on skin (uticaria or hives); swollen areas of skin; hay fever; wheezing (whistling sound from breathing through a narrowed airway); reddened eyes in the spring pollen season. Pattern of reaction to things in the air, foods, drugs, or things that contact skin.

Head: Headaches, history of blows to head, spinning sensation, fainting, seizures.

Eyes: Trouble with vision, color blindness, double vision, blow to an eye, inflammation of an eye, glasses. When were glasses last tested to see if correct?

Ears: Difficulty hearing; ringing in the ears; spinning sensation; discharge of fluid from the ears; pain; tenderness of the bone around the ear. History of hearing testing; history of operations; history of treatment of ear infections. Have tubes been placed in ears?

Nose: Colds, runny nose, pain in sinuses of bones of face; stopped-up nose; nosebleeds.

Mouth: Sore mouth or tongue; toothache.

Throat: Hoarseness, sore throat, inflamed tonsils, voice changes. Snoring? If snoring, are there periods without breathing? If so, how long? If snoring, is there daytime sleepiness?

(*continued*)

Table 4. (Continued)

Neck: Swelling; enlarged lymph nodes; enlarged thyroid; stiff neck; reduced range of motion in neck.

Breasts: Degree of development. Has milk come from breasts? Lumps in breasts; pains; discharge from nipples. Development of breast tissue in male.

Respiratory system: Pain in chest, shortness of breath, wheezing, trouble getting air in or out. Is this worse when in bed or lying down? Cough; coughing up sputum or mucus; coughing up blood; pain on taking a deep breath; contact with people who have tuberculosis.

Heart and blood vessels: Pounding of the heart; rapid heart beat; irregular-feeling heart beat; pain in chest; shortness of breath out of proportion to exertion; trouble breathing at night or when lying down; blue color of hands and feet and lips; swelling of ankles.

Digestive system: Change in appetite or weight; trouble swallowing; nausea; much burping or passing gas; pain in abdomen; vomiting; vomiting of blood; yellowing of skin or whites of eyes; change in color, frequency, consistency, odor, of stools. Are there bulges from anal region, as in hemorrhoids? Changes in bowel habits. Itching around anal region.

Genital, urinary, reproductive systems: Change in color of urine; increase or decrease in frequency or amount of urine; having to get up several times at night to urinate; pain on urination; inability to urinate; bedwetting; incontinence of urination in daytime; passage of kidney stones or gravel; discharge from penis; lesion of skin around the genitals. Age of onset of menstruation, frequency of periods, regularity, duration, pain, discharge of pus; date of last menstrual period and previous period. History of pregnancies, abortions, deliveries, complications of pregnancy.

Nervous system: Cranial nerves (the twelve nerves that come from the brain without going through the spinal cord). Trouble smelling, trouble with vision, numbness in face, difficulty chewing, weakness of the face, change in taste sensation, trouble with hearing, loss of balance, difficulty pronouncing words, trouble swallowing, limited motion in neck. *Motor system*: paralysis or weakness anywhere; any muscle getting smaller; involuntary movements; convulsions; change in gait; clumsiness. *Sensory system*: Pain, numbness, or reduced ability to feel pain anywhere. *Autonomic system*: Trouble controlling urination or defecation; usually great or little sweating; redness, blueness, or paleness of skin. *Brain*: Headaches; staring spells; smelling, hearing, seeing things that are not there; confusion and memory problems; doing things without remembering them; seeming to be in a daze and not responsive to people; aimless stereotyped movements; unexplained change in personality; exposure to substances toxic to the brain, including lead.

Note: For mental and behavioral status questions, see symptoms listed in Table 1.

frequently used laboratory tests? The tests I will mention are listed in Table 5.

We should think of an abnormal laboratory test as having a differential diagnosis just as a symptom or abnormal physical finding has. Much of the information below is abstracted from Wallach (1983).

The complete blood count (CBC) involves quantifying the various components of the blood. An anemia is a reduction in the number or functioning of the red blood cells that carry oxygen to the tissues. An anemia may be signaled by an abnormally low RBC (red blood cell count), Hgb (concentration of hemoglobin, the oxygen-carrying component of red blood cells), or hct (hematocrit, the percentage of the blood volume the red cells take up when the components are separated by centrifugation). As might be expected, these measures of red blood cell adequacy tend to be correlated with one another; they are not perfectly correlated, however, since the total volume of the red blood cells is determined by both the size and the number of these cells. In distinguishing certain anemias from others, it is useful to know the mean volume of the red cells (abbreviated MCV, for mean cellular volume) and the mean concentration of hemoglobin in the cells (abbreviated MCHC, for mean cellular hemoglobin concentration). Anemias caused by iron deficiency result in reduced MCV and MCHC. Lead toxicity, if severe enough, can cause an anemia with lowered MCV and MCHC. On the other hand, anemias caused by failure to absorb vitamin B_{12} or folate result in increased MCV and normal MCHC. As mentioned before, anemias are in the differential diagnosis of fatigue and energy loss and can be confused with depression; deficiency of vitamin B_{12} or folate can directly cause psychiatric symptoms. Sickle cell anemia, which occurs in one out of 625 American blacks, is characterized by normal MCV and MCHC.

The white blood cell count (WBC) is more complicated because there are several different sorts of white blood cells: granulocytes (or polymorphonuclear leukocytes, or "polys"), lymphocytes, and monocytes. A general increase in white blood cell count may be produced by a variety of disorders, including acute infections, poisonings, and tissue injury. Increased "polys" are found with most bacterial infections. Infectious mononucleosis, whose symptoms can overlap with those of depression, results in an increased number of lymphocytes, as does infectious hepatitis. Increased eosinophils are found with allergic diseases, such as bronchial asthma, hay fever, and drug allergy. Reduced white blood cell counts, as well as reduced red blood cell counts, can be produced if the patient's bone marrow is suppressed by the action of carbamazepine, chlorpromazine, or other drugs. The platelet count, which

Table 5. Some Frequently Obtained Laboratory Tests

Complete blood count (CBC) including among others:
- Red blood cell count (RBC)
- Hematocrit (Hct)
- Hemoglobin (Hgb)
- Mean cellular volume (MCV)
- Mean cellular hemoglobin concentration (MCHC)
- White blood cell count (WBC)
- Count of lymphocytes, monocytes, neutrophils, eosinophils, and basophils
- Platelet count

Urinalysis, including among others:
- Glucose
- Protein
- Microscopic examination for bacteria
- White blood cells and red blood cells
- Red blood cell casts
- Urobilinogen
- Ketones

Blood Chemistries, including among others:
- Serum glutamic-oxaloacetic transaminase (SGOT)
- Serum glutamic-pyruvic transaminase (SGPT)
- Gamma GTP Guanosine triphosphate)
- Alkaline phosphatase
- Bilirubin
- Lactate dehydrogenase (LDH)
- Albumin
- Globulins
- Total protein
- Blood urea nitrogen (BUN)
- Creatinine
- Cholesterol
- Sodium
- Potassium
- Bicarbonate
- Glucose
- Calcium

Other tests:
- Thyroid function studies
- Pregnancy test
- Blood lead level
- Free erythrocyte protoporphyrin (FEP)
- Electrocardiogram (EKG)
- Electroencephalogram (EEG)
- Computed tomographic (CT) scan; magnetic resonance imaging (MRI) scan of the brain

can also be suppressed in such cases, is important because without sufficient platelets, dangerous or fatal bleeding episodes are more likely to occur.

The urinalysis (UA) is another frequently given routine laboratory test. A wide variety of kidney diseases can cause abnormal urinalysis results. Because of the role of the kidney in getting rid of psychotropic drugs, particularly lithium, it is reassuring to have a normal urinalysis before starting such drugs. Glucose detected in the urine is a cause for suspecting diabetes mellitus, although this is not the only cause. Protein in the urine may be caused by a wide variety of illnesses, including kidney infections, other kidney diseases, systemic infections, and poisoning with metals. Bacteria in the urine, when the urine has been collected properly, give evidence of an infection somewhere in the urinary tract. White blood cells and red blood cells (more than one or two per "high power field" under the microscope) in the urine can also be caused by infections and a variety of kidney diseases. Red blood cell "casts," or, in other words, red blood cells molded together in the shape of one of the tubes of the kidney, indicate disease in the kidney. Urobilinogen in the urine can be an indicator of damage to the liver, as, for example, by acute hepatitis. Ketones in the urine can be positive with diabetes, or with a variety of metabolic diseases that can have central nervous system effects, such as phenylketonuria. Ketones in urine can also be caused by starvation or by diets with no or almost no carbohydrates.

The organ that for most drugs (other than lithium) is most important for getting rid of the drug is the liver, whose job it is to catalyze a variety of chemical reactions that render drugs inactive or excretable. Several blood tests look for enzymes that are present in liver cells, but which are not released in large amounts into the bloodstream unless the liver is damaged. Three liver function test enzymes are abbreviated SGOT (serum glutamic-pyruvic transaminase), SGPT (serum glutamic-oxaloacetic transaminase), and Gamma GTP (guanosine triphosphate). Inflammations of the liver that are due to infection or alcohol, for example, would cause elevations in these enzymes. Alkaline phosphatase, another enzyme present in the liver, is elevated with liver disease; however, this enzyme is also present in bone and is often elevated with bone disease or in periods of rapid bone growth in children and adolescents. Bilirubin, one of the by-products of the metabolism of worn-out red blood cells, is excreted by the liver; liver disease can increase bilirubin. In addition to showing up on laboratory values, increased bilirubin can cause a yellowing of the skin and whites of the eyes, called jaundice. Another enzyme, lactate dehydrogenase (LDH), is present in the liver as well as in various other organs including muscle, heart, and blood cells. It is increased with heart attacks, sickle cell crises, hepatitis, and various other diseases. It is possible to "fractionate" LDH to separate it out into the varieties present in various organs so as to detect more about what diseased organ is responsible for the increased LDH. In severe liver disease, the albumin, which is a protein produced by the liver, may be decreased. Other diseases, including hyperthyroidism, and long-standing severe kidney disease where albumin is lost in the urine, can produce lowered blood levels of albumin. The major contributor to the "total protein" in the blood, other than albumin, is the set of proteins called *globulins*. These are associated with the immune system of the body and are increased in some long-standing infections and in some diseases thought to be caused by the body's producing an immune reaction against itself, such as rhematoid arthritis and systemic lupus erythematosus.

Two blood chemistry tests provide a good measure of kidney functioning. The BUN, or blood urea nitrogen, and the serum creatinine, if normal, give us additional assurance that the kidney is functioning well enough to excrete a drug such as lithium. Of the two, the serum creatinine is the more sensitive and specific indicator of kidney functioning. Creatinine should be measured before starting treatment with lithium, and periodically during lithium treatment, since lithium is excreted by the kidney and also since lithium has been reported upon occasion to affect kidney functioning.

An abnormally high level of cholesterol in the blood may be due to hereditary factors. It also may be secondary to hypothyroidism, and, if so, should rapidly return to normal with treatment of the thyroid condition.

Now let us turn to the "electrolytes" in the blood, also often obtained in routine testing. The sodium in the blood may be rendered abnormal by excessive vomiting, diarrhea, or sweating, especially if the child is too sick to take in salt and water *ad lib* to replace whatever was lost. Addison's disease, or reduced function of the outer part of the adrenal gland, can also result in a low serum sodium; this disease is in the differential diagnosis of altered mental status. Serum potassium is increased in Addison's disease. Potassium is decreased in Cushing's syndrome, the opposite of Addison's, where there is overly great secretion from the outer part of the adrenal gland. Potassium may also be rendered abnormal by much vomiting or diarrhea. The serum bicarbonate is decreased by insults that tend to make the blood more acidic, such as toxicity from an acidic substance such as aspirin, the acidosis that results from untreated diabetes, and the failure to excrete accumulated acidic wastes that may be caused by longstanding kidney disease. Too much or too little calcium in the blood can cause altered mental status. Too much calcium can result from an excess of vitamin D intake, too much secretion of parathyroid hormone, and a variety of other conditions. Too little calcium can result from too little absorption of vitamin D, too little secretion of parathyroid hormone, and a variety of other conditions. To a chemist, glucose is not really an electrolyte, but it is often included in batteries of blood electrolytes. The glucose in the blood taken at a random moment may, if excessively high or low, be due to diabetes or the effects of diabetes treatment. Adrenalin tends to raise blood glucose, so levels taken in high excitement can be elevated. Blood glucose taken 2 hours after a meal is a better screening test for diabetes than a random test.

Thyroid function studies have their results reported beside a variety of symbols. T3 and T4 stand for the active hormones secreted by the thyroid gland. T3 as measured by radioimmunoassay is reported to be the most sensitive lab test for borderline hyperthyroidism (Wallach, 1983, p. 447). Thyroid stimulating hormone (TSH) is a hormone released by the pituitary that prompts the thyroid to secrete its hormone. If TSH is high and thyroid hormones are low, the problem is in the thyroid gland; if TSH is low and thyroid hormones are low, the problem is in the pituitary. Thyroid function studies should be done before and during therapy with lithium, since lithium can reduce the functioning of the thyroid gland.

A pregnancy test is advisable for females in the child-bearing years, especially if drug treatment is planned. Lithium has been found to cause birth defects, and the clinician would want to think twice about all other drugs if the patient is found to be pregnant.

As implied earlier, a test of blood lead level is useful in children who are hyperactive, who show cognitive decline, who have a tendency to eat nonfood items, or who are faced with such environmental risk factors as an old house with peeling paint. The free erythrocyte protoporphyrin is another test abnormally elevated in the face of lead toxicity; in some settings it may be easier to obtain than the blood lead level. It is not as specific as blood lead level, being elevated in iron deficiency anemia and in a hereditary disease of red blood cell metabolism as well as in lead toxicity.

The electrocardiogram (EKG) is often used with children who are candidates for tricyclic antidepressant therapy, since the tricyclics can complicate preexisting disorders of heart rhythm.

The electroencephalogram (EEG) is mainly useful in detecting seizure disorders. When many neurons fire at once, as they do in an epileptic seizure, they produce a "spike" visible on the EEG. Different sorts of seizures produce characteristic EEG patterns. As mentioned above, temporal lobe epilepsy is usually the sort most likely to be confused with a learned behavioral disturbance. The failure to find temporal spikes on an EEG does not rule out temporal lobe seizures, for two reasons: first, the epileptic discharge could be occurring at other times, but not the time when the tracing is taken; second, the discharge could be taking place at the time of the tracing, but could be taking place in brain structures too far from the electrodes to make spikes. In order to maximize the possibility of picking up seizure activity during the EEG, it is best that the patient be sleep deprived (i.e., only around three or four hours sleep the night before the test), and to be asleep at the time of the test.

The other major positive finding from the EEG is slowing of the average frequency of the waves. This finding can be caused by a drug that depresses the functioning of the brain, or any of a number of metabolic diseases that in effect put too much or too little of something into the blood that nurtures the brain. Although the finding of EEG slowing does not tell what is wrong, it is sometimes useful in distinguishing an organic disorder from a learned behavioral pattern.

The computed tomographic (CT) scan and the magnetic resonance imaging (MRI) scan of the brain use X rays and magnetic fields, respectively, together with computer technology, to take pictures of the brain at any desired depth or plane. Such scans are quite valuable in detecting tumors, subdural bleeds or bleeds elsewhere in the brain, abscesses, swelling or atrophy of the brain, and other conditions that produce alteration in the physical structure of the brain or part of it, as opposed to an alteration in the chemical environment bathing the brain. Garber, Weilburg, Buonanno, Manschreck, and New (1988) provide guidelines for the choice between these two scanning methods.

DRUG TREATMENT OF VIOLENT BEHAVIOR

The question of medical treatment for violent behavior is especially relevant to inpatient units, where such behavior is frequently the target of treatment and the most important symptom to eliminate in whatever way possible.

There is no widespread agreement upon a syndrome of violent behavior that should be treated with drugs. It stands to reason that a conscious, unemotional, rational choice to be violent (as, for example, in the professional hit man) is less susceptible to biologic influence than that prompted by explosive rage or another emotional state in which the person feels "out of control"; the latter variety seems to be the sort of aggression observed in studies reporting successful drug treatment (e.g., Sheard & Marini, 1978).

Despite the lack of agreement upon a drug-treatable violent disorder, an enormous number of studies have examined the effects of various drugs on aggression, both in animals and in human beings (these are extensively reviewed by Miczek, 1987). The three most promising classes of drugs for treatment of violent behavior are the neuroleptics, lithium, and the beta-adrenergic blockers.

The neuroleptic or dopamine-blocking drugs, such as haloperidol, fluphenazine, and chlorpromazine, are probably the most frequently used agents in the treatment of violent individuals, particularly in emergency situations. A number of studies have demonstrated that these drugs reduce aggression in schizophrenic patients, which is not surprising in that their primary use is to reduce the general irrationality of such patients. However, a few studies have also found an antiaggressive effect in conduct-disordered children (Alderton & Hoddinott, 1964; Campbell *et al.*, 1982, 1984; Cunningham, Pillai, & Blanchford Rogers, 1968; Schweikert, 1971).

A number of case studies have reported aggressive individuals' benefiting from lithium treatment (Miczek, 1987 p. 231). In addition, a double-blind study of 66 highly aggressive prisoners reported progressively fewer episodes of violence over time with lithium treatment over a 3-month interval, in treated individuals as contrasted with placebo-treated individuals (Sheard, Marini, Bridges, & Wagner, 1976). Many of the subjects were adolescents: all were between 16 and 24 years of age; average age was about 19. Several of these cases demonstrated an impressive change in behavior (Sheard & Marini, 1978). Campbell *et al.*, in a study reported in 1982 and in 1984, found both haloperidol and lithium clearly superior to placebo in reducing aggression in a double-blind, placebo-controlled study of 61 undersocialized aggressive conduct-disordered children, of average age about 9 years.

Given the role of adrenergic hormones in the "flight or fight" response, it makes sense that drugs blocking the actions of these hormones should be tried as antiaggressive drugs. Several case studies and two group studies suggest that drugs blocking beta-adrenergicc receptors have a place in the treatment of violent behavior. Greendyke, Schuster, and Wooton (1984) reported that in a study without a control group, seven of eight adult male patients with organic brain disease and assaultiveness decreased their assaultive episodes from six or eight per day to less than one per day after being treated with propranolol (a beta blocker) for 4 weeks. Williams, Mehl, Yudofsky, Adams, and Roseman (1982) reviewed the medical records of 30 children and adolescents with organic brain dysfunctions and uncontrolled rage outbursts who had been treated with propranolol; 24 of the subjects were reported to have experienced moderate to marked improvement.

Temporal lobe epilepsy (or complex partial seizures, or psychomotor epilepsy) is in the differential diagnosis of abnormal behavior, when that behavior is brief in duration (seconds to minutes), does not vary from episode to episode (i.e., is stereotypic), does not appear to be in response to the demands of the situation, and when the person does not remember what happened during the episode. Because rage outbursts resemble such episodes in occurring periodically and in representing a loss of control, researchers have wondered whether drugs like carbamazepine (the drug of choice for temporal lobe epilepsy) are useful in rage attacks. A couple of studies (Groh, 1978; Puente, 1978) suggest that the behavior of responding violently to minimal provocation may be successfully treated by carbamazepine; nevertheless, the methodologic difficulties in these studies led O'Donnell (1985) to conclude after reviewing the evidence, that "there is as yet no clear basis for treating even severely aggressive conduct disorders with anticonvulsants in the absence of clinical seizure disorder, with or without abnormal EEGs" (p. 274).

In examining drug effects on violence, mention should be made of some of the drugs that have *worsened* violent behavior. One of these is alcohol. Miczek (1987) summarized a series of animal studies with alcohol:

> Low doses of alcohol increased elements of aggressive behavior in isolated aggressive and timid mice . . . and dominant rats . . . whereas two to three times as high doses were necessary to decrease a large number of aggressive postures and movements . . . ; a further twofold increment in dose level produced sedation. (p. 238)

In summarizing human data on alcohol and violence, Miczek (1987) cited 9 studies supporting an association between homicide and alcohol consumption, and 15 studies supporting an association between alcohol consumption and physical assaults. Finally, at least 10 laboratory studies have found an effect of alcohol on the severity of shock that subjects choose to deliver to a supposed victim (Miczek, 1987, p. 243).

The benzodiazepines have effects similar to alcohol in many ways; a number of case reports and controlled studies have found increases in aggression with the use of these sedatives (Miczek, 1987). However other studies have also found decreases in aggressive behavior and have arrived at diametrically opposed conclusions.

The evidence on the effects of stimulants, such as dextroamphetamine or methylphenidate, on aggression is similarly mixed. On the one hand, several studies have found reduced aggression in hyperactive children treated with methylphenidate (Miczek, 1987, p. 274). On the other hand, Ellinwood (1972) summarized data on amphetamine abusers by postulating that amphetamines, more than any other group of drugs, may be related specifically to aggressive behavior. Ellinwood (1971) reported the histories of 13 persons who committed homicide while intoxicated with amphetamines. Effects of predisposing personality, psychiatric diagnosis, and dose of drug probably are responsible for the mixed results.

Explaining and reducing violence is one of the most complex tasks facing behavioral science, and space obviously does not permit looking at the phenomena of violence from all possible viewpoints. Thinking about the violent patient from the viewpoint of the medical model entails not only examining drug effects, but also thinking in terms of the other major topics that were discussed here: diagnosing psychiatric syndromes, not only for the identified patient but also for the family members; being aware of side effects induced by any drug treatment that is chosen; considering medical illness that could be masquerading as psychiatric illness; and gathering evidence regarding such medical illness by the medical history, including a review of systems, physical examination, and laboratory tests. When such medical thinking is used hand in hand with thinking about learning and situational factors, the chances of finding a way to help the patient are maximized.

REFERENCES

Alderton, H. R., & Hoddinott, B. A. (1964). A controlled study of the use of thioridazine in the treatment of hyperactive and aggressive children in a children's psychiatric hospital. *Canadian Psychiatric Journal, 9,* 239–247.

American Psychiatric Association. (1987). *Diagnostic and statistical manual of mental disorders* (3rd ed., rev.). Washington, DC: Author.

Barness, L. A. (1983). Nutrition and nutritional disorders. In R. E. Behrman, V. C. Vaughan, & W. E. Nelson (Eds.), *Nelson textbook of pediatrics* (12th ed.). Philadelphia: W. B. Saunders.

Brett, E. M. (1983). Epilepsy and convulsions. In E. M. Brett (Ed.), *Pediatric neurology.* New York: Churchill Livingstone.

Bukowskyj, M., Nakatsu, K., & Munt, P. W. (1984). Theophylline reassessed. *Annals of Internal Medicine, 101,* 63–73.

Campbell, M., Small, A. M., Green, W. H., Jennings, S. J., Perry, R., Bennett, W. G., Padron-Gayol, M., & Anderson, L. (1982). Lithium and haloperidol in hospitalized aggressive children. *Psychopharmacology Bulletin, 18,* 126–130.

Campbell, M., Small, A. M., Green, W. H., Jennings, S. J., Perry, R., Bennett, W. G., & Anderson, L. (1984). Behavioral efficacy of haloperidol and lithium carbonate: A comparison in hospitalized aggressive children with conduct disorder. *Archives of General Psychiatry, 41,* 650–656.

Chisholm, J. J. (1983). Increased lead absorption and lead poisoning. In R. E. Behrman, V. C. Vaughan, & W. E. Nelson (Eds.), *Nelson textbook of pediatrics* (12th ed.). Philadelphia: W. B. Saunders.

Cunningham, M. A., Pillai, V., & Blachford Rogers, W. J. (1968). Haloperidol in the treatment of children with severe behaviour disorders. *British Journal of Psychiatry, 114,* 845–854.

DeGowin, R. L. (1987). *DeGowin and DeGowin's bedside diagnostic examination* (5th ed.). New York: Macmillan.

Ellinwood, E. H., Jr. (1971). Assault and homicide associated with amphetamine abuse. *American Journal of Psychiatry, 127,* 1170–1175.

Ellinwood, E. H., Jr. (1972). Amphetamine psychosis: Individuals, settings, and sequences. In E. H. Ellinwood & S. Cohen (Eds.) *Current concepts on amphetamine abuse* (pp. 143–157). Rockville, MD: National Institute of Mental Health.

Fisher, D. A. (1978). Pediatric aspects (of hyperthyroidism). In S. C. Werner & S. H. Ingbar (Eds.), *The thyroid: A fundamental and clinical text* (4th ed.). New York: Harper & Row.

Garber, H. J., Weilburg, J. B., Buonanno, F. S., Manschreck, T. C., & New, P. F. J. (1988). Use of magnetic resonance imaging in psychiatry. *American Journal of Psychiatry, 145,* 164–171.

Gilman, A. G., Goodman, L. S., Rall, T. W., & Murad, F. (1985). *Goodman and Gilman's The pharmacological basis of therapeutics* (7th ed.). New York: Macmillan.

Graef, J. W. (1983). Environmental toxins. In M. D. Levine, W. B. Carey, A. C. Crocker, & R. T. Gross (Eds.), *Developmental-behavioral pediatrics.* Philadelphia: W. B. Saunders.

Greendyke, R. M., Schuster, D. B., & Wooton, J. A. (1984). Propranolol in the treatment of assaultive patients with organic brain disease. *Journal of Clinical Psychopharmacology, 4,* 282–285.

Groh, C. (1978). The psychotropic effect of Tegretol in nonepileptic children, with particular reference to the drug's indications. In W. Birxmayer (Ed.) *Epileptic seizures—Behavior—Pain.* Berne, Switzerland: Hans and Huber.

Herskowitz, J., & Rosman, N. P. (1982). *Pediatrics, neurology, and psychiatry—Common ground.* New York: Macmillan.

Hurwitz, E. S., Barrett, M. J., Bregman, D., Gunn, W. J., Pinsky, P., Schonberger, L. B., Drage, J. S., Kaslow, R. A., Burlington, B., Quinnan, G. V., LaMontagne, J. R., Fairweather, W. R., Dayton, D., Dowdle, W. R. (1987). Public Health Service study of Reye's syndrome and medications: Report of the main study. *Journal of the American Medical Association, 257,* 1905–1911.

Huttenlocher, P. (1987). Degenerative disorders of cerebral white matter. In R. E. Behrman, V. C. Vaughan, & W. E. Nelson (Eds.), *Nelson textbook of pediatrics* (13th ed., pp. 1314–1316). Philadelphia: W. B. Saunders.

Hyman, S. E., & Arana, G. W. (1987). *Handbook of psychiatric drug therapy.* Boston: Little, Brown.

Kidd, K. K., & Pauls, D. L. ((1982). Genetic hypotheses for Tourette syndrome. In A. J. Friedhoff & T. N. Chase (Eds.), *Advances in neurology: Vol. 35. Gilles de la Tourette syndrome.* New York: Raven Press.

Miczek, K. A. (1987). The psychopharmacology of aggression. In L. L. Iversen, S. D. Iverson, & S. H. Snyder (Eds.), *Handbook of psychopharmacology: Vol. 19. New directions in behavioral pharmacology* (pp. 183–328). New York: Plenum Press.

Needleman, H. L., Gunnoe, C., Leviton, A., Reed, R., Peresie, H., Maher, C., & Barnett, P. (1979). Deficits in psychologic and classroom performance of children with elevated dentine lead levels. *New England Journal of Medicine, 300,* 689–695.

Nuwer, M. R. (1982). Coprolalia as an organic symptom. In A. J. Friedhoff & T. N. Chase (Eds.), *Advances in neurology: Vol. 35. Gilles de la Tourette Syndrome.* New York: Raven Press.

O'Donnell, D. J. (1985). Conduct disorders. In J. M. Wiener (Ed.), *Diagnosis and psychopharmacology of childhood and adolescent disorders.* New York: Wiley.

Pearson, H. A. (1983). Diseases of the blood. In R. E. Behrman, V. C. Vaughan, & W. E. Nelson (Eds.), *Nelson textbook of pediatrics* (12th ed.). Philadelphia: W. B. Saunders.

Puente, R. M. (1978). The use of carbamazepine in the treatment of behavioral disorders in children. In W. Birxmayer (Ed.), *Epileptic seizures—Behavior—Pain.* Berne, Switzerland: Hans and Huber.

Riela, A. R., & Roach, E. S. (1983). Reye's syndrome: Twenty years in perspective. *North Carolina Medical Journal, 44,* 351–355.

Russell Jones, R., & Stephens, R. (1983). The contribution of lead in petrol to human lead intake. In M. Rutter and R. Russell Jones (Eds.), *Lead versus health.* New York: Wiley.

Rutter, M. (1983). Low level lead exposure: Sources, effects and implications. In M. Rutter & R. Russell Jones (Eds.), *Lead versus health.* New York: Wiley.

Scheinberg, I. H., & Sternlieb, I. (1984). Wilson's disease. In *Major problems in internal medicine:* Vol. 23, Philadelphia: W. B. Saunders.

Schweikert, W. (1971). Anxious-depressed adults and problem children treated with thioridazine in private practice. *Current Therapeutic Research and Clinical Experience, 12,* 162–168.

Sheard, M. H., & Marini, J. L. (1978). Treatment of human aggressive behavior: Four case studies of the effect of lithium. *Comprehensive Psychiatry, 19,* 37–45.

Sheard, M. H., Marini, J. L., Bridges, C. I., & Wagner, E. (1976). The effect of lithium on impulsive aggressive behavior in man. *American Journal of Psychiatry, 133,* 1409–1413.

Starko, K. M., Ray, C. G., Dominguez, L. B., Stromberg, W. L., & Woodall, D. F. (1980). Reye's syndrome and salicylate use. *Pediatrics, 66,* 859–864.

Stores, G. (1975). Behavioural effects of anti-epileptic drugs. *Developmental Medicine and Child Neurology, 17,* 647–658.

Strayhorn, J. M. (1987). Medical assessment of children with behavioral problems. In M. Hersen and V. B. Van Hasselt (Eds.), *Behavior therapy with children and adolescents: A clinical approach* (pp. 50–74). New York: Wiley.

Strohl, K. P., Sullivan, C. E., & Saunders, N. A. (1984). Sleep apnea syndromes. In N. A. Saunders & C. E. Sullivan (Eds.), *Sleep and breathing.* New York: Marcel Dekker.

Till, K. (1975). *Paediatric neurosurgery for paediatricians and neurosurgeons.* Oxford: Blackwell Scientific Publications.

Wallach, J. (1983). *Interpretation of pediatric tests: A handbook synopsis of pediatric, fetal, and obstetric laboratory medicine.* Boston: Little, Brown.

Weinberger, M., & Hendeles, L. (1980). Pharmacologic management. In C. W. Bierman & D. S. Pearlman (Eds.), *Allergic diseases of infancy, childhood, and adolescence.* Philadelphia: W. B. Saunders.

Williams, D. T., Mehl, R., Yudofsky, S., Adams, D., & Roseman, B. (1982). The effect of propranolol on uncontrolled rage outbursts in children and adolescents with organic brain dysfunction. *Journal of the American Academy of Child Psychiatry, 21,* 129–135.

II

Treatment of Children

4

Depression and Suicide

GRETA FRANCIS AND KATHLEEN J. HART

INTRODUCTION

The purpose of this chapter is to describe behavioral treatment approaches for depression and suicide in hospitalized youngsters. We have limited the scope of the chapter to a discussion of major depression, dysthymic disorder, and related suicidality. As such, we have not included information pertaining to bipolar affective disorder and suicidality related to nondepressive disorders, such as substance abuse and conduct disorder.

Inpatient psychiatric units serve a large number of children and adolescents who carry a primary diagnosis of major depressive disorder or dysthymia. Psychiatric hospitalization is most likely sought for depressed youngsters who have made a suicide attempt, been unresponsive to outpatient treatment, or experienced multiple social or family stresses. The goals of hospitalization typically include stabilization of the child's acute crisis, diagnostic assessment, short-term intensive treatment, and planning for appropriate outpatient care and/or placement.

GRETA FRANCIS • Department of Psychiatry and Human Behavior, Brown University School of Medicine, Emma Pendleton Bradley Hospital, East Providence, Rhode Island 02915. KATHLEEN J. HART • Department of Psychology, Xavier University, Cincinnati, Ohio 45207.

Inpatient Behavior Therapy for Children and Adolescents, edited by Vincent B. Van Hasselt and David J. Kolko. Plenum Press, New York, 1992.

Clinical Description

Over the course of the last decade, psychiatric and psychological research has led to general agreement that the essential features of *major depressive disorder* (MDD) and *dysthymia* are similar from childhood through adulthood. As defined in the most recent edition of the *Diagnostic and Statistical Manual of Mental Disorders* (DSM-III-R) (American Psychiatric Association, 1987), MDD is characterized by the presence of any five of the following symptoms for a 2-week period: (1) depressed mood (or irritability in children or adolescents); (2) diminished interest or pleasure in previously enjoyed activities; (3) significant weight loss or weight gain (in children below the age of 6 years, failure to make expected weight gains is considered symptomatic); (4) sleep problems as indicated by insomnia or hypersomnia; (5) psychomotor retardation or agitation (hypoactivity in children below the age of 6 years); (6) loss of energy or general fatigue; (7) feelings of worthlessness, or excessive/inappropriate guilt (which may be delusional); (8) diminished ability to make decisions or difficulty concentrating; and (9) suicidal or morbid ideation, death wishes, or suicide attempts. The criteria also specify that these symptoms do not constitute major depression if they can be attributed to other pathologies, such as organic mental disorder. Moreover, the affective state in MDD is not a normal grief reaction nor superimposed on schizophrenia or other psychotic disorders. In addition to the DSM-III-R criteria, depressed children and adolescents often exhibit other symptoms, such as anxiety, worry, and social withdrawal.

Although the distinction between MDD and dysthymia can be somewhat ambiguous, dysthymic disorders typically represent a more chronic and less severe form of mood disorder. In contrast to the criterion of 2-weeks duration of symptoms for MDD, the diagnosis of dysthymia is made if the symptoms (described below) have been present for at least 1 year for children and adolescents. The criteria required to make the diagnosis of dysthymia include depressed mood (or irritability in children and adolescents) and, during periods of depressed mood, at least two of the following symptoms must be present: (1) poor appetite or overeating; (2) insomnia or hypersomnia; (3) low energy level or chronic tiredness; (4) feelings of inadequacy, loss of self-esteem, or self-deprecation; (5) decreased attention, concentration, or ability to think clearly; and (6) pessimistic attitude toward the future (hopelessness). These symptoms may be relatively persistent or separated by periods of usual mood lasting a few days to a few weeks, but symptom relief cannot last more than 2 months at a time. Further, dysthymia is not diagnosed in the presence of an organic factor or chronic psychotic disorder.

Although in many cases MDD and dysthymia clearly warrrant intensive hospital management, these youngsters are frequently admitted for psychiatric hospitalization because of suicidal behavior. Robbins and Alessi (1985) characterized a large percentage of adolescent suicide attempters as clinically depressed. As such, a comprehensive clinical assessment of suicidality is critical. Assessment typically focuses on such factors as the *intention* of the individual making a suicide attempt (i.e., how seriously did the child want to die), and the *lethality* of the attempt (i.e., how serious was the attempt from a medical/toxicity perspective). Unfortunately, these issues can be difficult to assess in child and adolescent populations. Developmental-cognitive factors, such as an ignorance of the true lethality of the chosen method or the inability to understand the finality of death, raise questions as to the utility of these dimensions in the assessment of adolescent and child suicidality.

It has been documented that many psychiatric conditions coexist with MDD and dysthymia. Recent studies suggest that mild to moderate conduct problems are present in approximately one fourth to one third of children and adolescents who carry a primary diagnosis of affective disorder (Ryan *et al.*, 1987). Anxiety disorders (e.g., separation anxiety disorder) of sufficient severity to impair daily functioning also are evident frequently in this population. Indeed, it seems safe to speculate that comorbidity of two or more disorders may be the hallmark of the depressed psychiatric inpatient.

BEHAVIORAL AND PSYCHIATRIC ASSESSMENT

Assessment begins even before the child arrives on the unit. The referral source has provided at least enough information so as to secure admission. A number of variables should be evaluated when assessing a depressed child or adolescent. These include self- and significant-other reports of symptoms across affective, behavioral, cognitive, and physiological domains. According to Kazdin (1987), the most prudent strategy for evaluating childhood depression is to assess across different sources of information, methods, and areas of functioning. Such a multimethod evaluation package may include a diagnostic interview, an assessment of family functioning, family medical and psychiatric histories, physical examination and selected lab work, self-report inventories of depressive symptoms and related constructs (e.g., hopelessness, anxiety), and behavioral observations.

Diagnostic Interviews

As instruments designed to aid in the diagnosis of psychiatric disorders in children, a number of structured and semistructured, symptom-oriented interviews are available, including the Schedule for Affective Disorders and Schizophrenia for School Age Children (K-SADS) (Puig-Antich & Chambers, 1982), the Diagnostic Interview Schedule for Children (DISC) (Costello, Edelbrock, & Costello, 1985), the Interview Schedule for Children (ISC) (Kovacs, 1978), and the Diagnostic Interview for Children and Adolescents (DICA) (Herjanic & Reich, 1982). Using the K-SADS, for example, requires the clinician to interview the child and parent individually and then to make summary ratings of a large number of symptoms indicative of a wide range of psychiatric disorders. As such, the use of these diagnostic instruments allows for a comprehensive assessment of comorbidity.

Self-Report Instruments

There are a number of well-researched self-report inventories of depression and related constructs for use with children and adolescents. Depression self-rating instruments include the Children's Depression Inventory (CDI) (Kovacs, 1981), the Beck Depression Inventory (BDI) (Beck, Ward, Mendelson, Mock, & Erbaugh, 1961), and the Reynolds Adolescent Depression Scale (RADS) (W. M. Reynolds & Coats, 1986). These instruments tap behavioral, cognitive, and affective aspects of depression. Over the last few years, data have become available regarding the psychometric properties of these self-report inventories.

Questionnaires tapping related constructs, such as hopelessness, self-esteem, social behavior, and anxiety, also are available. For example, the Hopelessness Scale for Children (Kazdin, Rodgers, & Colbus, 1986) has been found to correlate with measures of depression and suicidality in children. Self-esteem inventories, such as the Self-Perception Profile for Children (Harter, 1982), and Piers-Harris Children's Self-Concept Scale (Piers, 1969) also are available. Social behavior can be assessed using the Matson Evaluation of Social Skills with Youngsters (MESSY) (Matson, Rotatori, & Helsel, 1983). The MESSY can be completed by the child, parent, or teacher and provides information regarding a wide variety of social skills, such as friendship-making skills and assertion. Helsel and Matson (1984) reported a relationship between scores on the MESSY reflecting social skills deficits and depression. The most commonly used and well-researched anxiety inventories for children include the Revised Children's Manifest Anxiety Scale (RCMAS) (C. R. Reynolds & Richmond, 1978) and the State-Trait Anxiety Inventory for Children (STAIC)

(Spielberger, 1973). A number of self-report inventories relevant to suicide potential recently have been developed. The Suicide Ideation Questionnaire (SIQ) (W. M. Reynolds, 1985) assesses the amount of suicidal ideation over the past month. The Suicide Intent Scale (SIS) (Beck, Schuyler, & Herman, 1974) is an interview measure of suicide intentionality.

Family Assessment

A large body of research has highlighted the relationship between affective disorders in children and their parents (e.g., Cytryn, McKnew, Zahn-Waxler, & Gershon, 1986). According to Emde, Harmon, and Good (1986), "a depressed and depressing parent often coexists with the development of a depressed and depressing child" (p. 137). As such, a comprehensive family assessment can provide important information as to the potential relationship between child and parent psychopathology.

The family therapist typically is the one to assess family functioning and gather information relevant to family psychiatric history. The parent is asked about the presence of major psychiatric disorders, suicidality, substance abuse, and psychiatric treatment in the child's first and second degree relatives. This information can be gathered in an unstructured clinical interview or by using structured instruments, such as the Schedule for Affective Disorders and Schizophrenia—Lifetime Version (SADS-L) (Endicott & Spitzer, 1978).

Family functioning is evaluated most efficiently by conducting a functional analysis. The goal is to formulate a "picture" of the way the family works. This may include questions as to the roles individuals assume within the family, how family members respond to the identified patient, how the child interacts with various family members, and the antecedents and consequences of the child's depressive behavior.

Medical Assessment

Although childhood depression rarely is found to be due to primary medical illness, there are a number of medical disorders and conditions which can exacerbate or mimic MDD and dysthymia. For this reason, a thorough medical evaluation is essential in the comprehensive assessment of the child presenting with depressive symptoms. Hypothyroidism is probably the most likely contributing or causative medical condition. For this reason, thyroid studies (T4 and TSH [thyroid-stimulating hormone], minimally) would be done as part of the initial medical workup along with a complete blood count, sedimentation rate, urinalysis, serology, and tests measuring electrolytes, blood nitrogens, calcium, and liver enzymes (Gourash & Puig-Antich, 1986). Other medical conditions which can contribute to depression in this population include mononucleosis, Wilson's disease, central nervous system (CNS) lesions or tumors, closed head injury, and syphilis. Despite normal lab results, it is generally advised that medical "clearance" is not written in stone, and medical conditions should be reconsidered in cases which follow an unusual course or do not respond to intervention (Gourash & Puig-Antich, 1986).

Behavioral Observations

Depressed youngsters evidence a variety of behaviors which are readily observed. For example, social withdrawal, sad affect, long response latency, limited verbalization, tearfulness, and poor eye contact have been reported in depressed children (e.g., Kazdin, Esveldt-Dawson, Sherick, & Colbus, 1985; Kazdin, Sherick, Esveldt-Dawson, & Rancurello, 1985). On an inpatient unit, behavioral observations can be conducted naturalistically by milieu staff in a variety of situations, such as during school, meals, or free playtime. Moreover, records can be kept of the child's sleep pattern and eating habits. These observational data are very valuable in assessing the child's response to hospitalization.

COGNITIVE-BEHAVIORAL TREATMENT

There is a paucity of data in the behavioral literature describing controlled outcome studies of depressed and/or suicidal youngsters. That which has been conducted has focused almost exclusively on the assessment of pharmacological agents such as imipramine (Kazdin, 1987). As such, we will discuss the use of existing adult-oriented behavioral treatment approaches with depressed children and adolescents. The most common behavioral approaches for the treatment of depression in adults are activity-increase strategies, social skills training, and cognitive therapies. In treating children, it is clear that parent-oriented and/or family-oriented strategies also will be needed. On an inpatient unit, treatment can be conducted via individual therapy, small or large group therapy, family therapy, and milieu therapy. Milieu therapy may consist of treatment aimed at the unit as a whole (e.g., token economy) or at the individual child (e.g., a contingency contract). One advantage of an inpatient setting is the opportunity to provide the round-the-clock treatment which is not possible on an outpatient basis. Moreover, the group of potential therapists is large and usually includes psychiatrists, psychologists, social workers, nurses, child care workers, and teachers. Treatment progress can be assessed across time using symptom interviews, self-report measures, staff observations, teacher ratings, and records of food intake and sleep patterns.

Activity-Increase Strategies

A highly structured milieu afforded by many inpatient settings provides the opportunity to conduct activity-increase treatment. The hospitalized youngster typically "normalizes" sleeping and eating habits, partly as a function of regular meal and bedtimes. Moreover, the daily schedule often is structured to include positive social (e.g., group meetings) and physical (e.g., gym) activities. The assumption underlying activity-increase strategies is that depressed children are not engaging in behaviors which are intrinsically reinforcing or likely to be reinforced in the environment. It is assumed that they possess the appropriate skills to perform such behaviors but are doing so at a greatly diminished rate. For example, depressed youngsters may know how to invite peers to play with them, but have decreased motivation to do so. In order to use activity-increase strategies, it is important to actively involve the child in identifying behaviors which have the potential for reinforcement (e.g., Emery, Bedrosian, & Garber, 1983). Target behaviors could include those which the child enjoyed prior to becoming depressed. The therapist would help the child schedule activities and then have the child rate the extent to which the activity was enjoyable. Moreover, the therapist can seek assistance from significant others in the child's life to provide tangible or social reinforcement for participation in activities.

According to Kolko (1986), although diminished activity level has been reported in clinical descriptions of depressed youngsters, there are no empirical data available to support this observation.

Social Skills Training

A number of studies have reported a relationship between depression and unpopularity in children (Francis & Ollendick, 1989; Strauss, Forehand, Smith, & Frame, 1986) as well as social behavior deficits in clinically depressed youngsters (Puig-Antich *et al.*, 1985). Depressed youngsters may evidence poor eye contact, long response latency, short response length, slouching posture, low voice volume, diminished rate of interaction, or lack of appropriately assertive responding. Social skills training is appropriate particularly for children who do not possess adequate friendship-making or friendship-maintaining skills. Social skills training also can be helpful for depressed and withdrawn youngsters who possess, but do not perform, adequate skills because it provides the opportunity to reinforce the performance of these skills.

Social skills training typically incorporates a social learning theory framework and includes the techniques of instruction, modeling, behavior rehearsal, feedback, and reinforcement. For example, the child is provided with information about appropriate nonverbal skills (e.g., it is important to look a person in the eye during a conversation); the therapist models inappropriate and appropriate use of skill; the child practices appropriate skill; the child receives feedback regarding performance; and the child receives reinforcement for appropriate responses. Treatment often is easiest when conducted in a group format because it allows youngsters to observe more naturalistic modeling and receive feedback from peers. Typical content areas include nonverbal behaviors (e.g., eye contact, response latency, response length, posture, voice volume), conversation skills, social initiation skills, affect recognition and expression, prosocial skills, and negative and positive assertion skills.

A small number of studies have reported positive results with the use of social skills training for depressed children (e.g., Calpin & Cincirpini, 1978; Calpin & Kornblith, 1978; Frame, Matson, Sonis, Fialkov, & Kazdin, 1982; Petti, Bornstein, Delamater, & Conners, 1980). For example, Frame *et al.* (1982) described a multiple-baseline design to evaluate the effectiveness of social skills treatment for a hospitalized, depressed 10-year-old boy. Assessments were conducted via a behavioral role-play test tapping a variety of components of social skill (e.g., eye contact, affect). At the end of treatment and at 3-month follow-up, improvements in target behaviors were observed. The extent to which treatment impacted on other of the child's depressive symptoms is not known.

Calpin and colleagues (Calpin & Cincirpini, 1978; Calpin & Kornblith, 1978) used social skills treatment to address social behavior deficits in a small number of hospitalized youngsters characterized by problems with aggression and depression. Target behaviors included verbal and nonverbal components of social skill. Results indicated an improvement in social skills following treatment.

Kolko (1986) described a social skill treatment package used with a 12.8-year-old hospitalized girl who presented problems with depression, school refusal, and social behavior deficits. Treatment consisted of social skills training, cognitive problem-solving training, and contingency contracting. At discharge, the girl was described as less dysphoric, more liked by peers, and more socially skilled.

In summary, social skills treatment appears to be helpful in remediating social deficits in depressed youngsters. However, the impact of social skills treatment on depression *per se* is not known currently.

Cognitive Therapies

According to Emery, Bedrosian, and Garber (1983), depressed youngsters may systematically distort experiences in ways similar to adults through cognitive errors, such as selective abstraction, overgeneralization, all-or-none thinking, and minimization of positives. The use of cognitive therapy allows the child to learn to identify and modify these maladaptive cognitions.

Maladaptive cognitions can be assessed via think aloud procedures or self-report inventories, such as the Children's Negative Cognitive Error Questionnaire (CNCEQ) (Leitenberg, Yost, & Carroll-Wilson, 1986) or the Children's Action Tendency Scale (CATS) (Kaslow, Rehm, & Siegel, 1984). The CNCEQ is a 24-item self-report measure that assesses cognitive distortions (e.g., overgeneralizing) in social, academic, and athletic situations. Leitenberg *et al.* (1986) found differences in cognitive distortions between depressed and nondepressed, anxious and nonanxious, and low and high self-esteem children. The CATS is a 48-item self-report inventory which assesses global, stable, and internal attributions in positive and negative situations. Depressed children have been found to make such attributions in response to negative situations more so than nondepressed children (e.g., Kaslow *et al.*, 1984).

Once maladaptive cognitions are identified, cognitive therapy consists of challenging these beliefs by examining the evidence, identifying alternative explanations, and examining the consequences (Emery *et al.*, 1983). Such challenges consist of teaching the child to address the following questions: (1) What is the evidence that this belief is true? (2) What is another way of explaining this? (3) Even if the belief is true, how bad is it? Emery and colleagues (1983) emphasized that although the child's level of cognitive development must be considered when implementing cognitive therapy, latency-age children typically possess the necessary level of development. Cognitive therapy can be enhanced when the young child is assisted by parents or significant others.

A small number of recent studies (e.g., W. M. Reynolds & Coats, 1986; Stark, Reynolds, & Kaslow, 1987) have demonstrated the efficacy of cognitive therapies (problem-solving and self-control) for the treatment of depression in children and adolescents. For example, W. M. Reynolds and Coats (1986) examined the efficacy of relaxation and cognitive-behavioral therapy in the treatment of adolescent depression. Subjects consisted of 30 high-school-aged adolescents who were assessed at four points in time: screening, pretreatment, posttreatment, and 5-week follow-up. Students were randomly assigned to one of three conditions: cognitive-behavioral, relaxation, or wait-list control. Assessment instruments included self-report depression, self-esteem, and anxiety inventories. Treatment was conducted in groups which ran for 10 sessions over a 5-week period. Cognitive-behavioral treatment consisted of training in self-control skills (i.e., self-monitoring, self-evaluation, self-reinforcement). Relaxation treatment consisted of training in progressive muscle relaxation. Results indicated that both relaxation and cognitive-behavioral therapy proved effective in reducing depressive symptoms. As the authors acknowledged, one limitation of this study is that subjects were not diagnosed as having major depression as defined in the DSM-III. The extent to which these results might replicate using clinic or hospital populations of depressed youngsters awaits empirical investigation.

Parent-Focused Treatment

In treating depressed youngsters, it may be necessary to modify maladaptive interactions between the child and the parent. For example, a lethargic or irritable depressed child may balk at completing daily household chores. This could lead to a negative cycle in which the parent incessantly nags the child, the child gets more irritable and continues to balk, and the parent ends up doing the chores for the child. Parents need to be educated regarding the potential outcome of such maladaptive interactions. Moreover, it often is necessary to refocus the parents' attention from negative to positive events because the parents may be as pessimistic as the child. For example, a parent may focus exclusively on what activities the child no longer participates in while ignoring the fact that the child has just begun to express interest in participating in a new activity. Helping parents shift their attention from symptomatic behavior to nonsymptomatic behavior can prove essential. Furthermore, the parent may model and reinforce catastrophic thinking. In our clinical experience, we frequently have heard the parents express catastrophic thoughts, such as "This is awful. Andrea dropped a grade in Math so we know she will never get into college" or "Frank will never make any friends since he stopped playing baseball." In working with these families, it is easy to see how cognitive behavior therapy may be needed simultaneously for the child and parent.

Treatment Specific to Suicidality

In the case of the suicidal patient, treatment initially is focused on prevention of continued suicidal behavior. Safety needs are of primary concern at the onset of hospitalization, and some degree of restriction in activity or mobility is typical. Ongoing treatment, however, requires that the youngster reintegrate into a less restricted environment. Ideally, these transitions from restricted living (e.g., frequent staff monitoring, restriction to room or unit) to less restricted living (access to dayroom facilities, release to school program or to other off-unit activities) are based upon staff observation of patient responsibility and the child's demonstration of "safe" behavior, such as following unit rules and maintaining contact with staff members. Such strategies as identification of specific target behaviors (e.g., the child stays with the group and does not isolate herself; the adolescent *tells* staff if he feels unsafe rather than harms himself) and reinforcement for performance of prosocial and safe behaviors can provide the concrete evidence that both the staff and patient need to accurately assess safety.

Overholser and Spirito (1990) described the treatment of a 17-year-old suicidal male using cognitive-behavioral treatment. The adolescent was hospitalized on a pediatric unit in a general hospital following an overdose. Initial treatment efforts focused on medical stabilization and providing a safe environment. Continued treatment focused on cognitive therapy aimed at challenging cognitive distortions, disrupting irrational beliefs, and reinforcement of reasons for living.

Combination of Behavioral and Pharmacological Intervention

Inpatient treatment allows for medication trials to be conducted with greater opportunity for evaluation of efficacy than typically is available via outpatient treatment. There are a number of uncontrolled studies which suggest that tricyclic antidepressants are helpful in alleviating depressive symptoms in children and adolescents (e.g., Nissen, 1984; Staton, Wilson, & Brumback, 1982). As such, tricyclic antidepressants appear to be a viable treatment option for hospitalized depressed youngsters. A reasonable approach is to evaluate the youngster's response to the inpatient milieu alone for a period of time and then add medication as needed. The case studies described below illustrate such an approach in which medication did not appear to be indicated given the decrease in symptoms observed with milieu-based treatments alone. Conversely, a child might not evidence adequate symptom relief even after a few weeks of hospitalization and, thus, the addition of a tricyclic antidepressant may prove beneficial.

CASE HISTORIES

Case 1

Douglas was a 7-year-old white male who lived with his parents and younger sister. He attended school regularly and was in the second grade. His mother worked as a store clerk and his father was an unemployed construction worker. Doug's mother was chronically depressed, and his father had significant alcohol problems. Neither parent was involved in treatment for their problems. The family had experienced a number of recent losses, including the deaths of Doug's paternal grandmother and maternal grandfather.

The first psychiatric contact for this youngster came after he attempted to choke himself at school and stated that he wanted to die. School personnel referred him for an emergency outpatient evaluation at a clinic specializing in the treatment of childhood depression. Doug was diagnosed with major depressive disorder and placed on imipramine. He and his mother attended weekly outpatient sessions that were focused on medication management and basic parent education. After 9 months of outpatient treatment, Doug was referred for admission to the hospital because of a worsening of symptoms reflecting lack of response to outpatient treatment efforts.

Upon admission, Doug and his parents were interviewed separately by a child psychiatrist and clinical child psychologist using the K-SADS. His teacher and outpatient therapist also provided information. It is important to note that initial assessment relied on reports from Doug's parents, school personnel, and outpatient therapist because Doug denied any and all problems. For example, he described himself as "mostly happy" even while tears were running down his face. On self-report measures of depression, anxiety, fear, self-esteem, and hopelessness, he also described himself as problem-free. The following symptoms were described by parents and significant others: pervasive sadness, extreme anhedonia, poor concentration, social withdrawal, decreased appetite with a 9-pound weight loss over the previous nine months, difficulty falling asleep, and hypersensitivity to criticism. Moreover, Doug evidenced significant separation anxiety symptoms, including frequent worry that his parents or sister would die, extreme distress when separated from the family, difficulty sleeping alone at night, and nightmares involving separation. Doug's separation anxiety was observed immediately upon his arrival on the unit. He cried on and off throughout the day and evidenced extreme and lengthy distress once his parents left. Moreover, Doug's mother demonstrated extreme anxiety about having to leave her child in the hospital, even though visiting had been arranged for the following day. There was no indication of disruptive behavior problems, psychosis, manic symptoms, or current suicidal ideation or intent.

The social worker met with the parents in order to gather the social history and family psychiatric history. A pediatric nurse practitioner also met with the family to collect information pertinent to Doug's medical and developmental history. Doug was assigned to a primary nurse. A series of lab tests and an electrocardiogram (EKG) were ordered. The child psychiatrist began to taper Doug off his imipramine so as to gather baseline information regarding his symptomatology and functioning.

During the first 2 weeks of hospitalization, a comprehensive assessment was completed. No medical problems were discovered, other than his recent weight loss. Intellectual and psychoeducational assessments revealed Doug to be a boy of above average intellectual ability with school performance at or above grade level. Doug was described best diagnostically as suffering from major depressive disorder superimposed upon long-standing separation anxiety disorder. His family was stressed both emotionally and financially. Unresolved issues included grief over the recent deaths of close family members, the mother's chronic depression and separation anxiety, the father's alcohol problems, and conflicting parenting styles between the mother and father.

Treatment was multifaceted and included activity-increase strategies, graded exposure, and social skills training for Doug. In addition, the family was involved in treatment that was focused on uniting the parents around the issue of child management, encouraging the parents to seek help for their individual problems, and resolving grief issues.

Activity-increase strategies were implemented via the behavioral milieu management program. Doug was provided with a series of daily expectations including appropriate hygiene, attendance at school, participation in unit activities, such as art, gym, and off-unit outings, adequate food intake at meals, and regular bedtime. In essence, Doug began to follow an activity-oriented daily schedule. He received stars for appropriate participation in, and completion of, activities and tasks. Each day he traded in his stars for preferred activities, such as later bedtime, videogame time, and one-to-one time with his primary nurse. Although reserved and inhibited at first, Doug was extremely compliant and met all expectations with apparent ease. He clearly possessed the skills necessary to exhibit the prosocial behaviors. Once he mastered the minimal expectations, he was encouraged to demonstrate higher level skills by initiating activities and assuming leadership tasks, such as helping to organize games or serving as the team captain during a kickball game.

As an adjunct to the activity-increase strategy, Doug participated in social skills training using a small group format. As noted above, although many of Doug's social behaviors were very appropriate, he was hesitant to initiate interactions and often behaved in a rather passive manner. As such, the goals of social skills training were to teach Doug to initiate social interactions with peers and adults and to provide him with an opportunity to receive positive feedback for his attempts. Another important aspect of social skills treatment was teaching Doug to identify and express affect. Over the course of the hospitalization, Doug became an active participant in the group. He was able to engage in spontaneous interaction with group members and occasionally provided feedback to others regarding their performance on role-play tasks. In addition, while initially Doug was hypersensitive to perceived negative feedback, he became better able to respond appropriately to constructive criticism. Finally, Doug made noticeable progress in his ability to label his emotions and let people know when he felt sad or scared.

Doug's concurrent separation anxiety was treated using graduated exposure in that he was actually separated from his family for large amounts of time. For approximately the first 2 weeks, his parents visited on a daily basis. Following this, they decreased their visiting frequency to four times per week. As expected, while Doug demonstrated initial nervousness with each change, eventually his anxiety diminished. Similarly, Doug's phone calls to and from parents decreased from many times per day to once a day with a concurrent decrease in distress. One of Doug's major complaints was a fear of sleeping alone. Although Doug had a roommate during most of his hospital stay, he did practice sleeping alone in a room a number of times. Finally, as Doug's discharge approached, he had a number of home visits which allowed him and his parents the opportunity to practice separating.

During the 6-week hospitalization, Doug demonstrated a number of positive changes. He gained back the weight he had lost and looked quite healthy. This was in sharp contrast to the pale, thin young boy observed at the time of admission. His activity level increased and his anxiety level had begun to decrease. Given these changes, it was felt that a trial of medication was not warranted. His parents utilized family therapy fairly well. They became more united in their approach to dealing with Doug, and the mother's separation anxiety improved. Both parents were hesitant to acknowledge their problems. The mother reluctantly agreed to seek individual therapy whereas the father refused. Upon discharge, referrals were made for individual therapy for Doug and his mother, and for family therapy.

Case 2

Sylvia was a 13-year-old white female who was admitted to a medical hospital because of a suicide attempt in which she ingested several prescription drugs and liquid household cleaners. Following medical stabilization, she was transferred to a psychiatric facility to receive treatment. Sylvia had been raised in a chaotic family environment; she lived for the first 10 years of her life in the natural home with an alcoholic mother who, at the time of the hospital admission, was no longer granted visitation rights or contact with Sylvia. From early childhood until approximately 10 years of age, Sylvia had been physically and sexually abused by her natural father. As a result of Sylvia's testimony, he was eventually convicted of those abusive acts. At the time of hospital admission, her father was serving time in jail for those charges. However, Sylvia expressed continued fear of her father and his anticipated revenge at her participation in his trial and conviction. Indeed, she had periodic dreams that he might escape and find her, and she lived in fear of the day he would be released from jail (anticipated to be close to Sylvia's 18th birthday) and seek revenge. Since her removal from the home at age 11, Sylvia initially lived with relatives and eventually was placed in a foster home. Over the years, she had become increasingly depressed as characterized by sadness, irritability, suicidal ideation, sleep and appetite change, and declining school attendance and performance. The precipitant for her suicide attempt was unclear, but appeared to be a result of escalating (and untreated) depression. A complete medical workup yielded no abnormal results.

Sylvia responded well to the structure of the milieu which focused on activity-increase strategies. Although she continued to complain of fatigue, she was able to participate in the school program and other milieu activities. In light of her rapid response to the milieu and relief of many of the vegetative symptoms, medication was not administered. Instead, individual treatment focused on cognitive therapy and problem-solving strategies to deal with her guilt over her participation in her father's conviction and her fears regarding his anticipated revenge. Over the course of the first 2 months of her hospitalization, suicidal ideation decreased significantly and positive participation in school and other activities increased. At the end of 3 months, the individual therapist felt that Sylvia had derived significant benefit from hospitalization, and plans for placement ensued. While awaiting placement, a new psychiatrist assumed Sylvia's case and was struck by her continued lethargy, particularly in light of the relief of many of her other symptoms. He ordered new thyroid studies which indicated mild to moderate hypothyroidism. Hormone treatment was initiated, and Sylvia enjoyed further improvement in mood, attitude, and energy level. Placement eventually was secured, and Sylvia was discharged.

Case 3

Jennifer was a 16-year-old white female who was admitted to an inpatient psychiatric unit after evaluation in the emergency room (ER). A school nurse learned that Jennifer had taken an overdose of Tylenol. Reports from the ER indicated that she spent 3 days planning her suicide attempt, and was assessed to be currently acutely suicidal. Jennifer reported a 2-month history of moderate dysphoria, sleep disturbance, decreased concentration, feelings of hopelessness, and suicidal thoughts.

Jennifer's history was marked by her parents' divorce when she was 3 years old. While the older sisters remained with the mother, Jennifer was left in her father's care. In actuality, Jennifer was raised by her father's stepmother, with whom she developed a very close relationship. This caretaker died when Jennifer was 12 years old requiring Jennifer to move in with her father and his new wife. The subsequent years reportedly were quite turbulent, primarily due to conflicts between the married couple. When the marriage eventually dissolved, Jennifer was left in the sole care of her father. Since he worked evenings, she was frequently left unattended and experienced a significant degree of loneliness. A family friend became aware of Jennifer's distress and offered to give her a home. Unfortunately, intense rivalry developed between Jennifer and the teenage children in the friend's family. It was at that time that Jennifer began to experience significant depressive symptoms that continued to intensify following the break-up with a boyfriend and the discovery that she was pregnant. When she was informed by the family friend that she would not be permitted to remain in the home if she was pregnant, Jennifer became more despondent and formulated the suicide plan which precipitated hospitalization.

Hospitalization provided a safe environment in which a comprehensive diagnostic assessment could be completed and a treatment plan could be developed. Jennifer's symptoms were described best as indicative of a major depressive disorder. She responded well to the schedule of the hospital routine and readily engaged in the school program and other available activities. This improvement seemed to be due, in great part, to the unit token economy, which targeted her decreased activity level and social withdrawal. Soon, her increased activity and socialization became reinforcing, and tokens were no longer the primary motivation for behavioral performance.

Pending her decision regarding the pregnancy, Jennifer was not medicated. Eventually, she elected to abort. Following the abortion, her mood further elevated and other symptoms quickly resolved. As such, pharmacological intervention was not conducted. Individual therapy was initiated to help Jennifer resolve previously unrealized grief issues, and to help her decide on her future residence. Although she initially hoped to return to the foster family, conflicts did not resolve, and Jennifer decided to return to the care of her father. After a period of continued hospitalization which focused primarily on preparing Jennifer and her father for her return and helping them develop appropriate expectations of one another, Jennifer was discharged.

PROBLEM AREAS

Although there are numerous advantages to inpatient treatment of depression and suicide in youngsters, problem areas do exist. Oftentimes a child's length of stay is contingent upon factors, such as adequate insurance coverage and accessibility of appropriate outpatient resources. Neither of these factors is under the direct control of the clinical treatment team. Another problem relates to generalization and maintenance of treatment gains. Inpatient treatment offers extremely specialized care which may be quite unlike the care which the child is to receive upon discharge. For example, it can be relatively easy to increase the activity level of a depressed child given access to a structured milieu. However, such behavior may not be so easily maintained when the child returns to an environment in which financial factors limit his or her access to enjoyable activities. Furthermore, a suicidal adolescent may find it easy to self-disclose when given frequent opportunity to do so and multiple caring clinicians to listen. Once the adolescent leaves the hospital, there likely will not be such immediate availability of support. As such, one important goal of hospitalization should be to identify and implement a system whereby generalization and maintenance are maximized.

Summary

In this chapter, we have provided an overview of behavioral treatment approaches to depression and suicide in hospitalized children and adolescents. Although research in this area currently is sparse, strategies such as those aimed at activity increase, social skills training, and cognitive therapy appear to be promising for use in the inpatient setting. Since depressed and suicidal youngsters constitute a sizable proportion of the inpatient psychiatric population, the need to develop and empirically evaluate treatment outcome clearly is necessary.

References

American Psychiatric Association. (1987). *Diagnostic and statistical manual of mental disorders* (3rd ed., rev.). Washington, DC: Author.

Beck, A. T., Ward, C., Mendelson, M., Mock, J., & Erbaugh, J. (1961). An inventory for measuring depression. *Archives of General Psychiatry, 4*, 561–571.

Beck, A. T., Schuyler, D., & Herman, I. (1974). Development of suicidal intent scales. In A. T. Beck, H. L. P. Resnick, & D. J. Lettieri (Eds.), *The prediction of suicide* (pp. 45–46). Maryland: Charles Press.

Calpin, J. P., & Cincirpini, P. M. (1978, May). *A multiple baseline analysis of social skills training in children.* Paper presented at the Midwestern Association for Behavior Analysis, Chicago.

Calpin, J. P., & Kornblith, S. J. (1978, November). *Training of aggressive children in conflict resolution skills*. Paper presented at the meeting of the Association for the Advancement of Behavior Therapy, Chicago.

Costello, E. J., Edelbrock, C. S., & Costello, A. J. (1985). Validity of the NIMH Diagnostic Interview Schedule for Children: A comparison between psychiatric and pediatric referrals. *Journal of Abnormal Child Psychology, 13*, 579–595.

Cytryn, L., McKnew, D. H., Zahn-Waxler, C., & Gershon, E. S. (1986). Developmental issues in risk research: The offspring of affectively ill parents. In M. Rutter, C. E. Izard, & P. B. Read (Eds.), *Depression in young people* (pp. 163–188). New York: Guilford Press.

Emde, R. N., Harmon, R. J., & Good, W. V. (1986). Depressive feelings in children: A transactional model for research. In M. Rutter, C. E. Izard, & P. B. Read (Eds.), *Depression in young people* (pp. 135–160). New York: Guilford Press.

Emery, G., Bedrosian, R., & Garber, J. (1983). Cognitive therapy with depressed children and adolescents. In D. P. Cantwell & G. A. Carlson (Eds.), *Affective disorders in childhood and adolescence: An update* (pp. 445–471). New York: Spectrum.

Endicott, J., & Spitzer, R. L. (1978). A diagnostic interview. The schedule for affective disorders and schizophrenia. *Archives of General Psychiatry, 35*, 837–844.

Frame, C., Matson, J. L., Sonis, W. A., Flakov, M. J., & Kazdin, A. E. (1982). Behavioral treatment of depression in a prepubertal child. *Journal of Behavior Therapy and Experimental Psychiatry, 3*, 239–243.

Francis, G., & Ollendick, T. H. (1989). *The validity of teacher nominations to identify social withdrawal in elementary school-aged children*. Unpublished manuscript.

Gourash, L., & Puig-Antich, J. (1986). Medical and biological aspects of adolescent depression. *Seminars in Adolescent Medicine, 2*, 299–310.

Harter, S. (1982). The Perceived Competence Scale for Children. *Child Development, 53*, 87–97.

Helsel, W. J., & Matson, J. L. (1984). Assessment of depression in children: The internal structure of the Child Depression Inventory (CDI). *Behaviour Research and Therapy, 22*, 289–298.

Herjanic, B., & Reich, W. (1982). Development of a structured psychiatric interview for children: Agreement between child and parent on individual symptoms. *Journal of Abnormal Child Psychology, 10*, 307–324.

Kaslow, N. J., Rehm, L. P., & Siegel, A. W. (1984). Social-cognitive and cognitive correlates of depression in children. *Journal of Abnormal Child Psychology, 12*, 605–620.

Kazdin, A. E. (1987). Assessment of childhood depression: Current issues and strategies. *Behavioral Assessment, 9*, 291–319.

Kazdin, A. E., Esveldt-Dawson, K., Sherick, R. B., & Colbus, D. (1985). Assessment of overt behavior and childhood depression among psychiatrically disturbed children. *Journal of Consulting and Clinical Psychology, 53*, 201–210.

Kazdin, A. E., Sherick, R. B., Esveldt-Dawson, K., & Rancurello, M. D. (1985). Nonverbal behavior and childhood depression. *Journal of the American Academy of Child Psychiatry, 24*, 303–309.

Kazdin, A. E., Rodgers, A., & Colbus, D. (1986). The Hopelessness Scale for Children: Psychometric characteristics and concurrent validity. *Journal of Consulting and Clinical Psychology, 54*, 241–245.

Kolko, D. J. (1986). Depression. In M. Hersen & V. Van Hasselt (Eds.), *Behavior therapy with children and adolescents: A clinical approach* (pp. 163–168). New York: John Wiley and Sons.

Kovacs, M. (1978). *Interview Schedule for Children (ISC)* (10th revision). University of Pittsburgh School of Medicine, Pittsburgh, PA.

Kovacs, M. (1981). Rating scales to assess depression in school-aged children. *Acta Paedopsychiatrica, 46,* 305–315.
Leitenberg, H., Yost, L. W., & Carroll-Wilson, M. (1986). Negative cognitive errors in children: Questionnaire development, normative data, and comparisons between children with and without self-reported symptoms of depression, low self-esteem, and evaluation anxiety. *Journal of Consulting and Clinical Psychology, 54*(4), 528–536.
Matson, J. L., Rotatori, A. F., & Helsel, W. J. (1983). Development of a rating scale to measure social skill in children: The Matson Evaluation of Social Skills with Youngsters (MESSY). *Behaviour Research and Therapy, 21,* 335–340.
Nissen, G. (1984). Somatogenic depression in children and adolescents. *Acta Paedopsychiatrica, 50,* 21–28.
Overholser, J. C., & Spirito, A. (1990). Cognitive-behavioral treatment of suicidal depression. In E. L. Feindler & G. R. Kalfus (Eds.), *Casebook in adolescent behavior therapy* (pp. 211–232). New York: Springer-Verlag.
Petti, T. A., Bornstein, M., Delamater, A., & Conners, C. K. (1980). Evaluation and multimodality treatment of a depressed pre-pubertal girl. *Journal of the American Academy of Child Psychiatry, 19,* 690–702.
Piers, E. V. (1969). *Manual for the Piers-Harris Children's Self Concept Scale.* Nashville, TN: Counselor Recordings and Tests.
Puig-Antich, J., & Chambers, W. (1982). *Schedule for affective disorders and schizophrenia for school-age children* (6–16 years)—Kiddie-SADS. New York: New York State Psychiatric Institute.
Puig-Antich, J., Lukens, E., Davies, M., Goetz, D., Brennan-Quattrock, J., & Todak, G. (1985). Psychosocial functioning in prepubertal major depressive disorders: I. Interpersonal relationships during the depressive episode. *Archives of General Psychiatry, 42,* 500–507.
Reynolds, C. R., & Richmond, B. O. (1978). What I think and feel: A revised measure of children's manifest anxiety. *Journal of Abnormal Child Psychology, 6,* 271–280.
Reynolds, W. M. (1985). *Suicide Ideation Questionnaire.* Unpublished manuscript, University of Wisconsin, Madison.
Reynolds, W. M., & Coats, K. I. (1986). A comparison of cognitive-behavioral therapy and relaxation training for the treatment of depression in adolescents. *Journal of Consulting and Clinical Psychology, 54,* 653–660.
Robbins, D. R., & Alessi, N. E. (1985). Depressive symptoms and suicidal behavior in adolescents. *American Journal of Psychiatry, 142,* 588–592.
Ryan, N. D., Puig-Antich, J., Ambrosini, P., Rabinovich, H., Robinson, D., Nelson, B., Iyengar, S., & Twomey, J. (1987). The clinical picture of major depression in children and adolescents. *Archives of General Psychiatry, 44,* 854–861.
Spielberger, C. D. (1973). *State-Trait Anxiety Inventory for Children.* Palo Alto, CA: Consulting Psychological Press.
Stark, K. D., Reynolds, W. M., & Kaslow, N. J. (1987). A comparison of the relative efficacy of self-control therapy and a behavioral problem-solving therapy for depression in children. *Journal of Abnormal Child Psychology, 15,* 91–113.
Staton, R., Wilson, H., & Brumback, R. A. (1982, October). *Differential effects of amitriptyline versus imipramine upon childhood psychological functioning.* Paper presented at the meeting of the American Academy of Child Psychiatry, Washington, DC.
Strauss, C. C., Forehand, R., Smith, K., & Frame, C. L. (1986). The association between social withdrawal and internalizing problems of children. *Journal of Abnormal Child Psychology, 14,* 525–535.

5

Mental Retardation and Psychiatric Disorders

Rowland P. Barrett, Anne S. Walters, Arthur F. Mercurio, Margaret Klitzke, and Carl Feinstein

Introduction

Systematic attempts to teach and habilitate mentally retarded children and adolescents began in the early nineteenth century, when Jean-Marc-Gaspard Itard (1775–1838), a French physician, attempted to educate Victor, the "wild" 11-year-old boy who was discovered by hunters in the forest of Aveyron. Using techniques similar in theory to current behavior modification methods, Itard aided Victor in developing adequate self-care, social skills, and receptive language ability over a 5-year period. Although Itard considered his approach a failure because Victor did not develop speech, his methods suggested that mentally retarded individuals could acquire and refine a variety of adaptive behaviors through systematic training. Edouard Séguin (1812–1880), who as a medical student had worked with Itard, continued developing his mentor's techniques, and by the mid-nineteenth century, had established educational

Rowland P. Barrett, Anne S. Walters, Arthur F. Mercurio, Margaret Klitzke, and Carl Feinstein • Department of Psychiatry and Human Behavior, Brown University School of Medicine, Emma Pendleton Bradley Hospital, East Providence, Rhode Island 02915.

Inpatient Behavior Therapy for Children and Adolescents, edited by Vincent B. Van Hasselt and David J. Kolko. Plenum Press, New York, 1992.

programs for mentally retarded individuals throughout Europe (cf. Tylenda, Hooper, & Barrett, 1987).

In modern Western culture, mental retardation is the most widespread and best known of the developmental disabilities. Conservative estimates have indicated that in the United States alone, 4 million people are mentally retarded (National Institutes of Health, 1989). This number increases dramatically when individuals with borderline intellectual functioning are included in prevalence estimates. Given such large numbers of afflicted individuals, it is not surprising that mental retardation continues to be of great interest to contemporary society and remains a focus of professional concern.

Indeed, societal interest and professional concern have spawned a large number of public and private agencies within the United States that are dedicated to improving the quality of life of mentally retarded citizens. Professional societies, such as the ten-thousand-member *American Association on Mental Retardation,* and parent-sponsored organizations (e.g., *National Association of Retarded Citizens*) are formidable advocacy groups which list chapters in virtually every state. Organizations such as these have been most influential in promoting the care and welfare of the mentally retarded population. All states in the United States have legislation which mandates the appropriation of funds and requires states to plan, develop, coordinate, and administer a complete, comprehensive, and integrated statewide program for its mentally retarded citizens. At the federal level, Public Law 94–142, the *Education for All Handicapped Children Act,* has ensured that mentally retarded children and adolescents have the right to receive the special education that is necessary to facilitate their optimal growth and development. Recent federal legislation in the form of Public Law 100–146, the *Developmental Disabilities Assistance and Bill of Rights Act,* provides funding for a national network of councils on developmental disabilities, legal protection and advocacy programs, and university-affiliated programs for each state.

Yet, despite the dramatic changes in social and political climates across the past 25 years that have facilitated understanding and care of the mentally retarded population, much work remains. In particular, there is more to learn regarding the assessment, diagnosis, and treatment of behavioral and emotional disorders in mentally retarded individuals. The study of psychopathology in the mentally retarded population has traditionally received little emphasis from clinicians and applied researchers who are associated with either field of study. As recently as 1985, for example, there were only four texts dedicated to examining emotional and behavioral disturbance in this population (Matson & Barrett, 1982; Menolascino & McCann, 1983; Sigman, 1985; Szymanski &

Tanguay, 1980). This long-standing lack of professional interest has been a rather unfortunate circumstance for the field of mental retardation, particularly in view of the findings of epidemiologic studies conducted during the past two decades. Such investigations have consistently uncovered rates of behavioral and emotional disturbance within the mentally retarded population as between two and six times greater than that observed in the intellectually nonimpaired population (Eaton & Menolascino, 1982; Reiss, 1990; Russell & Tanguay, 1981; Rutter, 1977; Rutter, Graham, & Yule, 1970). According to the National Institutes of Health (1989), approximately 160,000 mentally retarded individuals are treated annually for destructive behavior (i.e., aggression, self-injury) alone at a cost in excess of $3 billion. Of course, these data do not suggest that psychopathology is a fixed result of mental retardation. However, such findings firmly establish the prospect of emotional and behavioral disorders as a salient feature of mental retardation and validate continuing efforts to research better and more comprehensive approaches to assessment, diagnosis, treatment, and prevention for an undeniably at-risk population (Borthwick-Duffy & Eyman, 1990; Jacobson, 1990).

This chapter has been prepared with just such children and adolescents in mind—the so-called *dually diagnosed* children and adolescents who present with emotional and behavioral disorders, in addition to their mental retardation (Menolascino, 1965). The chapter focuses on the description of a moderately sized, behaviorally oriented, hospital-based program for mentally retarded children and adolescents with a wide range of emotional and behavior disorders. It is important to note, however, that this chapter describes this one program, and should not be considered a comprehensive review of all services available to mentally retarded children, adolescents, and their families. Further, the focus on providing an overview of behavior therapy in an inpatient setting should not be construed as a lack of emphasis on adjunctive treatment, such as family or communication disorders therapies. To the contrary, these therapies are viewed as an integral part of the treatment process. The interested reader is referred to Barrett (1986) for a review of therapies that are applicable to the dually diagnosed client.

PROGRAM DESCRIPTION AND STATEMENT OF PHILOSOPHY

Overview

The Developmental Disabilities Program (DDP) is one of several clinical service programs available on an inpatient basis at the 60-bed

Emma Pendleton Bradley Hospital, a children's psychiatric center located in East Providence, Rhode Island. The hospital also offers day treatment services to an additional 70 patients and maintains an active outpatient clinic. Founded in 1931 as the nation's first child psychiatric facility, Bradley Hospital has served since 1982 as the Division of Child and Adolescent Psychiatry for the Brown University Program in Medicine.

The DDP at Bradley Hospital offers the full range of inpatient, day patient, and outpatient services to mentally retarded, autistic, or otherwise developmentally handicapped children and adolescents, who present with varying degrees of emotional or behavioral disorder. The program is designed as a specialty hospital service for dually diagnosed children and adolescents who reside in the southern New England area. Although the majority of children and adolescents referred to the program are residents of Rhode Island, Massachusetts, and Connecticut, the program routinely has acted on referrals from the remaining New England states (Maine, New Hampshire, and Vermont), as well as many East Coast states (New York, Pennsylvania, New Jersey, Maryland, Delaware, and South Carolina), and a few from the Midwest (Nebraska) and the Far West (Colorado, Utah, and California).

The DDP is comprised of six clinical service areas, including an *Intake and Referral Service*, an *Inpatient Unit*, a *Day Treatment Program*, an *Outpatient Clinic*, a *Follow-Up Program*, and an *Aftercare Service* (see Figure 1).

In order to promote an integrated program and ensure an element of continuity of patient care, direct care and professional staff are shared among the various clinical service components. Although certain staff members may be assigned to a specific component of the program for a majority of their clinical duties, it is intended that they have active clinical or administrative responsibilities within all aspects of the program.

Staffing and Organizational Structure

The DDP employs a multidisciplinary staff of four clinical psychologists, a psychology technician who specializes in behavioral assessment, two child psychiatrists, four psychiatric social workers, five special education teachers, 11 psychiatric nurses, two communication disorders specialists, and 30 milieu therapists. The organizational structure of the program, as well as the administrative and clinical lines of authority, are presented in Figure 2.

Ancillary services, such as pediatrics, pediatric neurology, occupational therapy, orthopedics, physical therapy, ENT (ear, nose, throat)

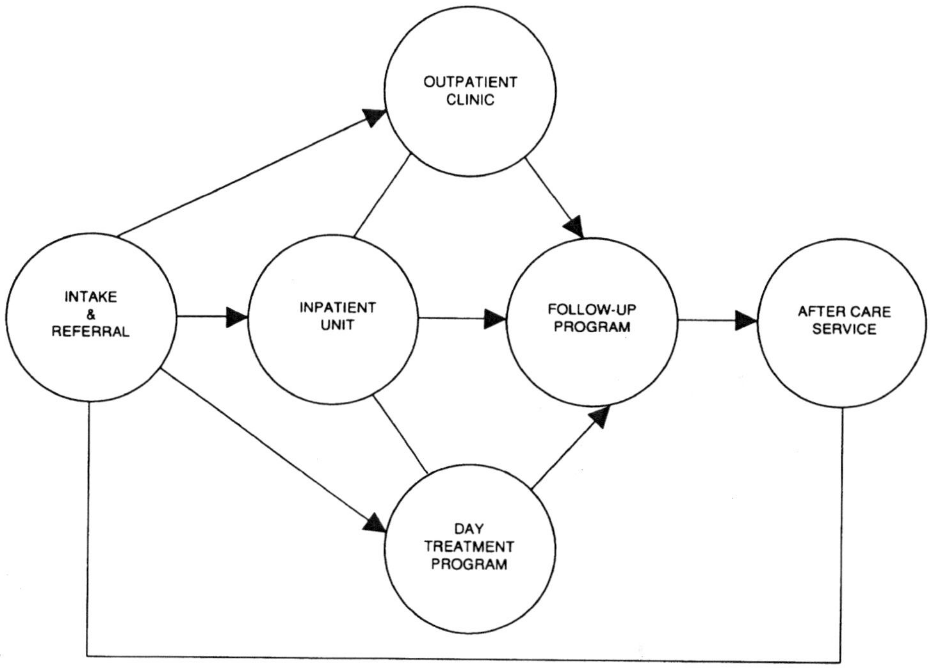

Figure 1. The six clinical service components of the Developmental Disabilities Program at Emma Pendleton Bradley Hospital. The arrows between clinical service areas connote possible patient flow activity.

and audiology, ophthalmology, cardiology, endocrinology, and dental medicine, are routinely available to the program through either in-house or contracted consultation.

The program is also actively involved in teaching and training by virtue of the hospital's affiliation with the medical school. All senior staff members have faculty appointments through the Division of Child and Adolescent Psychiatry to the Brown University Program in Medicine. The medical school affiliation allows the program to integrate a significant number of trainees from a variety of different professional disciplines within its organizational structure. The program supports several trainees on a continuing full-time basis, including a Post-Doctoral Fellow in Clinical Psychology (specializing in developmental disabilities), a 4th-Year Child Psychiatry Fellow, and pre-doctoral interns in clinical psychology, social work, and communication disorders. Student special education teachers, student nurses, pediatric residents, general psychiatry residents, and medical student clerks also receive training through the program on a regular basis.

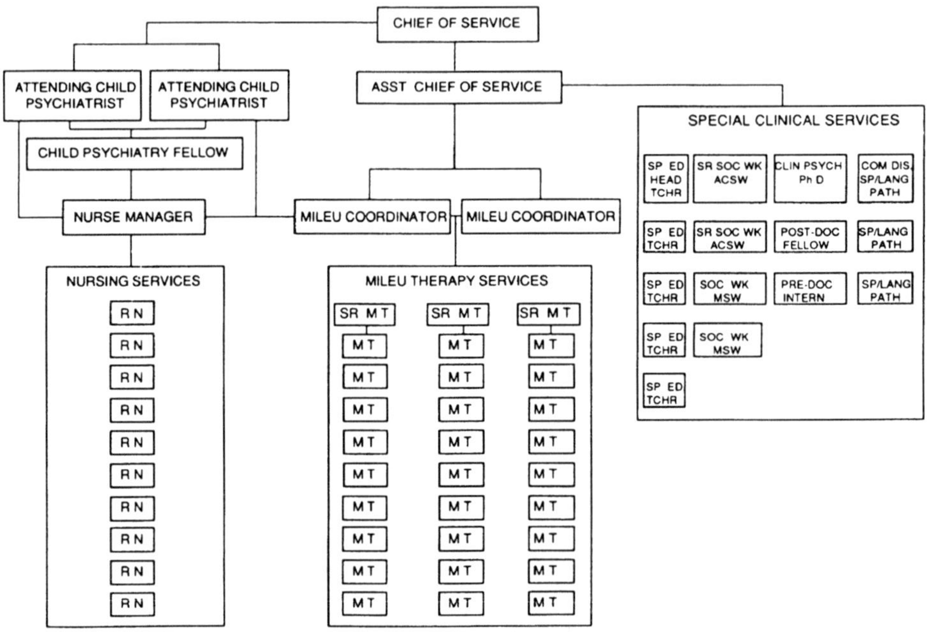

Figure 2. The administrative and organizational structure of the Developmental Disabilities Program at Emma Pendleton Bradley Hospital.

Statement of Philosophy

The majority of mentally retarded children and adolescents referred to the DDP are described as presenting with long-standing emotional and behavioral problems that have been resistant to conventional treatment. Most patients are referred following unsuccessful outpatient pharmacotherapy trials and/or a series of changes in school or residential placements. More than a few patients have been labeled "untreatable" upon referral.

The DDP takes exception to the commonly held belief that emotional and behavioral disorders in mentally retarded children and adolescents are "chronic," "untreatable," and an inevitable result of their developmental disability. Quite to the contrary, the program operates under the assumption that emotional and behavioral disorders coexisting with mental retardation are highly treatable in the vast majority of cases, regardless of the magnitude and irreversibility of the underlying developmental impairment.

Although the program's multidisciplinary nature allows for a variety of different approaches to be used in understanding and treating the emotional and behavioral disorders of its patients, the program seeks to employ a model of empirical clinical practice, whenever possible. In this regard, the empirically based practice of behavioral assessment (cf. Barrett, Ackles, & Hersen, 1986) structures the delivery of all clinical services offered by the program within the context of a *least intrusive treatment practices* model.

The least intrusive treatment practices model developed by the program and adopted for use in providing clinical care is designed to specifically address two approaches to treatment commonly applied to mentally retarded and developmentally disabled patient populations: behavior modification and pharmacotherapy. It is the philosophy of the program that any and all attempts to modify disordered behavior will be accomplished in such a manner as to be clearly and adequately perceived by the therapist and patient, and/or patient's parent(s), legal guardian(s), and advocate(s), as conforming to a standard of community practice commonly acknowledged as the least intrusive and least invasive means available for accomplishing the identified goals of treatment.

This model of clinical practice requires that the program commit itself to the use of positive reinforcement strategies as the principle agent for behavior change and pursue desired changes in aberrant behavior without the use of aversive techniques and behavior-modifying drugs. Although the philosophy of the program advocates strongly for the use of nonaversive, nondrug approaches to treatment as representative of its commitment to a least intrusive treatment practices model, it is important to note that the program is neither *anti*aversive nor *anti*drug when considering a patient's treatment needs. In cases where individual patients may require treatment involving either the use of an operantly based aversive approach to treatment or a behavior-modifying drug, such patients are not denied their right to access these types of interventions. Although it has been the history of the program to restrict aversive behavior modification practices to the use of those techniques commonly acknowledged as "mildly aversive" (e.g., time-out from positive reinforcement), and to generally avoid the use of neuroleptic drugs, on the occasions that these treatment practices are determined necessary, they are pursued only upon obtaining the informed consent of the patient's parent(s), legal guardian(s), and/or legal advocate(s), and documentation that (1) positive reinforcement approaches have failed to produce the desired therapeutic effect; (2) positive reinforcement approaches will be used systematically in combination with the identified (mildly) aversive approach or drug treatment; and (3) neither (mildly) aversive procedures nor drug treatments are being employed as a matter of convenience or method of restraint. It is the goal of diagnosis and treatment to impact directly on the individual patient's quality of life in a manner sufficient to allow discharge to a less restrictive environment where treatment that has been identified as effective may be continued and further progress ensured.

Finally, it is noteworthy that the program views its treatment mandate as extending to members of the patient's family. This includes the provision of family therapy, marital (or couples) therapy, and skills training in behavior management. Further, family members and others closely associated with the patient (e.g., school and agency personnel) are provided with an authoritative understanding of the emotional or behavioral disorder that led to treatment, and the techniques determined as effective in treating the disorder. The program maintains a strong commitment to parent and agency education and training as a method of supporting and assisting families, as well as ensuring the maintenance of hospital-based treatment gains. Family and agency work is assigned a high priority within the program and valued as a proactive means of combating recidivism and preventing future hospital-based treatment.

Clinical Service Areas

Intake and Referral Service

The Intake and Referral Service of the DDP is multipurpose and serves both as a clearinghouse for referrals made to specific clinical service areas within the program (i.e., inpatient, day treatment, outpatient), as well as a triage function for emergency referrals.

The program's Intake and Referral Service is staffed by one (or more) representatives of the seven professional disciplines (i.e., clinical psychology, child psychiatry, social work, special education, psychiatric nursing, milieu therapy, communication disorders) assigned to the program on a full-time basis. This team meets weekly to review existing referrals and to process new referrals to each of the program's clinical service areas, as well as to monitor the waiting list and schedule preadmission interviews for the inpatient and day treatment components of the program. When an emergency referral is received, a mini-team (clinical psychologist, child psychiatrist, psychiatric nurse, milieu therapy supervisor, and social worker) conducts a site visit and consults directly with the referral agency and family of the prospective patient.

Outpatient Services

The program maintains an active Outpatient Specialty Clinic in Developmental Disabilities that provides assessment, diagnostic, and treatment services to families of children and adolescents between the ages of 2 and 22 years. The Outpatient Clinic is staffed by members of the Day Treatment Program and Inpatient Unit, who contribute a weekly minimum of 2 hours of direct patient contact to the clinic. Psychological testing, psychopharmacology consultation, speech and language assessments, family therapy, and behavior therapy involving classroom-based school consultations and parent skill training in behavior management are the most frequently requested services.

The Outpatient Clinic also serves as the base of operations for the program's *Follow-Up Service* and *Aftercare Service*. Routine contact is maintained with the families and receiving agencies of children and adolescents who are discharged from either the Day Treatment Program or the Inpatient Unit for a minimum of 1 year. Depending upon the data obtained during scheduled follow-up interviews, an aftercare program consisting of the full range of outpatient clinical services is made available to former patients, their families, school programs, and other agencies involved in continuing care.

Day Patient Services

The partial hospital service, known as the Developmental Disabilities Day Treatment Program, is an intermediate term (1 to 2 years), behaviorally oriented program that provides assessment, diagnostic, and treatment services for 15 mentally retarded children and adolescents between the ages of 8 and 18 years. Patients referred to the Day Treatment Program present with emotional and behavioral disorders that preclude placement in the public school special education classroom, but are not severe enough to warrant admission to inpatient hospitalization. Patients enrolled in the Day Treatment Program live at home (or in local community group homes) and commute to the hospital on a daily basis for 230 school days each year. Transportation is provided by the patient's school system.

The Day Treatment Program is fully staffed by special education teachers and milieu therapists and shares access to the full range of ancillary clinical services available to the Inpatient Unit (i.e., clinical psychology, child psychiatry, pediatrics, psychiatric social work, communication disorders, psychiatric nursing, and occupational therapy).

The Day Treatment Program maintains an active relationship with the special education authorities for each patient, with the ultimate goal of reintegrating children and adolescents within their home school district. An added feature of the Day Treatment Program is its ability to serve as a "step-down" program for children and adolescents who have been discharged from the program's Inpatient Unit. Children and adolescents discharged to home or other community living arrangements within a 60-mile radius of the hospital have the option of commuting to the Day Treatment Program upon discharge from inpatient hospitalization. Patients who take advantage of the step-down component of the program typically have shorter lengths of stay as inpatients and are significantly more successful in maintaining their hospital-based gains than patients who are unable to access such programming.

Of course, the Day Treatment Program may also serve a "step-up" function and provide referrals to the Inpatient Unit, if patients should happen to show a deteriorating clinical course during partial hospitalization and require more intensive treatment. Indeed, the step-down and step-up components of programming have proven so valuable to discharge planning and the long-term success of treatment, that the hospital is actively pursuing the development of a locally based intermediate care residential program that will allow children and adolescents who are referred from out-of-state to benefit from this aspect of care in a manner similar to local patients.

Inpatient Services

Overview. The inpatient service, known as the Developmental Disabilities Unit (DDU), is a relatively short-term (45 to 120 days), behaviorally oriented hospital program that provides assessment, diagnostic, and treatment services for 15 children and adolescents. These patients range in age from 4 to 22 years and present with severe emotional and behavioral disorders in addition to mental retardation. Children and adolescents admitted to the DDU are usually no longer being safely or effectively managed either in their home and/or school settings.

The DDU operates at full census across the calendar year and, quite unlike most general inpatient psychiatric programs for children and adolescents, shows no evidence of seasonal variation in its referral pattern (i.e., full census during the school year followed by diminished referrals and admissions across the summer months).

Patient Data. Data obtained by consecutively reviewing 50 of the most recent admissions to the inpatient service show a patient mix of 30 males and 20 females with mean admission ages of $12\frac{5}{12}$ years and $15\frac{1}{12}$ years, respectively. The modal age for boys first admitted to the inpatient unit was 9 years, while girls were substantially older at 16 years of age. The age range for admissions to the inpatient unit was $3\frac{10}{12}$ years to $19\frac{3}{12}$ years for boys and $9\frac{9}{12}$ years to $21\frac{11}{12}$ years for girls. These data also indicate the presence of a wide array of DSM-III-R (American Psychiatric Association, 1987) multiaxial diagnoses.

Table 1 shows that for this group of 50 inpatients, a total of 102 diagnoses were made within 15 separate Axis I diagnostic categories and that 86 diagnoses were made across nine Axis II diagnostic categories. Twenty-one patients were diagnosed on Axis I with a form of affective disorder and 10 patients were diagnosed with attention deficit hyperactivity disorder. Additionally, 21 patients were given V-code diagnoses indicative of either a parent–child problem or chronic family disturbance. On Axis II, the full range of mental retardation subtype diagnoses were evident, although moderate mental retardation was the most frequent diagnosis. Seventeen of the 50 patients also were diagnosed with either autism or pervasive developmental disorder, not otherwise specified. Four patients were diagnosed with organic personality disorder and 15 patients presented with language and communication difficulties that could not be explained by their level of mental retardation.

A total of 98 diagnoses in 31 different diagnostic categories were listed on Axis III. Seizure disorders were diagnosed in 25 of the 50 inpatients reviewed. Chronic otitis media (8), hearing impairment (9), obesity (8), and asthma and allergies (8), were prominent physical disorder diagnoses as well.

The mean Axis IV score for this patient group was 4.8 and Axis V ratings ranged from 5 to 80. Approximately 80% of this patient group presented with Global Assessment of Functioning (GAF) scores of 25 or less, upon admission to hospitalization.

Additionally, it was noted that chief complaints upon admission to hospitalization showed 21 of the 50 patients to be referred specifically for treatment of aggressive behavior, whereas 11 of the 50 patients were referred for treatment of self-injurious behavior. "Irritability" (labile mood) and oppositional behavior (with or without aggression and/or self-injury) was noted as a chief complaint upon referral for admission in approximately 80% of the 50 inpatient cases reviewed.

Table 1. Frequency of Multiaxial Diagnoses for 50 Consecutive Admissions to a Psychiatric Inpatient Hospital Program for Mentally Retarded and Developmentally Disabled Children and Adolescents with Severe Behavior Disorders

DSM-III-R Categorical Diagnosis			
Axis I	Axis II	Axis III	
Oppositional Disorder (21)	Borderline Intellectual Functioning (7)	Seizure Disorder (25)	Microcephaly (2)
Chronic Family Disturbance (21)	Mental Retardation (43)	Generalized (12)	Hypogammaglobulinemia (1)
Attention-Deficit Hyperactivity	Mild MR (8)	Complex partial (8)	Ulcerative Proctitis (1)
Disorder (10)	Moderate MR (25)	Absence (4)	Herpes Stomatitis (1)
Major Depression (9)	Severe MR (6)	Lennox-Gaustaut (1)	Tardive Dyskinesia (1)
Bipolar Disorder (6)	Profound MR (4)	Hearing Impairment (9)	Primary Enuresis (1)
Late Luteal Phase	Receptive/Expressive Language	Chronic Otitis Media (8)	Atlanto-axial Instabilities (1)
Dysphoric Disorder (1)	Disorder (15)	Obesity (8)	Eczema (1)
Overanxious Disorder (3)	Autism (8)	Vision Impairment (7)	Hiatal hernia (1)
Intermittent Explosive Disorder (2)	Pervasive Developmental Disorder,	Asthma (5)	Congenital Blindness (1)
Post Traumatic Stress Disorder (7)	NOS (9)	Sleep Disorder (1)	Iron Deficiency Anemia (1)
Stereotypy/Habit Disorder (6)	Organic Personality Disorder (4)	Allergies (3)	Conjunctivitis (1)
Tourette's Disorder (4)		Scoliosis (3)	Arachnoid Cyst (1)
Obsessive-Compulsive Disorder (4)		Trisomy-21 (3)	Fecal Impaction (1)
Simple Phobia (1)		Fragile-X (3)	
Elective Mutism (1)		Acne Vulgaris (3)	
Pica (1)		Hemiplegia (2)	

BEHAVIOR THERAPY IN THE INPATIENT SETTING

Overview

Behavior therapy is central to each of the clinical services (inpatient, day treatment, outpatient) offered by the Developmental Disabilities Program and serves as the basis for the development and delivery of additional therapies, such as individual and group psychotherapy, family therapy, and pharmacotherapy. All patients admitted to the inpatient service receive behavior therapy that is individually tailored to their specific needs. Upon admission to the DDU, a hierarchy of problem behavior that led to the patient's hospitalization is constructed and a preliminary behavior therapy plan, including a behavioral assessment protocol, is prescribed. On the 10th day following admission, a *Comprehensive Evaluation Conference* is convened. At this meeting, diagnostic findings are reviewed, the case is formulated, and a *Master Treatment Plan* is developed that integrates behavioral assessment and behavior therapy with other existing diagnostic and treatment protocols. Importantly, maladaptive and inappropriate behavior that is not viewed as having directly led to the patient's hospitalization is not targeted for treatment. The caution here is a simple one: Inpatient work with mentally retarded children and adolescents who present with severe emotional and behavioral disorders is highly labor intensive. An enormous amount of staff energy and time may be consumed by the assessment and treatment of benign inappropriate behavior that is quite incidental to the reason for hospitalization and best reserved for treatment in a less restricted (and less costly) setting (e.g., partial hospitalization, outpatient clinic) upon discharge. In an inpatient setting, the visibility of inappropriate behavior is not automatically equated with treatment.

Behavioral Assessment

As noted earlier, the Developmental Disabilities Program places a heavy emphasis on the concept of empiricism and its role in the determination of diagnostic accuracy and treatment effectiveness. Simply put, our model involves a quantifiable or data-based approach to clinical decision-making that is heavily weighted by objective observation and yields information that is verifiable through replication. The most common paradigm of the empirical model, as it pertains to the diagnosis and treatment of the mentally retarded population, is represented by the behavioral assessment approach. Such an approach consists of gathering information from a wide variety of sources in a number of different ways, but typically from within a framework that includes four basic methods: (1) behavioral interviewing, (2) traditional standardized psychological testing, (3) behavioral checklists and psychiatric rating scales, and (4) direct behavioral observation (cf. Barrett *et al.*, 1986). These strategies are described in the sections below.

Behavioral Interviewing. On the DDU, as well as in the Day Treatment Program and Outpatient Clinic, behavioral interviewing is the initial step in an evaluation process designed to yield a conceptualization of the patient and the circumstances that have led to the development of problem behavior and, subsequently, to hospitalization. Correspondingly, the program employs an assessment format that involves interviewing third-party informants who are considered most knowledgeable of the patient (e.g., parents, siblings, relatives, and teachers) as well as directly interviewing (or observing) the patient. Information gathered across multiple interviews with those closely associated and most familiar with the patient and his or her problem behavior has proven valuable to initial case formulation and preliminary treatment planning.

Behavioral interviewing, as opposed to its traditional counterpart, contributes to initial case formulation and preliminary treatment planning by conducting a *functional analysis* of the patient's disordered behavior. Behavioral excesses or deficits that led to referral are operationally defined in observable and measurable terms and information is obtained about reliably occurring antecedent and consequent conditions that may be serving both to cue the occurrence of the problem behavior and to maintain its presence, respectively.

In the behavioral assessment literature, this approach is known as the *A-B-C* format. Antecedents (A) are identified that reliably precede or cue the occurrence of the problem behavior (B) which, in turn, may be strengthened or maintained according to the consequence (C) that is contingently applied (Bijou, Peterson, & Ault, 1968).

Establishing a functional relationship between reliably occurring antecedents, disordered behavior, and reliably occurring consequences is an essential first step toward understanding the patient and the dynamics underlying the presentation of disordered behavior. Even in cases where reliable antecedent or consequent conditions are unable to be identified and organic factors are equally evasive, we have found the process of interviewing the most knowledgeable third-party informants to be highly valuable. The interviewing process provides a way of formally recognizing what parents and teachers (for example) describe as the problem behavior, their conceptualizations as to the causes or reasons for its occurrence, and their speculations as to how the behavior may best be treated during hospitalization. Further, it serves to communicate to parents, teachers, and other agency personnel that they are valued members of the patient's treatment team. Although many patients will respond favorably to the highly structured and professional care of the inpatient setting, the ultimate criterion for a successful hospitalization is the continuation of a favorable clinical course upon discharge. Typically, environmental changes (i.e., development of a structured daily routine, implementation of behavioral programming) will need to occur in the patient's home and special education setting in order to ensure the maintenance of hospital-based treatment gains. This requires establishing good and respectful working relationships with parents, teachers, and other agency personnel who are charged with the long-term care of the patient so that necessary modifications to the home and school environments will be forthcoming upon discharge from hospitalization.

Psychological Testing. The second element of the behavioral assessment package involves the use of standardized psychological tests, such as verbal and nonverbal intelligence tests, assessments of social and adaptive ability, psychoeducational and achievement tests, and neuropsychological test batteries. Standardized testing is recommended as the next step beyond behavioral interviewing because it allows for a brief period of direct observation of the patient. Specifically, it provides an opportunity to directly observe the patient under situationally demanding and possibly stressful conditions relative to task performance, which may be serving to cue the occurrence of the problem behavior that led to hospitalization. As such, both sets of observations may be helpful in confirming prior data obtained using the A-B-C interview format or, if such data do not exist, in confirming third-party conceptualizations.

We have found the results of tests, such as the Stanford-Binet Intelligence Scale—Fourth Edition, the Wechsler Intelligence Scales (WISC-R, WPPSI-R, WAIS-R), the McCarthy Scales of Children's Abilities, the Leiter International Performance Scale, the Bayley Scales of Infant Development, the Kaufmann Assessment Battery for Children, the Vineland Adaptive Behavior Scale, the AAMD Adaptive Behavior Scale, the Woodcock-Johnson Psycho-Educational Test, and the Peabody Individual Achievement Test, among others less frequently employed, to be valid in terms of identifying the relative intellectual, adaptive, social, and educational strengths and weaknesses of patients. These tests are useful for treatment planning as well since certain aspects of cognitive development will eventually manifest themselves in terms of adaptive skills (or skill deficits) and are relevant to the type of behavioral intervention selected.

Although the data yielded by a standardized test battery should certainly play a role in the assessment of problem behavior and the selection of subsequent treatment forms, they are by no means the final determinant in either process. In the proper sense, test data should be used to augment information gained through the initial interviewing stage and function as a steering mechanism to suggest further and more discrete forms of assessment (e.g., behavioral checklists, psychiatric rating scales).

Behavioral Checklists and Psychiatric Rating Scales. A third frequently used strategy in the behavioral assessment process is the problem-oriented checklist and rating scale. There are several reasons for the popularity of these instruments as follow-up devices to A-B-C interviewing and standardized psychological tests. First, they are quick to administer. Usually, a checklist may be completed in 20 minutes, making it a viable daily assessment form. Abbreviated forms may take even less time. Second, they are efficient and provide a relatively comprehensive survey of problem behavior. The majority of preferred checklists and rating scales have been subjected to factor analysis and contain normative data, as well as estimates of reliability and validity. Moreover, such instruments yield quantifiable data and may be used effectively for both the assessment of a presenting problem and the objective evaluation of the treatment program designed to address it.

Checklists and rating scales range from assessments of broadly defined psychopathology, such as the parent and teacher forms of the Child Behavior Checklist (CBCL) (Achenbach & Edelbrock, 1983), to scales that focus on a specific syndrome (e.g., hyperactivity) (Conners, 1974; Goyette, Conners, & Ulrich, 1979). It is important to point out, however, that many scales, including the above have excluded the mentally retarded population during normative sampling and, as such, show limited clinical utility with these patients. Despite this shortcoming, several of these scales are routinely employed with higher functioning patients to evaluate behavioral and pharmacotherapy outcomes.

Other scales, such as the Aberrant Behavior Checklist (Aman & Singh, 1983), the Self-Injury Trauma Scale (Iwata, Pace, Kissel, Nau, & Farber, 1990), the Affective Behavior Checklist (Barrett, Tylenda, Kaminer, & Feinstein, 1986), and the Emotional Disorders Rating Scale (Feinstein, Kaminer, Barrett, & Tylenda, 1988), were developed exclusively for use with mentally retarded patients and appear most promising for use in behavioral research as well as in the course of daily clinical practice.

We have found the Aberrant Behavior Checklist particularly valuable in the behavioral assessment of patients with moderate, severe, and profound mental retardation. Although full-scale scores are most useful in objectively determining a patient's overall response to treatment, the scale is equally useful in the objective evaluation of selected behavior therapy and pharmacotherapy trials. For example, we routinely employ full-scale scores of the Aberrant Behavior Checklist as a measure of autistic children's responsiveness to treatment with fenfluramine. The inclusion of "social withdrawal," "hyperactivity," and "irritability" subscales within the Aberrant Behavior Checklist also permits the objective evaluation of social skills training protocols, stimulant drugs trials, and the effect of anticonvulsant drugs (i.e., phenobarbital) on mood, respectively. Similarly, we have found the Self-Injury Trauma Scale (Iwata *et al.*, 1990) useful in quantifying the magnitude of self-injurious behavior beyond what has traditionally been available in terms of behavioral assessment (i.e., time- or event-sampled frequency counts) and useful in monitoring the effectiveness of ongoing behavior therapy and pharmacotherapy.

The two remaining scales, the Affective Behavior Checklist (Barrett, Tylenda, *et al.*, 1986), a modified and collective version of the Children's Depression Rating Scale (Poznanski, Cook, & Carroll, 1979) and Hamilton Rating Scale (Hamilton, 1960), and the Emotional Disorders Rating Scale (Feinstein *et al.*, 1988) were developed by the program and are routinely employed. Both scales were developed because of the need for a reliable method of evaluating disorders of mood and affect in the developmentally disabled population. Although little research other than that generated by program staff is available to attest to the clinical utility of these scales, we have found them to fill a huge void in the area of behavioral assessment, particularly with respect to: (1) evaluating mood and affect in nonverbal autistic and/or mentally retarded patients, and (2) objectively quantifying their response to behavioral and drug treatments that target emotional disorders as areas of concern.

In conclusion, it is important to note that, as with the use of the A-B-C interview format and standardized psychological tests, behavioral checklists and psychiatric rating scales are not sufficiently precise to be used alone either in diagnostic assessment or in the evaluation of treatment progress. The utility of these scales is derived from their ability to objectively quantify third-party information as well as to confirm (or fail to confirm) behavior observed during the brief sampling periods afforded by testing. The role of the behavioral checklist and psychiatric rating scale is to objectively assess the problem area(s) under consideration for treatment and to provide clinicians with an empirical foundation upon which further, more narrowly defined, and precise assessments may be designed.

Direct Behavioral Observation. The most widely used and accepted strategy in behavioral assessment is direct behavioral observation. Indeed, all forms of information gathering that have been discussed to this point serve merely as precursors to this method, which stands as the cornerstone of empirically based assessment. It is a basic tenet of the program's commitment to empirical clinical practice that assessment must eventually rely upon direct observation techniques to be sufficiently precise.

Similar to the A-B-C interview format, direct observation consists of measuring the behavior selected for treatment (response assessment) and the antecedent and consequent conditions (stimulus assessment) that may be serving to both cue and maintain its presence. Response assessment is necessary to objectively determine the magnitude of the behavior targeted for treatment and to control for the occurrence of reactive changes in the target behavior that may be attributable to the assessment process (cf. Nelson & Hayes, 1979). Essentially, a patient's behavior may change because he or she is aware of being systematically observed and not as the result of treatment *per se*. Similarly, it is important to accurately assess the stimulus conditions (both antecedent and consequent) reliably associated with the target behavior. This is necessary in order to objectively ascertain the functional relationship between the problem behavior and the stimulus events that surround it and to document the effect of a stimulus manipulation, such as a change in consequence, on the behavior targeted for treatment.

The best known strategies for conducting response and stimulus assessments are *event-sampling* and *time-sampling* procedures. These procedures are used routinely on the DDU and in the Day Treatment Program to monitor various aspects of a wide variety of patient behavior. Both methods require that the behavior under assessment be clearly observable, definable, and measurable. That is, observations must be made without reference to inner states or hypothetical mechanisms, response definitions must be without ambiguity, and a final quantitative product must be obtained.

Event-sampling is a procedure wherein the frequency or duration of a specific behavior is measured for a given period of time. The yield of such an assessment is concrete and specific (e.g., eight attempts to hit another patient between 7:00 A.M. and noon; 180-min latency to sleep following completion of bedtime routine at 11:00 P.M.). As a measurement technique, event-sampling is appropriate only if the behavior in question is discrete or has a clearly observable beginning and end.

In cases of nondiscrete behavior, where it is difficult to judge when a separate response ends and another begins, time-sampling may provide the clinician with more meaningful information about the strength of the response and its reaction to treatment. Time-sampling is an assessment technique based on units of time rather than events. A common form of time-sampling is *interval recording*. In interval recording, behavior is observed for a given block of time (e.g., 20 min) with the time block further divided into shorter observation units or intervals (e.g., 10 sec). The behavior being observed is then scored as having occurred or not occurred within each of the separate intervals of observation. Target behaviors are noted as occurring only once per interval and, therefore, may be readily expressed as a percentage of occurrence across the total number of observation intervals comprising the larger time block. For example, if a patient engages in self-injurious rubbing and scratching in 60 of the 120 10-sec intervals contained in a 20-min observation period, it can be stated that the target behavior was performed 50% of the time while under observation. Repeated assessments of this type will allow for an accurate measurement of response strength and a base rate against which posttreatment comparisons may be made.

Although time-sampling formats utilizing 10-sec interval recording are preferred owing to their concise and circumscribed nature, such discrete units of observation work best in the laboratory setting and may be too cumbersome and labor intensive for the applied or natural environment, such as the special education classroom or residential milieu. In these settings, it is likely to be more convenient for staff to have specified times (e.g., every 15 min) where they engage in momentary observation of the patient and record the target behavior as having occurred or not occurred on a prescribed data sheet. It should be noted that the use of the term *momentary* is somewhat arbitrary. We have variously employed 5-sec, 15-sec, 1-min, and 2-min periods of constant observation in operationally defining the term momentary, depending on the patient being observed, the type of behavior being assessed, and other circumstances relative to the setting in which the time-sampling is being obtained.

Although such an approach to time-sampling is much less intense than the previously discussed methods of conducting 120 separate 10-sec observations within a 20-min time block, it allows for the collection of data across an entire day. Across successive days, this will prove to be (theoretically) as accurate as the shorter, labor-intensive assessments in terms of measuring response strength and the impact of treatment. At worst, "momentary" time-sampling may produce a serious underestimate of the true magnitude of targeted behavior; this is the risk with all forms of time-sampling. Typically, however, marked underestimates are quite obvious and reported by staff. When this occurs, adjustments to the assessment procedure are made. At best, a daylong ledger of a target behavior is produced, including an accurate depiction of "peak" and "lag" periods that allow for the more intensive study of the stimulus conditions potentially contributing to the differential rate of responding.

Although only a few direct observation techniques have been discussed here, techniques for event- and time-sampling are limited only by the creativity of the clinician who is interested in understanding the patient's behavior.

Reliability and Interobserver Agreement. The concept of reliability is fundamental to any discussion of an empirical approach to clinical practice. Recall that the basic tenet of the empirical approach is objectivity. If a single clinician completes a rating scale or engages in direct observation techniques designed to yield frequency, duration, or time-sampled measures of behavior, such data are reduced to subjective impression if, in fact, they are not reliably obtained by an additional, independent observer. Similar to the earlier assertion that direct behavioral observation serves as the cornerstone of behavioral assessment, the notion of *quality assurance*, whereby obtained patient data are established as reliable, serves as the foundation to the empirical approach in its entirety. Indeed, it may be stated unequivocally that behavioral measurements must be fully and objectively documented as acceptably reliable in order to meet the basic criterion underlying the empirical approach to clinical practice.

The most popular and, perhaps, straightforward method of obtaining quality control of observational data is represented by the concept of *interobserver agreement*. Essentially, two (or more) observers measure a targeted behavior in an independent fashion and compare their findings by adhering to various percentage agreement formulas with estimates of "reliability" demonstrated on a continuum between 0.00 (no agreement) and 1.00 (absolute agreement). The rule of thumb in behavioral assessment is to accept values of 0.80 and greater as indicative of acceptable agreement.

Calculation of agreement values differs according to the observation format used to collect data. For example, when employing a frequency measure, percentage agreement is computed by dividing the smaller of two independently obtained frequency counts by the larger count and multiplying the dividend by 100:

$$\frac{\text{(smaller } f \text{ count)}}{\text{(larger } f \text{ count)}} \times 100 = \% \text{ agreement}$$

Percentage agreement for duration data may be calculated in similar fashion, using the time in minutes or seconds in place of the frequency values:

$$\frac{\text{(less time duration)}}{\text{(greater time duration)}} \times 100 = \% \text{ agreement}$$

Applications of the percentage agreement formula to time-sampled data vary somewhat from the above examples; however, the essential features remain unchanged (see Rojahn & Schroeder, 1983).

Discussion of interobserver agreement as a quality control method in behavioral measurement should be tempered by the fact that the products yielded by such agreement formulas do not constitute actual reliability estimates. In the purest psychometric sense, reliability must (1) provide for measures of data consistency and stability, (2) assume an underlying observed score and true score variance component, and (3) address the issue of agreement between observers strictly by chance. That interobserver agreement formulas meet none of these criteria is the most commonly cited shortcoming to their use. Although spuriously high levels of what may be mistermed as "reliability" are the risks of employing such measures, these formulas adequately address the issue of quality control of data obtained in the course of routine clinical practice.

Single-Subject Experimental Designs. The use of empirical case studies employing single-subject experimental designs represents the final step of the behavioral assessment process that began with the use of the A-B-C interviewing format upon a patient's referral to hospitalization. Each of the behavioral assessment techniques reviewed to this point have focused on producing a reliable determination that a problem behavior existed, how the problem behavior may best be measured, the extent or magnitude of the disorder, and whether the behavior in question was being influenced by reliably occurring stimulus events (i.e., antecedents and consequences).

Single-subject case studies are routinely employed by the Developmental Disabilities Program as the final method of studying changes in targeted behaviors following the introduction of treatment. Consequently, any change in the targeted response may be unequivocally related to the intervention being applied. In this regard, the program takes full advantage of the available single-subject experimental designs as strategies for evaluating the effectiveness of treatment (see Hersen & Barlow, 1976).

Behavior Therapy

The Developmental Disabilities Program has adopted the traditional position of behavioral psychology that human behavior is learned and is a function of environmental transactions among stimulus, organismic, and response variables. If a patient has been successful in learning undesirable behavior, there is a high probability of the patient's learning desirable behavior, particularly if the contingencies leading to the development of undesirable behavior are properly understood and managed in such a way as to be effectively modified. Importantly, however, the program recognizes that merely understanding and managing contingencies, while a necessary condition, is not sufficient for changing patient behavior (Russo, 1990). We strongly support the position that an equally critical variable in changing human behavior is the person (i.e., parent, teacher, staff member) who manages the contingencies and the interpersonal relationship established with the patient. Designing stimulus conditions that allow patients to respond with desirable behavior is a key component of effective behavior management.

Children and adolescents admitted to the DDU require a comprehensive behavior therapy proogram to address chief complaints in the typical areas of oppositional responding, aggression, disruptive (tantrum) behavior, destructive behavior, motivational deficits, and poor social skills. Consistent with the program's philosophical commitment to change undesirable behavior through positive reinforcement strategies, a heavy emphasis is placed on the use of systematic attention (scheduled positive reinforcement) and planned ignoring (extinction). "Time-in with positive reinforcement" and "time-out from positive reinforcement" are the cornerstone strategies for all behavior therapy procedures within the program (cf. DiLorenzo & Ollendick, 1986; Williams, Schroeder, Eckerman, & Rojahn, 1983).

Time-in and Time-out

Understanding the use of *time-in* and *time-out* requires a thorough appreciation of its underlying principles: positive reinforcement and extinction. The application of these two basic concepts is fundamental to behavior therapy. Behavior occurs as a function of stimulus conditions (antecedent and consequent) in the environment and a change in stimulus conditions can produce a change in behavior. It is the principle of reinforcement that behavior rewarded contingent upon its presence will recur with increased frequency and become successively strengthened. As a corollary to this principle, previously reinforced behavior that is contingently ignored (or is unreinforced) will recur with decreased frequency and become successively weakened (Skinner, 1938).

The complementary use of time-in and time-out is predicated on the behavioral theory that human behavior does not occur in a vacuum. Rather, it is learned and developed across a continuum of environmental experience that results in the selective retaining of responses that gain access to preferred goal states (rewards) and the selective omission of previously learned responses because they are no longer reinforced.

Time-in. All children and adolescents admitted to the DDU (as well as those enrolled in the Day Treatment Program) have a formal time-in program that is integrated within their Master Treatment Plan. Time-in may take one of several forms designed to develop a variety of helpful, prosocial behavior by specifically targeting desirable adaptive behavior within three general prosocial behavioral categories: personal responsibilities (e.g., completion of self-care activities), compliant behavior (e.g., following directions, accepting limits), and social-community responsibilities (e.g., respecting peers and property). Response definitions within these general classes of prosocial behavior are altered to reflect the level of cognitive and adaptive ability of the individual patient. Specifically, different levels of expectation translate into different criteria for success according to an individual patient's ability. Similarly, time-in protocols are individualized in terms of the schedule of reinforcement. Some patients may receive time-in on a fixed ratio basis of once per adaptive response: other patients may receive it on a fixed interval basis of 5, 10, 15, 20, 30, or 60 minutes. Still other patients may have time-in protocols that involve token reinforcement conditions requiring them to complete a series of hourly behavioral contracts that may be cashed-in for back-up reinforcers at specified times throughout the day and evening.

Importantly, targeted responses contained in the time-in program are incompatible with the undesirable behavior typically listed among the chief complaints of the patient upon hospitalization (e.g., motivational deficits, oppositional responding, aggression, disruptive tantrums, property destruction, social skills deficits). Of equal importance, it should be noted that time-in programs do not merely reinforce the absence of undesirable behavior (e.g., the absence of aggression or property destruction); they target an observable response that is incompatible with the presenting problem (e.g., respects peers and property). Thus, patients are given an opportunity to successfully perform a concrete adaptive response that leads to a reinforcer. This approach is viewed as superior to the alternative of being reinforced for simply "omitting" an undesirable behavior. After all, the goal of time-in (as a positive reinforcement program) is to actively teach specific prosocial behavior.

Our experience strongly suggests that a greater durability of favorable clinical response is obtained by differentially reinforcing prosocial behavior that is specifically incompatible (DRI) with a problem behavior, such as aggression, as opposed to differentially reinforcing other (DRO) behavior that may not be prosocial in nature, but involves the omission of an aggressive response. Teaching a child or adolescent the rewards of interacting with peers, teachers, and family members in a helpful and prosocial manner is decidedly different from teaching them simply not to throw a punch or a tantrum.

Time-out. Time-out from positive reinforcement is among the most heavily researched behavioral approaches to treatment (cf. DiLorenzo & Ollendick, 1986; Leitenberg, 1965; Williams *et al.*, 1983). This procedure requires that access to positive reinforcement be contingently removed upon the occurrence of a response that is targeted for suppression. Correspondingly, it becomes obvious that time-out cannot be effective in the absence of a companion time-in program where positive reinforcement conditions are in effect.

Time-out may take one of two forms: *nonexclusionary* or *exclusionary* tactics. Applications of nonexclusionary time-out include the contingent removal of preferred activities and/or contingent removal of attention for a specified period of time (e.g., Foxx & Shapiro, 1978; Spitalnik & Drabman, 1976). The principal advantage in using nonexclusionary approaches to time-out is that it allows the patient to remain within a particular setting (e.g., the special education classroom) and to continue to be engaged in instruction. Termination of a nonexclusionary time-out period is contingent upon the expiration of a brief specified period of time (e.g., 10 min), the absence of the behavior that led to the restriction of access to reinforcement (e.g., absence of disruptive classroom behavior), and the performance of an adaptive objective relevant to the setting (e.g., completion of an academic task). A significant limitation to the use of nonexclusionary time-out is the lack of control over potential sources of reinforcement that may occur as the direct result of retaining the patient within the setting (e.g., peer and teacher attention derived from continued disruptive behavior).

The traditional form of time-out involves removal of the patient from the setting in which the behavioral transgression has occurred and placement to a second setting devoid of the potential for reinforcement. Exclusionary time-out from positive reinforcement may include contingent removal to an isolated (but supervised) area of a particular setting (a so-called time-out area), or contingent removal to a seclusion room. Criteria for release from exclusionary time-out is contingent upon the expiration of a brief specified period of time (2 to 59 min) and the absence of disruptive behavior within the time-out setting. The principal benefit of exclusionary time-out is that it guarantees control over potential sources of reinforcement that are operational within the time-in setting. In principle, exclusionary time-out ensures that the patient will be ignored. Importantly, exclusionary time-out also prevents a patient from being continually disruptive in the time-in setting at the expense of peers. Disadvantages of exclusionary time-out are almost exclusively related to the use of the seclusion format and involve the potential for injury to both staff and patient during transport, the potential for overuse and abuse, the unknown effects of imposing social isolation on a (mentally retarded) youngster, and the potential for self-injury within the seclusion room (Williams *et al.*, 1983).

The full range of nonexclusionary and exclusionary time-out from positive reinforcement approaches are employed with patients of the Developmental Disabilities Program. Importantly, time-out procedures are considered within the framework of the program's *Least Intrusive Treatment Practices* model for the delivery of clinical services. Therefore, they must be a part of the patient's written treatment plan and be accompanied by a companion time-in program.

Compliance Training

As noted earlier, oppositional behavior is ranked highly among the presenting problems of children and adolescents referred to the Developmental Disabilities Program. Parents and teachers routinely complain that the patient is unwilling to follow directions or accept limits on behavior.. Typically, they report that noncompliance is pervasive, frequently escalates to include aggressive and/or self-injurious behavior, and has withstood a variety of treatment efforts. Almost invariably parents and teachers report that if they were successful in enlisting the patient's cooperation in following directions and accepting limits, progress in many areas (e.g., aggression, self-injury) would be forthcoming.

We have been successful in employing a 7-point treatment program for oppositional behavior that provides a good working example of what is meant by the statement that the application of the principles of time-in and time-out comprises the cornerstone of behavior therapy for our program. An outline of the program is as follows:

1. Whenever the patient has been observed to be helpful or pro-social, this behavior should be reinforced with substantial praise and attention. (Recall that all patients also have a "Social-Community Responsibilities" criterion to meet within their larger time-in program.)
2. Whenever the patient has been observed to be helpful, cooperative, and compliant, this behavior should be rewarded with substantial praise and attention. (Here, too, patients have criteria to meet in terms of "Personal Responsibilities" and "Compliance" within their larger time-in programs.)
3. Whenever a patient fails to comply with a request:
   (a) *Use one additional verbal prompt* (e.g., "I have asked you once to please stand up and walk with the group. Please stand and come with me now"). If the patient complies, see Step 2.
   (b) If the patient fails to respond to the use of an additional verbal prompt, say nothing more. *Use one physical prompt* that completes the first step of the request (e.g., guide or lift the patient to a standing position and gesture for him to proceed with the group). If the patient complies, acknowledge the cooperation ("Thank you"), but do not apply a credit to the patient's time-in program.
   (c) If the patient fails to respond to the physical prompt, *manually guide* the patient through the completion of the request (e.g., physical prompting, as necessary, until the patient has rejoined the group). Importantly, make no comments to the patient. Carry out the physical prompting procedure in a casual, matter-of-fact manner.
   (d) If the patient aggresses, tantrums, or becomes otherwise disruptive in response to the manual guidance procedure (or at any time during the Compliance Training procedure), implement the patient's formal time-out program.
   (e) Once the patient has met the criterion for release from time-out, require the patient to perform as originally directed and revert to Step 2 (and all succeeding steps) of this program until the compliance objective is achieved.

Of course, modifications to the Compliance Training Program must be made to allow for the participation of autistic, language disabled, and nonverbal patients; however, the essential components of time-in and time-out remain unchanged.

Visual Screening

Another frequently used behavior therapy program by the Developmental Disabilities Program that employs the principle of time-out is visual screening (see McGonigle, Duncan, Cordisco, & Barrett, 1982). This procedure requires a therapist to briefly shield a patient's eyes with the hand contingent upon the observed occurrence of a targeted undesirable behavior. Visual screening or "visual time-out" has been used effectively to suppress a wide variety of maladaptive and inappropriate responses in mentally retarded and autistic children, including self-injury (Barrett, Matson, Shapiro, & Ollendick, 1981; Lutzker, 1978; Rincover & Devany, 1982; Singh, 1980; Singh, Beale, & Dawson, 1981; Zegiob, Alford, & House, 1978), disruptive behavior (Barmann & Murray, 1981; Zegiob, Jenkins, Becker, & Bristow, 1976), and stereotypic responding (Barrett, Staub, & Sisson, 1983; McGonigle *et al.*, 1982; Rincover, 1978; Rincover, Cook, Peoples, & Packard, 1979; Rincover, Newsome, & Carr, 1979).

Visual screening has a number of advantages in addition to its well-documented effectiveness as a response suppressor. First, it is an easy procedure for parents, teachers, and staff members to learn. Second. the procedure is typically quite brief with application times ranging from 2 seconds to 1 minute. Third, the procedure does not require the patient to leave the setting and, as such, has many of the same advantages attributed to the use of nonexclusionary time-out. Fourth, and finally, it requires no special equipment and may be conveniently applied in virtually every type of setting. Disadvantages are similar to those reviewed for exclusionary time-out, including the risk of injury to patient and/or the person applying the procedure. Importantly, the risk of injury with this procedure appears to be directly proportional to the amount of time a patient is expected to spend in the visual screening contingency (i.e., brief visual screening serves to minimize the risk of injury to all parties). A second disadvantage is that the procedure lacks utility with most adolescents. Because visual screening is not intended as a means of physically managing a patient, it is relatively easy to escape the procedure. Escape proficiency is related to patient strength and, for most adolescents, it is a simple matter to remove the therapist's hand at will. Despite its limitations, we have found visual screening to be a valuable behavior therapy procedure, particularly when used in combination with a well-formulated time-in program.

Individual and Group Psychotherapy: Social Skills Training

The capacity to establish and maintain relationships is a significant area of deficit among dually diagnosed, developmentally disabled children and adolescents. Further, these deficits have profound effects on the ability of these children and adolescents to be reintegrated into the community. Many researchers have suggested that longevity in community-based programs among developmentally disabled adults is inextricably linked to the level of support these adults receive from their social networks. Indeed, the relationship between impoverished social supports and reduced social/adaptive functioning has been established in a variety of populations ranging from psychiatric patients to recent immigrants to the United States (Flaherty, Gaviria, Black, Altman, & Mitchell, 1983; Flaherty, Kohn, Golbin, Gaviria, & Birz, 1986; Tolsdorf, 1976).

For these reasons, the ability to establish and make use of relationships with others is an essential component of adaptive functioning in developmentally disabled individuals. Although much of the attention paid to this area has been in the form of social skills training, our own approach is more expansive. We view social skills training, individual psychotherapy, group psychotherapy, and family psychotherapy as broadly addressing the issue of relationship disturbances among developmentally disabled children, adolescents, and their families. Just as the form of the disturbance may vary, so too will the treatment approach.

For example, children with pervasive developmental disorders or autistic spectrum disorders are likely to display deficits in the area of social skills that may be best addressed through social skills training (see Frankel, Leary, & Kilman, 1987). Within this category, the treatment focus for a socially aloof 5-year-old is likely to be quite different from that for a socially interested but deviantly relating 15-year-old. In the first case, treatment may consist of activities designed to build social "interest," perhaps in conjunction with speech and language therapy. In the second case, a more traditional form of social skills training that provides remediation in areas such as initiating and responding to conversation is more likely to be recommended. Developmentally disabled, nonautistic spectrum children and adolescents provide still another profile. The difficulties of a mildly mentally retarded adolescent with a seizure disorder and conflict with the parents may be best addressed through individual, group, and family psychotherapy. Correspondingly, decisions are made at the initial diagnostic and master treatment planning conference about the particular combination of therapies most appropriate for the individual child or adolescent and the family.

Individual psychotherapy has less often been a focus in the treatment of developmentally disabled children (Hurley, 1989). This is perhaps due to the fact that many professionals suffer from a lack of exposure during training to the psychotherapeutic needs of the population as well as from a bias that developmentally disabled children do not have the verbal skills necessary to benefit from psychotherapy. In cases where this is true, it is possible to devise other means of exploration (e.g., play or art therapy) that may accomplish the same end (Jakab, 1982). We view individual therapy as addressing two broad goals: (1) to explore and ameliorate patterns of dysfunctional relating in the child's life, and (2) to increase the range of the child's coping abilities. These goals place our treatment approach in the category of "supportive" rather than "insight-oriented" psychotherapy (Rockland, 1989).

Within the Developmental Disabilities Program, therapists (clinical psychologists, social workers, child psychiatrists, and trainees in these disciplines) meet with patients two to three times a week. As with psychotherapy with normally developing children, the goal is to develop a therapeutic alliance within which the themes of the therapy can evolve. Naturally, such themes vary with the patient's diagnosis and level of functioning. The psychotherapist also plays a role with respect to interpreting the child's behavior in the context of weekly treatment team meetings and to helping direct-care staff to cope with their reactions to the child, in making decisions about treatment approaches within the milieu, and in informing direct-care staff with regard to therapy goals.

Group psychotherapy has also been a useful adjunct, particularly with adolescents. Many dually diagnosed, developmentally disabled adolescents have become isolated from their peer groups. This is perhaps a function of the extent of their psychiatric difficulties. Correspondingly, they are accustomed to seeking support from adults rather than from their peers (Zigler & Burack, 1989). Group psychotherapy provides experience with peers as resources for support, as well as a forum within which to explore feelings about such shared issues as forming and maintaining friendships, growing up as a disabled person, separation from their families (including hospitalization), and reintegration into the community. Our groups range in size from 4 to 12, depending on the patient composition of the unit. They are usually led by a male–female therapist team. We have found it useful to have patients themselves define the nature and rules of the group. This is done in an effort to foster both a sense of group cohesiveness and increased self-efficacy in patients who are accustomed to following adults for guidance.

The theoretical background of social skills training on the unit is drawn from the fields of developmental psychology and psychopathology. That is, areas of focus are extracted from previous clinical and investigative endeavors on the nature of social relatedness in both normally developing and developmentally disabled individuals (particularly autistic individuals). Examples of these areas of focus include attachment and social interest, affective communication, regulation of mutual gaze, and initiation of social contact (see Walters, Barrett, & Feinstein, 1990). Although these areas will not be affected in all developmentally disabled children, they provide a guideline for assessing social relatedness and for developing a treatment approach. Within these guidelines, we have made use of a variety of commercial programs for planning sessions.

Social skills training is conducted by clinical psychologists, speech and language therapists, special education teachers, and milieu therapists. Although most patients receive an hour of formal group social skills per week from speech and language/special education or clinical psychology/speech and language teams, efforts are made to ensure that the focus of these groups is carried into the classroom activities of individual patients on a daily basis.

Behavior Therapy in Combination with Pharmacotherapy

Pharmacotherapy is a common prescription for mentally retarded children and adolescents who present with behavior disorders. Indeed, it may be among the first treatment approaches employed with this population upon the observance of problematic behavior. Unfortunately, drug therapy is often prescribed unwisely with this group of patients. A recent review by Bates, Smeltzer, and Arnoczky (1986) estimated that between 39% and 54% of psychoactive drugs administered to mentally retarded individuals were inappropriately prescribed.

As noted earlier in this chapter, the vast majority of patients referred to the Developmental Disabilities Program, particularly the DDU, have a substantial history of unsuccessful drug treatment. Many patients present with polypharmacy being listed among their chief complaints. Pharmacotherapy protocols within our program begin with carefully titrating patients off all behavior-modifying drugs and establishing basal magnitudes of the behavior(s) that led to treatment across a 2-week drug-free period. Behavior therapy protocols are then initiated and, as indicated, pharmacotherapy is restored. Importantly, pharmacotherapy within the Developmental Disabilities Program is subjected to the same stringent analysis as behavior therapy and involves the routine use of double-blind, placebo-controlled methodology and single-subject experimental designs that allow for the partitioning of relative therapeutic effect (Ackles, 1986).

When used responsibly within the framework of empirical clinical practice, a variety of pharmacotherapy approaches have been shown as impacting favorably on the treatment of dually diagnosed patients (e.g., Rivinus, Grofer, Feinstein, & Barrett, 1989).

MONITORING OF PATIENT CARE

The routine and careful monitoring of patient care is an indispensable feature of a comprehensive Quality Assurance Program and critical to the success of day-to-day program operations. Mentally retarded children and adolescents with severe emotional and behavioral disorders are a diagnostically complex and challenging population. As noted earlier, virtually every patient enrolled in the program presents with multiple Axis I, II, and III diagnoses with the majority of patients presenting with significant parent and family difficulties as well. The Developmental Disabilities Program employs a model that entails several standing meetings that occur on a weekly basis and allow multidisciplinary staff the advantage of consulting across disciplines while remaining current with respect to case formulations and treatment protocols. These weekly meetings, which are reviewed below, serve to ensure that the patient care delivered by the Developmental Disabilities Program is frequently monitored in a thorough and effective manner.

Intake, Referral, and Discharge Meeting

This meeting is held weekly for 1 hour and is attended by staff assigned to the program's Intake and Referral Service. As mentioned previously, staff attending this meeting review existing and new referrals to all areas of clinical service provided by the program, including inpatient, day treatment, and outpatient services. They also monitor the waiting lists for admission to either the DDU or Day Treatment Program and perform triage functions with respect to emergency referrals. Importantly, discharges are also planned at this weekly meeting with the dual objective of facilitating a smooth patient transition to the next placement, as well as allowing for the advanced coordination of prospective admissions. Planned discharges and planned admissions serve to greatly stabilize program operations. If staff are aware in advance of patient discharges and admissions, as well as the timing of changes in patient composition, surprises are minimized and staff morale does not suffer.

Pediatric Rounds

This meeting is held weekly for 1 hour and is attended by as many representatives as possible from all disciplines assigned to the program on a full-time basis. It is chaired by a hospital-based pediatrician assigned to the program. The 15 inpatients and 15 day patients enrolled in the program are reviewed each week by the program nursing staff with respect to well child care. Patients with Axis III diagnoses are either monitored or receive active treatment for their physical disorders. Special attention is directed to the possibility that medical disorders might be masquerading as behavior disorders and vice versa (see Gourash, 1986). Pediatric neurology, neuropsychology, dietary, orthopedic, ophthalmologic, ENT and audiologic, internal medicine, cardiology, gynecology, dermatology, genetic, and dental consults obtained from outside of the hospital are reviewed with all staff at this meeting.

Medication Review

This meeting is held for 1½ hours each week immediately following pediatric rounds. It is chaired by the attending child psychiatrists for the DDU and Day Treatment Program. The purpose of the meeting is to review drug-assessment and treatment protocols for all patients enrolled in the program. Special attention is paid to the evaluation of treatment protocols that involve the use of behavior modifying drugs in combination with behavior therapy (see Ackles, 1986). As with other forms of intervention, it is the intent of the program to empirically evaluate the effectiveness of pharmacotherapy. As indicated, drug trials are completed in double-blind, placebo-controlled fashion with protocols constructed in collaboration with the hospital pharmacists (e.g., Barrett, Feinstein, & Hole, 1989).

Treatment Review Meetings

Upon admission to either inpatient or day hospitalization, patients are assigned to one of five multidisciplinary treatment teams. These treatment teams meet on a weekly basis to formally review all aspects of patient care. Four of the treatment review teams are designated for inpatients, with each team performing reviews on approximately four patients each week. The day patient treatment review team also meets and reviews approximately four patients on a rotating basis each week. In this manner, all 15 day patients are reviewed by the treatment team once each month.

Administrative Quality Improvement Meeting

This meeting is held biweekly for one hour. The agenda includes announcements (e.g., staff vacations, position vacancies), clinical issues (e.g., on-call schedule, impending discharges and admissions, Individual Education Program [IEP] meetings), and quality assurance/quality improvement items (i.e., current status of activities designed to improve patient services and ensure patient and staff safety). Minutes of this meeting are distributed to all staff.

Because of the large number of nursing and child care personnel assigned to the Developmental Disabilities Program, additional direct-care staff meetings, similar in nature to the program-wide Administrative Quality Improvement meeting, are conducted bimonthly.

Behavior Clinic

This meeting is held weekly for 2 hours and serves as the final forum for clinical decision-making in any given week. Inpatients and day patients are selectively placed on the clinic docket throughout the course of the week when it is apparent that more discussion is necessary or further data are required before a clinical decision can be accomplished. Any staff member may refer a patient for review in this clinic. All staff members working with a patient referred to the clinic are required to attend this meeting. The most difficult clinical decisions with respect to patient care are made here. It is the culmination of the week's clinical activity and a meeting that is essential to program operations.

SUMMARY

This chapter reviewed selected aspects of the Developmental Disabilities Program of the Emma Pendleton Bradley Hospital located in East Providence, Rhode Island. This unique program is one of only four similar programs in the United States that are affiliated with medical schools and that offer specialty inpatient, day treatment, and outpatient services to mentally retarded, autistic, or otherwise developmentally handicapped children and adolescents who present with emotional and behavioral disorders. The program is committed to a model of empirical clinical practice and is strongly oriented toward the use of behavioral assessment and behavior therapy.

The program is composed of six clinical service areas, including an Intake and Referral Service, an Inpatient Unit, a Day Treatment Program, an Outpatient Specialty Clinic, a Follow-Up Program, and an Aftercare Service. The inpatient unit serves as the hub in this clinical scheme and supports the five remaining ancillary services in terms of revenue generation and staffing.

REFERENCES

Achenbach, T. M., & Edelbrock, C. S. (1983). *Manual for the Child Behavior Checklist and Revised Child Behavior Profile.* Burlington: University of Vermont, Department of Psychiatry.

Ackles, P. K. (1986). Evaluating pharmacological-behavioral treatment interactions. In M. Hersen (Ed.), *Pharmacological and behavioral treatment: An integrative approach* (pp. 54–86). New York: Wiley.

Aman, M., & Singh, N. N. (1983). *Aberrant Behavior Checklist.* Canterbury, New Zealand: University of Canterbury.

American Psychiatric Association. (1987). *Diagnostic and statistical manual of mental disorders* (3rd ed., rev.). Washington, DC: Author.

Barmann, B. C., & Murray, W. J. (1981). Suppression of inappropriate sexual behavior by facial screening. *Behavior Therapy, 12,* 730–735.

Barrett, R. P. (Ed.). (1986). *Severe behavior disorders in the mentally retarded: Nondrug approaches to treatment.* New York: Plenum Press.

Barrett, R. P., Matson, J. L., Shapiro, E. S., & Ollendick, T. H. (1981). A comparison of punishment and DRO procedures for treating stereotypic behavior of mentally retarded children. *Applied Research in Mental Retardation, 2,* 247–256.

Barrett, R. P., Staub, R. W., & Sisson, L. A. (1983). Treatment of compulsive rituals with visual screening: A case study with long term follow-up. *Journal of Behavior Therapy and Experimental Psychiatry, 14,* 55–59.

Barrett, R. P., Ackles, P. K., & Hersen, M. (1986). Strategies for evaluating treatment. In R. P. Barrett (Ed.), *Severe behavior disorders in the mentally retarded: Nondrug approaches to treatment* (pp. 323–357). New York: Plenum Press.

Barrett, R. P., Tylenda, B., Kaminer, Y., & Feinstein, C. (1986). *The Affective Behavior Checklist: A behavioral assessment tool for use in mentally retarded children and adolescents with mood disorders.* Unpublished manuscript. Brown University Program in Medicine.

Barrett, R. P., Feinstein, C., & Hole, W. (1989). Effects of naloxone and naltrexone on self-injury: A double blind, placebo controlled analysis. *American Journal on Mental Retardation, 93,* 644–651.

Bates, W. J., Smeltzer, D. J., & Arnoczky, S. M. (1986). Appropriate and inappropriate use of psychotherapeutic medications for institutionalized mentally retarded persons. *American Journal of Mental Deficiency, 90,* 363–370.

Bijou, S. W., Peterson, R. F., & Ault, M. H. (1968). A method to integrate descriptive and experimental field studies at the level of data and empirical concepts. *Journal of Applied Behavior Analysis, 1,* 175–191.

Borthwick-Duffy, S., & Eyman, R. K. (1990). Who are the dually diagnosed? *American Journal on Mental Retardation, 94,* 586–595.

Conners, C. K. (1975). Rating scales for use in drug studies with children. *Psychopharmaology Bulletin* (Special Issue on Children, 24–42.

Developmental Disabilities Assistance and Bill of Rights Act Amendments of 1987. Public Law 100–146; U.S.C. (Jan. 6, 1987).

DiLorenzo, T. M., & Ollendick, T. H. (1986). Behavior modification: Punishment. In R. P. Barrett (Ed.), *Severe behavior disorders in the mentally retarded: Nondrug approaches to treatment* (pp. 27–60). New York: Plenum Press.

Eaton, L., & Menolascino, F. J. (1982). Psychiatric disorders in the mentally retarded: Types, problems, and challenges. *American Journal of Psychiatry, 139,* 1297–1303.

Education of All Handicapped Children Act of 1975 and Federal Regulations. Public Law 94–142; 20 U.S.C. §§ 1401–1461.

Feinstein, C., Kaminer, Y., Barrett, R. P., & Tylenda, B. (1988). The assessment of mood and affect in developmentally disabled children and adolescents: The Emotional Disorders Rating Scale. *Research in Developmental Disabilities, 9,* 109–121.

Flaherty, J. A., Gaviria, F. M., Black, E. M., Altman, E., & Mitchell, T. (1983). The role of social support in the functioning of patients with unipolar depression. *American Journal of Psychiatry, 140,* 473–476.

Flaherty, J. A., Kohn, R., Golbin, A., Gaviria, M., & Birz, S. (1986). Demoralization and social support in Soviet-Jewish immigrants to the United States. *Comprehensive Psychiatry, 27,* 149–158.

Foxx, R. M., & Shapiro, S. T. (1978). The time-out ribbon: A nonexclusionary time-out procedure. *Journal of Applied Behavior Analysis, 11,* 125–136.

Frankel, R. M., Leary, M., & Kilman, B. (1987). Building social skills through pragmatic analysis: Assessment and treatment implications for children with autism. In R. Cohen, A. Donnellan, & R. Paul (Eds.), *Handbook of autism and pervasive developmental disorders* (pp. 333–359). New York: Wiley.

Gourash, L. F. (1986). Assessing and managing medical disorders. In R. P. Barrett (Ed.), *Severe behavior disorders in the mentally retarded: Nondrug approaches to treatment* (pp. 157–205). New York: Plenum Press.

Goyette, C. H., Conners, C. K., & Ulrich, R. F. (1979). Normative data on revised Conners' parent and teacher rating scales. *Journal of Abnormal Child Psychology, 6,* 221–236.

Hamilton, M. (1960). A rating scale for depression. *Journal of Neurology, Neurosurgery, and Psychiatry, 23,* 56–62.

Hersen, M., & Barlow, D. H. (1976). *Single case experimental designs: Strategies for studying behavior change.* New York: Pergamon Press.

Hurley, A. D. (1989). Individual psychotherapy with mentally retarded individuals: A review and call for research. *Research in Developmental Disabilities, 10,* 261–275.

Iwata, B. A., Pace, G. M., Kissel, R. C., Nau, P. A., & Farber, J. M. (1990). The self-injury trauma (SIT) scale: A method for quantifying surface tissue damage caused by self-injurious behavior. *Journal of Applied Behavior Analysis, 23,* 99–110.

Jacobson, J. W. (1990). Do some mental disorders occur less frequently among persons with mental retardation? *American Journal of Mental Retardation, 94,* 596–602.

Jakab, I. (1982). Psychiatric disorders in mental retardation: Recognition, diagnosis, and treatment. In I. Jakab (Ed.), *Mental retardation* (pp. 270–322). New York: Kargan.

Leitenberg, H. W. (1965). Is timeout from positive reinforcement an aversive event? A review of the experimental evidence. *Psychological Bulletin, 64,* 428–451.

Lutzker, J. R. (1978). Reducing self-injurious behavior in three classrooms by facial screening. *American Journal of Mental Deficiency, 85,* 510–513.

Matson, J. L., & Barrett, R. P. (Eds.). (1982). *Psychopathology in the mentally retarded*. New York: Grune & Stratton.

McGonigle, J. J., Duncan, D. V., Cordisco, L., & Barrett, R. P. (1982). Visual screening: An alternative method for reducing stereotyped behavior. *Journal of Applied Behavior Analysis, 15*, 461–468.

Menolascino, F. J. (1965). Emotional disturbance and mental retardation. *American Journal of Mental Deficiency, 70*, 248–256.

Menolascino, F. J., & McCann, B. M. (Eds.). (1983). *Mental health and mental retardation: Bridging the gap*. Baltimore: University Park Press.

National Institutes of Health. (1989). Treatment of destructive behaviors in persons with developmental disabilities. *National Institutes of Health Consensus Development Conference Statement, 7*, 1–14.

Nelson, R. O., & Hayes, S. (1979). Some current dimensions of behavioral assessment. *Behavioral Assessment, 1*, 1–16.

Poznanski, E. O., Cook, S. C., & Carroll, B. J. (1979). A depression rating scale for children. *Pediatrics, 64*, 442–450.

Reiss, S. (1990). Prevalence of dual diagnosis in community-based day programs in the Chicago metropolitan area. *American Journal of Mental Retardation, 94*, 578–585.

Rincover, A. (1978). Sensory extinction: A procedure for eliminating self-stimulatory behavior in developmentally disabled children. *Journal of Abnormal Child Psychology, 6*, 299–310.

Rincover, A., & Devany, J. (1982). The application of sensory extinction procedures to self-injury. *Analysis and Intervention in Developmental Disabilities, 2*, 67–81.

Rincover, A., Cook, R., Peoples, A., & Packard, D. (1979). Sensory extinction and sensory reinforcement principles for programming multiple adaptive behavior change. *Journal of Applied Behavior Analysis, 12*, 221–233.

Rincover, A., Newsome, C. D., & Carr, E. G. (1979). Using sensory extinction procedures in the treatment of compulsivelike behavior of developmentally disabled children. *Journal of Consulting and Clinical Psychology, 47*, 695–701.

Rivinus, T. M., Grofer, L. M., Feinstein, C., & Barrett, R. P. (1989). Psychopharmacology in the mentally retarded individual: New approaches, new directions. *Journal of the Multihandicapped Person, 2*, 1–23.

Rockland, L. H. (1989). *Supportive psychotherapy: A psychodynamic approach*. New York: Basic Books.

Rojahn, J., & Schroeder, S. R. (1983). Behavioral assessment. In J. L. Matson & J. A. Mulick (Eds.), *Handbook of mental retardation* (pp. 227–243). New York: Pergamon Press.

Russell, A. T., & Tanguay, P. E. (1981). Mental illness and mental retardation: Cause or coincidence? *American Journal of Mental Deficiency, 85*, 570–574.

Russo, D. C. (1990). A requiem for the passing of the three-term contingency. *Behavior Therapy, 21*, 153–165.

Rutter, M. (1977). Brain damage syndrome in children: Concepts and findings. *Journal of Child Psychology and Psychiatry, 18*, 1–22.

Rutter, M., Graham, P., & Yule, W. (1970). *A neuropsychiatric study of childhood*. London: Heinemann.

Sigman, M. (Ed.). (1985). *Children with dual diagnosis: Mental retardation and mental illness*. Orlando: Grune & Stratton.

Singh, N. N. (1980). The effects of facial screening on infant self injury. *Journal of Behavior Therapy and Experimental Psychiatry, 11*, 131–134.

Singh, N. N., Beale, I. L., & Dawson, M. J. (1981). Duration of facial screening and suppression of self-injurious behavior: Analysis using an alternating treatments design. *Behavioral Assessment, 3,* 411–420.

Skinner, B. F. (1938). *The behavior of organisms.* New York: Appleton-Century-Crofts.

Spitalnik, R., & Drabman, R. (1976). A classroom time-out procedure for retarded children. *Journal of Behavior Therapy and Experimental Psychiatry, 7,* 17–21.

Szymanski, L. S., & Tanguay, P. (Eds.). (1980). *Emotional disorders of mentally retarded persons.* Baltimore: University Park Press.

Tolsdorf, C. C. (1976). Social networks, support, and coping: An exploratory study. *Family Process, 15*(4), 407–417.

Tylenda, B., Hooper, S. R., & Barrett, R. P. (1987). Developmental learning disorders. In C. L. Frame & J. L. Matson (Eds.), *Handbook of assessment in childhood psychopathology: Applied issues in differential diagnosis and treatment evaluation* (pp. 187–217). New York: Plenum Press.

Walters, A. S., Barrett, R. P., & Feinstein, C. (1990). Social relatedness and autism: Current research, issues, directions. *Research in Developmental Disabilities, 11,* 303–326.

Williams, J. L., Schroeder, S. R., Eckerman, D. A., & Rojahn, J. (1983). Time-out from positive reinforcement with mentally retarded persons: An ecological review and analysis. In S. E. Breuning, J. L. Matson, & R. P. Barrett (Eds.), *Advances in mental retardation and developmental disabilities* (Volume 1, pp. 199–236). Greenwich, CT: JAI Press.

Zegiob, L. E., Jenkins, J., Becker, J., & Bristow, A. (1976). Facial screening: Effects on appropriate and inappropriate behaviors. *Journal of Behavior Therapy and Experimental Psychiatry, 7,* 355–357.

Zegiob, L. E., Alford, G. S., & House, A. (1978). Response suppression and generalization effects of facial screening in multiple self-injurious behavior in a retarded boy. *Behavior Therapy, 9,* 688.

Zigler, E., & Burack, J. A. (1989). Personality development and the dually diagnosed person. *Research in Developmental Disabilities, 10,* 225–240.

6

Inpatient Behavior Therapy with Autistic Youth

STEPHEN C. LUCE AND WALTER P. CHRISTIAN

INTRODUCTION

In comparison to other disabilities, autism is a very rare life-long disability that is typically observed prior to a child's third birthday. Afflicting only about one in 3,000 live births, this disorder has received a level of scrutiny and interest that far exceeds its prevalence. One might conclude from such a high level of attention that there would be a well-established approach to questions on etiology, assessment, and treatment. Unfortunately, little agreement exists on any of these issues. Unlike some of the other developmental disabilities, the cause of autism is unknown, its characteristics are similar to those of other diagnostic categories (e.g., mental retardation, schizophrenia), and its troubling behaviors have been shown to be largely unresponsive to traditional medical interventions and psychotherapeutic approaches.

DIAGNOSIS

Kanner (1943) first described the syndrome based on his analysis of 11 case studies that he had compiled largely from his clinic at the Johns

STEPHEN C. LUCE AND WALTER P. CHRISTIAN • The May Institute, Inc., 100 Sea View Street, Chatham, Massachusetts 02633.

Inpatient Behavior Therapy for Children and Adolescents, edited by Vincent B. Van Hasselt and David J. Kolko. Plenum Press, New York, 1992.

Hopkins University. He differentiated the autistic patients along three general categories: (1) disturbances in interpersonal relationships, (2) disturbances in the development of language, and (3) an insistence in sameness. Over the years, the diagnosis has become more general and less precise (Newsom & Rincover, 1981) to the point that many who are now receiving the diagnosis are patients that Kanner had not intended for this category. Indeed, the diagnostician has been forced to interpret the descriptions of the syndrome from the literature, and, to a great extent, there has been little agreement between them.

Recently, the American Psychiatric Association (1987) has inserted the term *Autistic Disorder* under the rubric of Pervasive Developmental Disorder. Characteristics of the disorder include impairment of social interaction, lack of verbal skills, and a restriction of interests. To validate the diagnosis, the individual must exhibit at least half of the 16 specific descriptors across the general areas. Although most previous diagnostic criteria required an early age of onset, the current manual now simply specifies infant versus childhood onset in the same category, thereby including under the same diagnosis persons who were previously distinguished from the autistic classification.

When we discuss the therapeutic approach to autistic youth, it becomes evident that, unlike most medical diagnoses, those descriptions used with individuals exhibiting autistic behaviors require highly individualized treatment without a great deal of regard to psychiatric diagnosis. This is due in part to the fact that while some researchers have tried to distinguish autism as a distinct disease entity (Rutter, 1978), it is increasingly obvious that it is a description of a syndrome consisting of a myriad of behavioral deficits and excesses (Koegel & Schreibman, 1982).

For the practitioner, the most practical description of autism contains functional behavioral characteristics. Lovaas, Ackerman, and Taubman (1983) provided just such a description: (1) six behavioral deficits, (2) two behavioral excesses, and (3) several behaviors that develop normally or approximate those exhibited by age-matched peers.

Behavioral Deficits

Presented roughly in their order of appearance in normal children, several deficiencies develop in autistic children or are lost soon after development. Behaviors characteristic of receptive sensory deficits (including abnormal responses to painful, auditory, or visual stimuli) are first to appear. Unlike in normal peers, eye contact and orientation toward parents does not develop in autistic children. Second, general emotional attachment to other persons in their environment does not develop. For example, when held, an autistic child does not mold to the body of the caretaker and often resists physical contact altogether. Further, if language develops (many autistic children remain mute), it is usually characterized by out-of-context, meaningless, or repetitive statements, such as in echolalia. In addition, toy play is usually severely delayed and infrequently practiced, and peer interactions are very infrequent. Finally, it is common for autistic children to develop very few of the self-care and social skills that their age-matched peers acquire with very little help from others.

Behavioral Excesses

Autistic children tend to exhibit two classes of behaviors in frequencies and/or with intensities that are abnormally high. One class of these behavioral excesses includes tantrums that can be quite severe and difficult to attribute to any antecedent. Aggressive behavior (toward self or others) is prevalent in some autistic persons. Self-injurious behaviors, in particular, appear to be related to the language and communication deficits described above (Carr & Durand, 1985).

The other class of behavioral excesses includes repetitive, stereotypic responses, such as rocking, spinning objects, and compulsively organizing objects in a ritualistic way. These self-stimulatory behaviors are often controlled by sensory events inherent in the activity (Rincover, 1982). For example, a ritualistic behavior, such as continuously flipping the pages of a telephone book, may be maintained by the sound of the pages, the way the pages look while being manipulated, or the tactual stimulation the autistic person receives.

Normally Developing Behaviors

Many of the behaviors exhibited by autistic persons develop quite normally or require skills that are particularly well developed in comparison to their overall level of functioning. These behaviors serve as an aid to the diagnostician to differentiate the autistic person from the mentally retarded. Those designated as mentally retarded tend to acquire skills more uniformly behind schedule. For example, motor skills are often age-appropriate in autistic individuals who are far behind in most other areas developmentally. In addition, the person exhibiting autism often has a very good memory, sometimes exceeding the expectations of people who are familiar with them. Some autistic persons may recite long conversations or repeat commercials heard, several days earlier, on television despite the fact that they may have little or no other useful language. In others, very strong technical interests may develop (e.g., a fascination with mechanical objects may promote skills that are surprisingly complex). If these splinter skills are particularly well established, as in the calculation of four-digit multiplication problems without the aid of paper or pencil, they are referred to as "autistic savant" (Rimland, 1984). Finally, some autistic clients exhibit idiosyncratic fears or pleasures that are inconsistent with their pervasive aloofness of the environment but are sometimes seen in the development of normal children.

ETIOLOGY

There have been two prominent etiological theories of autism that have proffered since initial recognition of the diagnosis in the 1940s. The *psychogenic hypothesis* relates autism to internal disturbances that come about as a result of environmental factors. Many researchers who promote this explanation have targeted parental mental health as a cause of the syndrome. Bettelheim (1967) has been cited as a major proponent of this theory which may have been derived from some of Kanner's early portrayals of the parents of autistic children as cold or "refrigerator types." Currently, this is not a widely supported theory.

Ferster (1961) supported a social environmental viewpoint to explain the development of autistic behaviors. Based on reinforcement theory, he believed that many of the responses that distinguish autistic persons are also exhibited by normal children and are remarkable only in their rate or frequency. He believed that the abnormal rate of the autistic behaviors was due to inadvertent reinforcing consequences in the social environment.

The theory adhered to by most investigators in the area is referred to as the *biogenic theory* of causation. This theory attributes autism to physical disorders of the brain or central nervous system. Support for this theory is derived from the fact that (1) autism is first seen quite early in a child's development; (2) most autistic people have normal siblings; (3) many of the characteristics of the syndrome (e.g., disturbed developmental rates, dysfunctional responses to stimuli, poor language development) are indicative of neurological dysfunction.

Despite the wide acceptance of the biogenic theory, specific causes of the physical disorder need to be identified before any definitive conclusion concerning etiology can be drawn. At this point, correlational data (Coleman, 1976) suggest many diverse potential causes for the behaviors evident in autism as well as several subgroups of the syndrome (e.g., individuals exposed to toxic substances neonatally, birth trauma, and family histories of dysfunctional traits).

Parents of Autistic Youth

Any program addressing the needs of autistic youth must include their families. Lovaas, Koegel, Simmons, and Long (1973) compared two groups of children for whom intensive treatment resulted in significant gains. One group of parents was also trained in the use of therapeutic techniques and one was not. Results showed that the experimental group developed many new skills and maintained improvement over the year; the control group exhibited poor skill maintenance. Other investigations also have demonstrated that parents of autistic youth can become extremely effective behavior change agents for their children (e.g., Anderson, Avery, DiPietro, Edwards, & Christian, 1987; Koegel, Schreibman, Britten, Burke, & O'Neill, 1982).

Parents of autistic children have been studied closely for many years. Most research has been an attempt to ascertain a cause for the syndrome. Early studies (Eisenberg, 1968; Kanner, 1943; Polan & Spencer, 1959) suggested that parents with autistic children were dissimilar from parents of normal children; however, more recent efforts have found fewer differences. Further, these disparities have proved irrelevant to the selection of a therapeutic approach.

Behavioral interventions must be individually tailored to the unique and diverse needs of each individual family. Since the requisite skills are rather complex and specialized, some parents will acquire them faster than others. In many cases, additional support will be needed to train parents to accommodate cultural or language differences between the therapist and themselves.

For the behavior therapist working with youth in an inpatient facility, parent training is also complicated by geographic obstacles. The incidence of autism is low; the incidence of the level of autism that warrants residential services is so low that families are likely to span hundreds of miles. Czyzewski, Christian, and Norris (1984) described an outreach parent-training model that has demonstrated its effectiveness and that addresses the problems associated with long distance (e.g., infrequently having the autistic youth at home, and difficulty arranging home visits).

Anderson and Schwartz (1986) compiled and reviewed several topics and skills that appear to be essential for maintenance of parent's skills. Essentially, they suggested that parents should have a working knowledge of (1) arranging a training environment, (2) providing effective antecedents and consequences, (3) shaping, (4) chaining, (5) prompt fading, and (6) behavior reduction strategies, such as differential reinforcement of other behaviors and acceptable aversive techniques (e.g., response cost, overcorrection). (For a more extensive review, see Koegel, Rincover, & Egel, 1982.)

Parents of autistic youth should be taught fundamental techniques that enable them to generalize their skills to future problems and issues after current difficulties have been ameliorated. Since basic techniques are first tested on specific current problems, the therapist must avoid the temptation of training only those skills that are useful for training at the child's current level of functioning. Baker and Brightman (1989) provided an excellent curriculum for parents that anticipates long-term training needs of special children.

As mentioned earlier, some inpatient admissions are precipitated by family or parent shortcomings. If, for example, inpatient care is based on the loss of a parent or to protect a youth from a parent who cannot provide proper care, it may be necessary to develop alternative family resources. One such alternative involves the careful selection and training of foster parents. These individuals can serve as interim or temporary parents with whom a child can acquire and demonstrate skills needed for community adjustment. In other cases, such support may be arranged for the long-term care of the child.

Characteristics of Autistic Youth in Need of Inpatient Services

Although we have already described the general characteristics of the autistic syndrome, it is important to note that the behaviors of those who are served in residential or inpatient facilities have an impact on the kind of services provided. As was evident from the description and diagnosis sections above, each autistic youth displays unique behaviors and traits that make it difficult to describe the entire group of persons falling within the syndrome. As a result, it is sometimes useful to speak in terms of the "degree of autism," or, more accurately, the number of autistic behaviors exhibited and the degree to which the person exhibits them (Christian, 1984).

Inpatient treatment of autistic youth has recently been reserved for those displaying the most severe behaviors. This is a result of legislation designed to minimize the dependence that has historically been placed on large centralized residential facilities which have provided insufficient care (Lakin, Bruininks, & Sigford, 1981). Consequently, clients placed in residential facilities for inpatient care are more likely to exhibit characteristics that are intolerable in the community. They are also more likely to have complications within their families that may or may not be related to the autistic behaviors. Specifically, clients in residential care may have more severe behavioral deficits and excesses. In addition, it is becoming increasingly apparent that the autistic client found in residential care will function at a level where savant skills are usually absent. In addition, those behaviors that develop normally are often hard to recognize because of the deficits. Inpatient autistic clients, therefore, are more likely to be from the "more severe" (Coleman, 1976) or the "lower" (DeMyer, 1979) subgroups of autistic persons. Since disruptions in the family configuration (e.g., loss or incompetence of one or more parents) sometimes necessitate inpatient placement, family problems are more likely to be present in the residential client.

In her study of autistic children and their families, DeMyer (1979) found that many parents sought residential care as their child became stronger and more difficult to manage. Fifty-eight percent of the autistic children she studied with a mean age of 15 years were in residential care. It has been suggested that as many as 75% of those clients with a diagnosis of autism are placed in full residential care; of the remaining 25%, extensive community support is necessary and often includes short-term inpatient placement.

THE ROLE OF INPATIENT TREATMENT WITH AUTISTIC YOUTH

Legal mandates (e.g., *Halderman v. Pennhurst*, 1977; *Wyatt v. Stickney*, 1972) and legislation (e.g., Rehabilitation, Comprehensive Services, and Developmental Disabilities Amendments of 1978, Public Law 95–602) have served as catalysts in improving the care of autistic youth. However, the need for inpatient options is still apparent. Some advocacy organizations (e.g., the Association for the Severely Handicapped, 1980) have suggested that all segregated facilities should be abolished. Such a move would include most inpatient services. Despite these vigorous and well-intentioned efforts, it would appear that we are far from abolishing inpatient treatment for autistic youth (DeMyer, 1979).

The traditional practice of routinely placing autistic youth in residential settings clearly was unnecessary. It is also true that many inpatient facilities provide insufficient care and little or no functional training to autistic youth. It is a mistake, however, to conclude that all inpatient care is inappropriate. Unfortunately, some patients, especially the chronic severely disabled, have not been adequately prepared for less restrictive settings. In other cases, no alternatives may exist as in the case of the autistic youth who has no family resources and is too severe for the available community programs. Historically, much of our knowledge concerning the treatment of autistic youth has been garnered from investigations conducted in residential facilities (Luce, 1979). Recently, researchers have begun to study facets of inpatient care that have been distressing and are trying to determine how long-term, wide-scale change can be achieved (Christian, 1984; Coughlin *et al.*, 1984).

In light of the obvious need for residential care combined with recent research demonstrating its efficacy with autistic youth, several investigators have recommended that inpatient treatment be included in a continuum of service options for autistic youth. When inpatient facilities are backed-up by less restrictive options, and the care of the youth in the inpatient component of the agency is geared toward the *transition* of youth through the continuum to less restrictive settings, the advantages of residential care are maximized.

Bird (1984) noted that some mental health professionals have focused primarily on the physical arrangements of the service setting. Specifically, a group home in the community would normally be considered less restrictive than a psychiatric hospital. Unfortunately, such a designation does not consider the ongoing programming in the setting. Many group homes are less therapeutic and more restrictive than larger settings. Consideration of a service continuum, therefore, must account for many factors beyond "bricks and mortar" (Christian & Hannah, 1983).

To be a functional component of a continuum of services, inpatient care must be *transitional*. That is, the objectives sought while in the relatively restrictive settings must be based on those skills needed to survive in the less restrictive settings (Luce, Anderson, Thibadeau, & Lipsker, 1984). Those objectives containing skills that are attained prior to the time of transition are referred to as *transitional priorities*. It is around these priorities that an inpatient program must revolve. Unfortunately, most transitional priorities include training systems that are very difficult to establish. For example, on occasions when a child is not able to stay in a community placement, the behaviors that resulted in unsuccessful placement were not being addressed.

Ideally, problem behaviors that place a client at risk for a more restrictive placement would be targeted at the less restrictive level (i.e., in the community) making admission as an inpatient unnecessary. The reason why certain problems (e.g., disruptions occurring at night) might not be addressed in the community are numerous (e.g., they are relatively rare; it is unusual to find public school personnel who are knowledgeable about remedial procedures). Unfortunately, once the client is placed in residential care, these same problem behaviors continue to be neglected. In fact, staff working in the classrooms of most residential programs have attained a higher level of training, are better paid, are better staffed, and are expected to design a more therapeutic program than residence personnel working afternoons, weekends, or at night. In an examination of factors in inpatient placement, Anderson, Luce, Newsom, Gruber, and Kennedy-Butler (1983) found that transitional priorities of a group of residentially placed autistic youth consisted of behaviors that are often overlooked (e.g., independent play) and did not involve areas that are usually emphasized in residential programs (e.g., academic and vocational skills). It was evident that despite significant deficits in academic and vocational skills, transition to the next less restrictive option was contingent on frequently neglected behavioral deficits and excesses.

BEHAVIORAL ASSESSMENT

The purpose of behavioral assessment in an inpatient setting is to determine what needs to occur before the patient can return to the community. Autistic youth exhibit numerous abnormal behavioral characteristics; therefore, selection of responses relevant to transition (*transitional priorities*) is sometimes difficult. It is important to realize that not all abnormal behaviors are transitional priorities. In some cases, the natural environment might require modification to accommodate a returning youth.

As a rule, applied psychologists have cautioned clinicians about the use of traditional standardized intelligence and aptitude assessment instruments with autistic youth (Newsom & Rincover, 1981). Since they do not discriminate abnormalities that are relevant from those that are irrelevant to transition, they are not particularly useful in decisions concerning transitional programming.

Ideally, effective assessment assists the clinician in selecting transitional priorities. Brown *et al.* (1979) stressed the importance of pursuing relevant goals with the severely handicapped. At the time, it was common for curricula geared toward the disabled to include activities designed to train behaviors that would be of minimal value to clients in the future. A clinician attuned to a client's subsequent needs would probably teach color discrimination with items of clothing (e.g., matching socks) rather than objects with little function (e.g., inch cubes). Clients would also improve balance with a bicycle or by walking to stores and restaurants, rather than by walking a balance beam in a school gymnasium. By directly teaching the functional skills, there is a greater likelihood that the skill actually needed for adequate community functioning would be mastered. In addition, there is no evidence to suggest that functional skills, such as riding a bicycle (for some disabled individuals the only means of transportation available), are improved or are more easily mastered by autistic youth after learning a nonfunctional skill such as balancing on the beam (Donnellan, 1980).

Brown *et al.* (1979) stressed the notion of the "criterion of ultimate functioning" in their effort to reduce the number of wasted teaching hours created by the pursuit of skills that are not useful to the student in the future. The inpatient clinicians are at a distinct disadvantage since they are treating clients in an artificial environment. We have discussed how, in such settings, there may be a tendency that clinicians will develop inappropriate skills; it may also be more difficult to determine transitional priorities in such artificial environments. There are several sources of information from which the clinician must ascertain transitional priorities. These include (1) the findings of previous research in the area, (2) the former environment, (3) the future environment, and (4) the direct observation of the client.

Before reviewing these sources, it is important to note that the priorities developed for each client are different. Two similar clients may have very disparate transitional priorities. These differences may be based on the overall level of functioning of the client. More often, however, they relate to the characteristics of the client's future environment. For example, a client placed in an urban setting may require different skills (e.g., using public transportation) than a similar client who will eventually reside in a rural setting.

Previous Findings

Several correlational studies provide pertinent information regarding transitional priorities. Although the level of experimental rigor prohibits a functional analysis of the factors, numerous skills and deficits appear to be instrumental in community adjustment or dysfunction. The methodology most often employed has been to survey large numbers of clients who were successfully (e.g., Edgerton & Bercovici, 1976) or unsuccessfully (e.g., Eagle, 1967; Eyman & Call, 1977; Sternlicht,

1978) transitioned to the community. Most clients surveyed were adults who resided in large centralized institutional settings prior to deinstitutionalization.

Since autistic youth exhibit some of the behaviors exhibited by that population, results of these studies may be generalizable to them. Specifically, it would appear that health concerns, particularly those that require assistance from a nondisabled person, significantly limit community options. If, for example, a community transition is dependent upon the use of a medication (e.g., for seizure control or health maintenance), the future site would probably have to include some supervision, thereby restricting community placement to a supervised apartment or specialized foster home. In addition to the medical needs of the client, previous research suggests that some dysfunctional behaviors limit transitional options more than others. For example, sexually aberrant and self-abusive behaviors can severely limit placement options in the community; however, some withdrawal responses or mildly unacceptable vocal habits restrict transition to only the least restrictive options, such as independent living (Hannah & Christian, 1984).

An Assessment of the Previous Environment

When a referral is made for inpatient care, a transitional clinician must determine the specific problems that led to the referral. In many cases, as with most child referrals, the past environment is identical to the future environment (i.e., the child is with his or her parents while enrolled in a local school). Therefore, in the process of identifying factors that led to inpatient referral, the transitional priorities needed for the future environment become apparent. In some instances, referrals are made because of factors that are irreversible or unrelated to the development or behavioral status of the client. For example, as parents become older, their ability to care for an autistic child becomes more limited. An inpatient referral may be initiated at that point despite the fact that the client's progress may have been adequate. Catastrophic events, such as the death or serious illness of a parent or guardian, may result in an inpatient referral in which transitional priorities are designed to develop skills needed in an alternative community setting.

All factors related to the causes for the referral must be determined and analyzed. Parents, guardians, or other care providers managing the child at the time of the referral must be thoroughly questioned. Using this procedure, the referring agents (parents, school, and mental health professionals) are immediately made aware of the fact that inpatient care is a temporary placement geared toward transition to less restrictive living arrangements. This is an important step since many people seeking residential care are interested in a long-term or indefinite inpatient placement. If the previous caretakers are to have a role in the future, they must be prepared to play an active role in the treatment of the youth and his or her transition. Some caretakers who are pursuing long-term inpatient care for autistic youth are unaware of the fact that autistic youth need not be permanently taken out of the community.

The data gathered from the survey of the former environment should include: (1) demographic information; (2) a developmental and medical history; (3) an assessment of current skills; (4) a review of all ongoing behavioral, educational, and medical treatment; (5) the client's family characteristics; (6) the level of social service support; and (7) a brief survey of community services available. An individualized assessment should also survey behavioral characteristics that are most influential in the decision to place the youth residentially (Anderson & Schwartz, 1986).

Future Environment Survey

As discussed above, the past and future environments may be similar. In most cases, they overlap. For example, since most inpatient youth transitioned to the community return to their homes, many of the community resources assessed in the survey of the past environment are also relevant to the future environment. Clinicians should be aware, however, that if inpatient care is to exceed one year, resource changes might occur. Some changes in community programs may be due to the age of the youth at discharge; such as in the case of the young adult who exceeds school age. Other changes may be related to differences in the funding or in the personnel in local mental health and educational agencies. Unfortunately, with the budget constraints confronting most of the social services in the community, the development of community services may not be favorable.

The future environment survey must reveal the skill level required for a child to function in the less restrictive site. If the anticipated future environment is serving autistic or similarly disabled youth at the time the survey is conducted, the future environment information can be gathered by observing the youth currently succeeding in that program. A visit to a classroom, home, or workshop already serving autistic youth can illuminate important training issues for the clinician who is preparing another youth to enter the same setting. Because issues related to client confidentiality prevent the future environment surveyor from fully assessing clients in prospective sites, on-site observations do provide a wealth of information.

Often the designated future environment of an autistic youth does not exist at the time of a referral or does not currently serve similar youths. In these situations, a qualified informant is needed to assess the future environment. It is possible to assess similar environments (e.g., foster homes) to an approximate estimate of the skills that a client may need to be placed. Scenarios of this kind make future environment assessment more difficult. Yet they create an opportunity for the clinician to shape the environment to improve the successful transition of the youth.

A number of standardized behavior checklists are available for the assessment of the future environment (e.g., Hannah & Christian, 1984; Nihira, Foster, Shelhaas, & Leland, 1974; Westaway & Apolloni, 1978). Clients who are currently succeeding in the future environment can be rated or an authority in the future environment (e.g., the manager of the agency developing a group home; a foster parent) can serve as an informant. A profile derived in the future site and that of the client can be compared to determine discrepancies. Those profile items of the target client that fall significantly short of, or are more severe than, well-adapted clients should be considered for the list of transitional priorities.

Direct Observation

Direct observational methods are also useful in evaluating the transitional needs of a client. Some therapists may rely almost entirely on direct observation. However, without the perspective of the prior and future environments, the actual behaviors exhibited by the youth may not be so revealing. Some behaviors may be exhibited more or less frequently in the assessment context than in other settings. For example, in a structured environment with a high frequency of demands, an autistic youth may emit more disruptive behaviors than would be evident in the community if those settings were more relaxed. There are also fluctuations in rates of responding in the early stages of inpatient placement until clients become oriented. Therefore, stable rates of behaviors, which are derived prior to and after inpatient placement, should first be established before change strategies can be implemented. To the extent that informant measures are obtained, care should be taken to assure measurement reliability. This can best be accomplished by soliciting evaluations from two informants independently (e.g., teacher and a parent).

Specifying Transitional Priorities

Once the assessment phase has been conducted, the dissemination of specific transitional priorities and their corresponding goal levels must be set. The transitional priorities must be specified to include the exact behavioral deficits and/or excesses and the terminal level needed for transition into the next environment. For example, a terminal objective for a transitional priority on aggresssion may be as follows: John (the *client*) will exhibit less than five responses per day (the *terminal rate*) of hitting, kicking, biting, or scratching where each individual event is counted (the *defined behavior*), for 60 consecutive days (the *maintenance criterion*) in all settings (the *generalization criterion*). Another example for a behavioral deficit may specify that Ralph will exhibit at least 90% of the steps of a 12-step showering chain with only verbal prompts for 30 consecutive days both in the group home and while at his parents home on weekends. The second showering objective would indicate that in the next environment, Ralph would be able to be supervised to a certain extent during self-care routines, such as showering. Perhaps he is going to a group home or his parents are able to continue training him toward greater independence (e.g., without any prompts).

Virtually everyone in contact with the client should have access to the transitional priorities. Clearly, all prospective caretakers in the residential and future environment should be aware of the levels of behavior to be attained in residential care. Parents and family members must also be familiar with the objectives to understand the prospective levels of behavior to be attained when their child comes home. In the continual pursuit of the transitional priorities, the inpatient staff members assure that time is spent in functional activities.

As the transitional priorities are developed for a group of inpatient autistic youths, it will become immediately apparent that the primary training arena for some skills is not a classroom setting during day hours. Some children randomly exhibit dysfunctional behavioral excesses (e.g., wandering) throughout the day; however, such problems become more serious at different periods (e.g., at night while parents are asleep). Others exhibit skill deficits (e.g., a lack of self-care skills) that are primarily exhibited and most efficiently taught in home settings (Reid, 1983).

PREPARING THE INPATIENT FACILITY

It is apparent that the kind of inpatient care being described here differs greatly from that commonly found 20 years ago when most autistic youth, regardless of functioning level, had no other options. The recommended assessment techniques are significantly different from those conventionally employed. It should come as no surprise, therefore, that there are several other aspects of the inpatient facility that must be engineered before full transitional programming can be implemented.

Behavioral practitioners have successfully established transitional programming in a variety of settings (e.g., Anderson *et al.*, 1987; Christian, 1984; Christian & Zampini, 1988; Phillips, Fixen, Phillips, & Wolf, 1979). These investigators have documented the steps they employed to reorganize or develop progressive services. Further, they have demonstrated that it is possible to make significant and comprehensive changes in a variety of human service agencies. The empirical evidence suggests that wide-scale changes can be implemented regardless of the condition of the agency prior to reorganization. Additional work is necessary in order to fully evaluate the essential components of institutional change (Reid & Whitman, 1983). However, enough is currently known to allow behavior therapists to proceed in the interest of providing improved services for disabled clients.

Preparing the Staff

Inpatient care is provided by the staff members who are in greatest contact with the clients. These direct-care staff play a vital role in the process of returning the autistic youth to less restrictive settings. Since the procedures employed by direct-care staff must be carried out with precision, adequate preparation and training are essential. The first step in preparing the staff is to understand that the terminal behavior of a proficient direct-care staff member in a behavioral setting is the product of a complete *orientation* and a form of *training* that is comprehensive and thorough. The two processes are distinct.

During orientation, therapists acquire a working knowledge of the basics of their jobs. It is usually conducted in a didactic format in which the staff members are acquainted with their position and the roles of others on the team. The orientation process is similar to the kind of inservice or workshops often conducted in human service settings. Although therapeutic techniques are discussed, they usually are not practiced. On occasions when they are, role-playing or other mechanisms are used to artificially create a situation in which a technique can be rehearsed.

Results obtained from an orientation process of this kind are usually confined to verbal performance. For example, when pre- and posttests are administered to orientation participants, their answers to questions about reinforcement techniques and to whom they should go for support on certain matters (e.g., for a question about their paycheck) should improve. Dyer, Schwartz, and Luce (1984), however, found that despite the fact that staff members could answer questions correctly about the advantages of functional materials, functional tasks, and age-appropriate activities, the actual tasks they were presenting to autistic children did not change until specific feedback was delivered to staff members in their work sites.

Unfortunately, many regulatory agencies use "the number of inservice orientation sessions held" as documentation of training. Occasionally, participants are required to pass an exam containing questions about the content of the workshop. Such an approach may have little or no relationship to on-the-job performance.

Orientation is essential but insufficient for comprehensive training. Training leads to performance changes that can be observed on the job while a therapist is working with the clients. The form of training we recommend (Larsson, Luce, & Christian, 1989) was derived from several studies in which staff members exhibited improved job performance only after receiving specific feedback. For example, Dyer *et al.* (1984) improved the quality of the tasks that children were presented in residential settings by providing staff with specific feedback explaining how their planned activity check or *pla-check* (Doke & Risley, 1972) scores could have been perfect. Egan, Luce, and Hall (1988) improved the record keeping of direct-care staff by providing them with written instructions on how their data books could have met several preset criteria. Both of these investigations and several others (e.g., Avery, Thibadeau, & Luce, 1984; Leidholt, Lipsker, Luce, & Christian, 1981) have demonstrated that if specific directives (i.e., feedback) are provided to direct-care staff while they are performing a task (or shortly after the completion of a task), performance can be significantly improved to exceed previous levels.

In response to these findings, we recommend the use of task-analyzed checklists that were developed for use in a preschool setting by Herbert-Jackson, O'Brien, Porterfield, and Risley (1977) and in a large institutional setting by Lattimore, Jones, and Calvert (1978). Recently, such a system has been implemented agency-wide in several residential and day treatment centers serving autistic youth and other individuals who exhibit severe developmental disabilities (Larsson *et al.*, 1989). Briefly, the task-analyzed training involves presenting a staff member with 7 to 24 checklists that outline the specific steps expected for mastery of the essential skills required for their job. Trainees are monitored in the performance of their jobs by working supervisors who previously mastered these skills and attained proficiency in a number of supervisory skills (e.g., giving feedback, organizing the environment). A trainee is provided feedback and is observed on all skills required for the job until mastery is attained. Once mastered, the level of feedback required to maintain this level is determined by periodic job performance evaluations.

Providing Adequate Supervision

The complexity of the task of preparing autistic youth for a return to the community is great enough to justify an employee-to-supervisor ratio of high density (3:1 to 8:1). Most direct-care personnel come to inpatient facilities inadequately prepared to carry out the tasks of their job; therefore, extensive training is usually required. In our experience, the rate of turnover among direct-care staff is relatively high, making it likely that in most work environments (e.g., home or classroom) there are staff members in training. The training system recommended above allows for this as well as the fact that supervisors are likely to be relatively new to the task of training and supervision. That is, the steps of a task are itemized to assure a clear description of job responsibilities and to ensure that no steps are missed by supervisors.

To improve supervision, we recommend *working* supervisors who also have direct-care responsibilities and work along with those they supervise. Typically, house managers of group homes have to work "day" hours (e.g., 9:00 A.M. to 5:00 P.M.) even when the staff they supervise are not on duty until the waning hours of their shift. Such a system is inappropriate and assures poor supervision.

Selection of supervisors should come from among the most proficient direct-care staff or from those who have already had successful supervisory experience in an identical agency. Since such supervisory experience is rare, the former criteria are usually employed. Unfortunately, some very skillful therapists are poor supervisors. Consequently, to the extent that supervisors are selected for their skills with clients, supervisor training will be more taxing and supervisor selection errors will be more likely. For that reason, selected supervisors will need to be put on probation until their skills are demonstrated in a manner that is identical to that used with their trainees. Specific supervisory skills must be task analyzed and taught via the checklist training system described above. Simply designating a supervisor from among a group of staff members will not necessarily improve performance even in cases where a supervisor is added to the staff, thereby improving the staff-to-client ratio (Leidholt *et al.*, 1981).

Maintenance of Client Rights

Many of the inpatient systems we recommend in this chapter serve to provide clients with the safest and most effective treatment available. A full description of legal safeguards relevant to inpatient care of autistic youth cannot be provided in this chapter; however, several comprehensive reviews are available (Martin, 1975; Timbers, Jones, & Davis, 1981; McClannahan & Krantz, 1981).

The autistic youth, usually represented by parents and/or another legal advocate (Luce *et al.*, 1984) must be afforded several client rights. Specifically, (1) they must be able to refuse unwanted interventions or ones they or their guardians are not aware of (*Kaimowitz v. Michigan Department of Mental Health*, 1973); (2) they must be treated in the least restrictive environment (*Dixon v. Weinberger*, 1975; *Lake v. Cameron*, 1966); (3) they must be exposed only to treatments that minimize harm to themselves (*New York State Association for Retarded Children, Inc. v. Carey*, 1975); and (4) they must be provided adequate care thaat is effective (*Donaldson v. O'Connor*, 1974; *Rouse v. Cameron*, 1966; *Wyatt v. Stickney*, 1972). Clearly, there can be disputes requiring "judgment calls" in the care of autistic youth. For example, in their efforts to provide efficacious treatment, some professionals have been accused of exposing clients to harm. Inpatient facilities must therefore establish a number of protective devices that are designed to protect clients and their families. Indeed, internal and external monitoring must be carried out. In addition to the internal systems described in this chapter, a human rights committee should be formed to assure that systems prescribed by law are followed. Systems must include informed consent and the development of individualized education or treatment plans (Education of All Handicapped Children Act, 1976). Local and national regulations are also designed to enforce the same and similar safeguards (e.g., Joint Commission on Accreditation of Hospitals, 1978) and must be addressed by inpatient facilities. Despite these rather extensive regulatory systems employed by most inpatient systems, violations of client rights (e.g., Bible & Snead, 1976) and regulatory system failures (Favell, Favell, & Risley, 1981) continue to occur.

Normalized Environments

The case for normalized environments has been made in the chapter and elsewhere (e.g., Wolfensberger, 1972). Many of the systems and routines presently described are designed to approximate those in the normal community. Some important obstacles found in human service systems cannot be eliminated by administrative reorganization or improved training and treatment practices (Wolfensberger, 1972). Architectural problems can create serious problems that can impede transition. Unnatural environments can make training impossible or create behaviors that do not generalize (Stokes & Baer, 1977). Autistic youth, noted for poor generalization (Koegel *et al.*, 1982), must be trained in environments that share common stimuli with their future environments (Welch & Pear, 1980).

IMPLEMENTING EFFECTIVE PROCEDURES

Strategies that have proven to be effective with autistic youth are more widely disseminated than those aspects of inpatient care that relate to service delivery. Perhaps because the earliest examples of applied behavior analysis were often conducted with autistic youth (e.g., Ferster, 1961; Lovaas, 1969; Risley & Wolf, 1967), most behavior analysts are familiar with the contingencies that have historically been successful with this population. In this chapter, we will briefly review only inpatient agency practices and program evaluation issues that are not as widely discussed elsewhere. Readers interested in a more complete description of useful, experimentally analyzed and peer-reviewed procedures with autistic youth should consult the several publications available for the novice practitioner (e.g., Carr, 1982; Favell & Greene, 1981; Koegel, 1982; Koegel & Schreibman, 1982; Lovaas, 1981; Luce & Christian, 1981; Mithaug, 1981; Rincover, 1982; Romanczyk & Lockshin, 1981) or trained behavior therapist (Lovaas, 1981; Koegel, Rincover & Egel, 1982; Sulzer-Azaroff & Mayer, 1977).

Events Preceding the Behavior

Several antecedent procedures can be used to promote desirable behaviors through environmental management or the careful use of prompts or cues. *Physical prompts* involving touching the child are useful in language development (Lovaas, 1969), but can be used to occasion a number of behaviors that are unlikely to occur without assistance. *Verbal prompts* and *cues* are usually considered less obtrusive and may be able to remain in effect in future environments (e.g., lines are drawn on home appliance dials to indicate the correct settings for a stove, a dryer, etc.). Despite the general tendency of autistic children to be inattentive to others, Egel, Richman, and Koegel (1981) demonstrated that these children successfully acquired discrimination performance through modeling (i.e., observing the reinforced responses of nonhandicapped peers). There is evidence that *task variation*, a process where antecedent stimuli are varied, represents an important manipulation that can improve performance (Dunlap & Egel, 1982). Usually, this entails working on several tasks simultaneously and alternating by trials. With varied or unvaried trials, shortening the interval between the consequence for one trial and the discriminate stimulus for the next one is most effective (Koegel, Dunlap, & Dyer, 1980).

Whenever antecedent manipulations are not easily maintaained in the future environment, *fading*, the process where the artificial antecedent event is changed to be identical to those found in the natural environment, must be used. Fading is particularly important with autistic youth who have a tendency toward overselectivity (i.e., responding to limited or obscure details in stimuli that are not reliably found elsewhere). Overselectivity, therefore, limits generalization (Lovaas, Litrownik, & Mann, 1971; Rincover & Koegel, 1975) and can create problems with antecedent and consequence procedures. If a task involves a series of behaviors (e.g., toothbrushing), *chaining* is sometimes used where the discriminative stimulus for one behavior (e.g., brushing teeth) is the completion of another (e.g., putting the toothpaste on the brush).

Recently, it has been suggested that an additional antecedent manipulation useful with autistic youth is to provide them with greater control over activities and outcomes (Dyer & Peck, 1987) or *choices*. For example, Koegel, Dyer, and Bell (1987) demonstrated a decrease in social avoidance and Peck (1985) reported an increase in social/communicative responses when child-preferred activities were employed.

Reinforcing Stimuli

Examples of reinforcement that was used with autistic youth are numerous in the behavioral literature. *Shaping*, for example, is useful for gradually changing a behavior so that it resembles one normally exhibited by a proficient person. Perhaps the clearest demonstrations of shaping (where successive approximations of a desired behavior are reinforced) are on film (Lovaas, 1969; 1981).

The choices of what food, privilege, or event to use as a reinforcer for autistic youth are diverse. It should be noted that an array of reinforcers is usually required, especially for ongoing inpatient work. Reinforcer variety is more powerful than a reliance on one reward (Egel, 1981). In addition, frequent *reinforcer assessment* has recently been shown to be an important tool for behavior therapists (Dyer, 1987). *Edibles* are valuable especially in the early stages of training, but they are prone to problems of satiation if they are relied on exclusively. Because of the reinforcing power of food, meals often become important therapeutic events in residential settings. It is important to note, however, that meals can be structured to be more therapeutic (Halle, Marshall, & Spradlin, 1979), although withholding of meals is forbidden (*Wyatt v. Stickney*, 1972). *Social reinforcers*, such as contingently using praise, affection, or other means of social contact, are very important and may be acquired by even the most withdrawn autistic child usually through pairing with other reinforcing events. Many community training sessions are reinforcing and can be used as a *privilege* to reinforce other behaviors (Blew, Schwartz, & Luce, 1985). In some cases, a privilege may be based on *sensory reinforcement* (Rincover, 1978). Often revealed through the observation and analysis of self-stimulatory behavior, this form of reinforcement can be a very effective reinforcer (Rotholz & Luce, 1983).

Suppressive Strategies

Many strategies can be used to suppress the behavioral excesses associated with autism. The most common approaches involve *differentially reinforcing other behaviors*. This may be accomplished by (1) reinforcing any behavior except the target behavior at the end of an interval (differential reinforcement of other behaviors—DRO); (2) reinforcing periods of time in which a specified rate of behaviors is exhibited (differential reinforcement of a low rate of behavior—DRL); or (3) reinforcing specific incompatible behaviors (differential reinforcement of incompatible behavior-DRI). The most encouraging novel application of differential reinforcement involves the uses of communicative responses used to suppress seriously disruptive, self-injurious, and aggressive behavior (Carr & Durand, 1985; Carr, Newsom, & Binkoff, 1980).

In those cases where the consequences maintaining a behavior can be interrupted, *extinction* can be used. Some of the earliest behavioral studies with autistic youth utilized extinction to successfully (Wolf, Risley, & Meese, 1964) or unsuccessfully (Corte, Wolf, & Locke, 1971; Lovaas & Simmons, 1969) reduce the rate of a dysfunctional behavior in autistic youth. Since many forms of self-stimulatory behavior are maintained by sensory reinforcers, the interruption of these stimuli (*sensory extinction*) is useful with autistic youth (Rincover, 1982).

Time-out involves removing the child from the environment that contains the reinforcers. In many cases, this can be accomplished by moving the child only a short distance away from an activity, such as with *contingent observation* (Porterfield, Herbert-Jackson, & Risley, 1976) or *activities time-out* (Luce & Christian, 1981). It is interesting to note that the most common form of time-out found in the literature employs the use of a small room with a closed door (Wolf *et al.*, 1964), a form of time-out that is unacceptable in many jurisdictions. Time-out failures often relate to the fact that autistic youth can engage in preferred activities, such as self-stimulatory behavior, during its administration and/or the fact that the environment from which they are removed is inadequately stimulating (Solnick, Rincover, & Peterson, 1977).

Most other reductive strategies utilize consequences that suppress the rates of the behaviors they follow. This is a class of procedures referred to as *punishers* or *aversive procedures* (Sulzer-Azaroff & Mayer, 1977). However, the term *aversive* is increasingly reserved for the subgroup of procedures that "are noxious, uncomfortable, or painful to an individual" (Lovaas & Favell, 1987, pg. 313). This lack of consistency in the behavioral literature is uncharacteristic and problematic, especially since it is often confusing to the practitioner in trying to decide to which procedures advocates are objecting. Essentially, while many of the painful and noxious procedures (e.g., electric shock) have been carefully analyzed, they are inaccessible to most practitioners, especially those working in residential treatment centers for autistic youth.

Other aversive procedures should be accessible to the inpatient clinician when careful safeguards are established. These should include *contingent effort* and social punishment or *verbal reprimands*. The former comprises a group of procedures that require some effort contingent upon a dysfunctional behavior when the result is a decrease of that behavior (Luce, Christian, Lipsker, & Hall, 1980). Of greatest utility to inpatient clinicians are the procedures that include correction, overcorrection, and positive practice (Foxx & Axrin, 1972); however, in some cases, forms of effort are used that are topographically unrelated to the inappropriate behavior or its appropriate counterpart. For example, brief contingent exercise easily prompted with voice prompts or pointing cues was used to reduce bizarre verbal and aggressive behavior in autistic and schizophrenic children (Luce, Delquadri, & Hall, 1980; Luce & Hall, 1981).

Verbal reprimands (Van Houten, 1980), sometimes called *social punishment* (Doleys, Wells, Hobbs, Roberts, & Cartelli, 1976), have been successfully applied with autistic youth. In its most acceptable form, the reprimand is sometimes referred to as a "negative feedback" which simply informs the youth that he or she has responded incorrectly. If properly implemented, the potentially reinforcing attention that results can be minimized, and the interaction can be carried out in a manner that is considered appropriate by onlookers (Van Houten, 1980).

EVALUATING BEHAVIORAL TREATMENT

The procedures described above are of little use to the individual client who is placed in an agency without a thorough system of program evaluation and behavior analysis. There are at least two levels of program evaluation needed in an inpatient facility. One level that evaluates the systems in place to ensure effective program implementation is of utmost importance to the behavioral clinician (Christian & Hannah, 1983). For example, Christian (1984) evaluated an inpatient program for autistic youth by analyzing 16 dependent variables using a variety of methods of measurement. Through the direct evaluation of documents, such as personnel records, financial reports, and client records, he obtained frequencies (e.g., number of staff employed), durations (e.g., the mean length of stay for clients discharged), and time samples (e.g., the number of clients receiving psychotropic medication on a given date) that reflected the condition of the agency.

Planned activity checks (Doke & Risley, 1972), described earlier in the section on behavioral assessment, are very useful indices of program implementation that can be taken as infrequently as 3 to 5 times per week (Dyer *et al.*, 1984) or several times per hour (Avery *et al.*, 1984). Normally, levels of engagement are tabulated (e.g., percentage of clients in a group home engaged in therapeutic activities).

On another level of program evaluation using similar methods of measurement, the focus is on the individual clients served in the facility. The most useful behavioral measure for this kind of evaluation consists of repeated measures or time series data (Campbell & Stanley, 1966). For every goal, there should be at least one program containing (1) a clearly defined behavior; (2) a baseline (preintervention) time series assessment of behavior; (3) a systematic intervention with a defined procedure or contingency designed to bring the behavior toward the desired levels; (4) a postintervention time series measure of the behavior; and (5) an assessment of response maintenance. Behavior therapists interested in contributing to the research literature or in utilizing restrictive procedures (Lovaas & Favell, 1987) will need to extend the program evaluation to replicate treatment effects using a design, such as a multiple baseline or reversal (Baer, Wolf, & Risley, 1968). The minimal format (an

AB design) is useful to document changes in behavior. And with an accumulation of several small group or single-subject AB programs, one obtains convincing evidence in support of a contention that the procedure introduced (and not an uncontrolled variable) is responsible for behavior change (Sidman, 1960). This method of procedural verification is useful in dissemination of information to other professionals, especially those who work with the client after discharge.

Measurement Reliability

Since most indices of client change are based on human observation, it is important to assess measurement reliability frequently. Usually, this is accomplished by having two observers assess the same behavior, while using identical methods, independently and simultaneously (Hall & Van Houten, 1983). To the extent that both observers record the same level of behavior, the measures are considered reliable. This method of measuring reliability, called *interobserver agreement,* should be conducted frequently with autistic youth. Even with precise definitions and clear and systematic intervention techniques, observer biases and drift can occur. Interobserver agreement checks are ideally conducted in about 30% of the sessions or observations recorded, but at least monthly. In cases where conditions frequently change (e.g., a program where a client advances through steps rapidly), at least two checks of interobserver agreement per phase are necessary (Luce, 1986).

Conducting Applied Research

Some behavior therapists may be surprised by the rigorous level of measurement and design recommended here (Luce, 1987). The inpatient clinician should never lose sight of the fact that his or her primary role in most facilities is service provision. Research dissemination is not a major emphasis for an agency serving autistic youth. Yet, many sound research practices must be employed when implementing behavioral programs. For example, the practice of obtaining reliable pre- and postintervention time series data on clients is essential to work effectively with autistic youth; this also approximates the research requirements needed for publication.

Lovaas and Favell (1987) recommend that in the treatment of very severe behavior problems (those potentially requiring aversive procedures), the clinician should carry out all the steps expected of the applied researcher. The purest and most unbiased form of peer review available to the behavioral clinician is that conducted by the editors of journals in their consideration of a manuscript for publication. Utilizing this process of safeguards, the behavioral inpatient clinician will be less likely to deviate from the mainstream view of acceptable practices.

SUMMARY

Autism represents one of the most mysterious and intriguing syndromes afflicting children. We have attempted to present the facts that are most pertinent to the delivery of effective inpatient services for autistic youth. With their general characteristics, it is understandable that historically, most autistic youth who were placed in residential settings have remained there for the rest of their lives. Indeed, the long-term, seemingly irreversible nature of inpatient care has led many advocacy groups to recommend that it should no longer be a treatment option for autistic youth. Increasingly, however, it has been shown that care of that kind is useful for a number of chronic conditions including autism. It is important to note that inpatient care can be delivered without many of the characteristics found objectionable by client advocates. Advantages of inpatient care include improved security and continuous observation that is not available for all youth in the community. Further, there is evidence that inpatient care can be transitional and community-based. When such an approach is utilized, those youth who would have been terminally placed in residential settings in the past can learn the skills they need and rapidly return to their own families or careproviders in the community.

We have attempted to highlight those techniques that have been shown to be helpful in transitional programs. Great strides have been made, but additional work is needed for widespread implementation of these strategies across inpatient treatment facilities. The efficacy of the techniques we covered have been documented empirically. Further, these strategies have been disseminated across many agencies with which we have had contact. It is anticipated that continued refinement and dissemination of these promising procedures will occur in the future.

REFERENCES

American Psychiatric Association. (1987). *Diagnostic and statistical manual of mental disorders* (3rd ed., rev.). Washington, DC: Author.

Anderson, S. R., & Schwartz, I. S. (1986). Transitional programming. In F. J. Fuoco & W. P. Christian (Eds.),*Behavior analysis and therapy in residential programs* (pp. 76–100). New York: Van Nostrand Reinhold.

Anderson, S. R., Luce, S. C., Newsom, C. D., Gruber, B. K., & Kennedy-Butler, K. (1983, May). *Individualized treatment planning for autistic youth*. Paper presented at the meeting of the Association for Behavior Analysis, Milwaukee.

Anderson, S. R., Avery, D. L., DiPietro, E. K., Edwards, G. L., & Christian, W. P. (1987). Intensive home based early intervention with autistic children. *Education and Treatment of Children, 10*, 352–366.

Association for the Severely Handicapped. (1980). TASH adopts resolution calling for abolition of institutions. *Newsletter of the Association for the Severely Handicapped, 6*, 1.

Avery, D., Thibadeau, S. F., & Luce, S. C. (1984, May). *The effects of man-to-man versus zoned supervision of severely handicapped children*. Paper presented at the tenth annual conference of the Association of Behavior Analysis, Nashville.

Baer, D. M., Wolf, M. M., & Risley, T. R. (1968). Some current dimensions of applied behavior analysis. *Journal of Applied Behavior Analysis, 1*, 91–98.

Baker, B. L., & Brightman, A. J. (1989). *Steps to independence: A skills training guide for parents and teachers of children with special needs*. Baltimore: Paul H. Brookes.

Bettelheim, B. (1967). *The empty fortress: Infantile autism and the birth of the self*. New York: Free Press.

Bible, G. H., & Snead, I. J. (1976). Some effects of an accreditation survey on program completion at a state institution. *Mental Retardation, 14*, 14–15.

Bird, B. L. (1984). The community-based service continuum. In W. P. Christian, G. T. Hannah, & T. J. Glahn (Eds.), *Programming effective human services: Strategies for institutional change and client transition* (pp. 113–138). New York: Plenum Press.

Blew, P. A., Schwartz, I. S., & Luce, S. C. (1985). Teaching community skills to autistic children using normal peer tutors. *Journal of Applied Behavior Analysis, 18*, 337–342.

Brown, L., Branstion-McClean, M. B., Baumgart, D., Vincent, L., Falvey, M., & Schroeder, J. (1979). Using the characteristics of current and subsequent least restrictive environments in the development of curriculum content for severely handicapped students. *Journal of the Association for the Severely Handicapped, 4*, 407–424.

Campbell, D. T., & Stanley, J. C. (1966). *Experimental and quasi-experimental designs for research*. Chicago: Rand McNally.

Carr, E. G. (1982). *How to teach sign language to developmentally disabled children*. Austin, Texas: Pro-ed.

Carr, E. G., & Durand, V. M. (1985). Reducing behavior problems through functional communication training. *Journal of Applied Behavior Analysis, 18*, 111–127.

Carr, E. G., Newsom, C. D., & Binkoff, J. A. (1980). Escape as a factor in the aggressive behavior of two retarded children. *Journal of Applied Behavior Analysis, 13*, 101–118.

Christian, W. P. (1984). A case study in the programming and maintenance of institutional change. *Journal of Organizational Behavior Management, 5*, 99–153.

Christian, W. P., & Hannah, G. T. (1983). *Effective management in human services*. Englewood Cliffs, NJ: Prentice Hall.

Christian, W. P., & Zampini, A. J. (1988). *Annual Report: Progress of organizational analysis and development in a state hospital facility*, Unpublished manuscript.

Coleman, M. (Ed.). (1976).*The autistic syndromes*. Amsterdam: North-Holland Publishing.

Corte, H. E., Wolf, M. M., & Locke, B. J. (1971). A comparison of procedures for eliminating self-injurious behavior of retarded adolescents. *Journal of Applied Behavior Analysis, 4*, 201–213.

Coughlin, D. D., Maloney, D. M., Baron, R. L., Dahir, J., Daly, D. L., Daly, P. B., Fixsen,

D. L., Phillips, E. L., & Thomas, D. L. (1984). Implementing the community-based teaching family model at Boys Town. In W. P. Christian, G. T. Hannah, & T. J. Glahn (Eds.), *Programming effective human services: Strategies for institutional change and client transition* (pp. 63–82). New York: Plenum Press.

Czyzewski, M. J., Christian, W. P., & Norris, M. B. (1984). Preparing the family for client transition: Outreach parent training. In W. P. Christian, G. T. Hannah, & T. J. Glahn (Eds.), *Programming effective human services: Strategies for institutional change and client transition* (pp. 177–202). New York: Plenum Press.

DeMyer, M. K. (1979). *Parents and children in autism.* New York: Wiley.

Dixon v. Weinberger, 405 F. Supp. 974 (D.D.C. 1975).

Doke, L. A., & Risley, T. R. (1972). The organization of day care environments: Required vs. optional activities. *Journal of Applied Behavior Analysis, 5,* 405–420.

Doleys, D., Wells, K. C., Hobbs, S. A., Roberts, M. W., & Cartelli, L. M. (1976). The effects of social punishment upon compliance: A comparison of time out and positive practice. *Journal of Applied Behavior Analysis, 9,* 471–482.

Donaldson v. O'Connor, 493 F. 2nd 507 (5th Cir. 1974).

Donnellan, A. M. (1980). An educational perspective of autism: Implications for curriculum development and personnel development. In *Critical issues in educating autistic children and youth* (pp. 53–58). Washington, DC: U.S. Department of Education, Office of Special Education.

Dunlap, G., & Egel, A. L. (1982). Motivational techniques. In R. L. Koegel, A. Rincover, & A. L. Egel (Eds.), *Understanding and educating autistic children* (pp. 106–126). San Diego: College-Hill Press.

Dyer, K. (1987). The competition of autistic stereotyped behavior with usual and specially assessed reinforcers. *Research in Developmental Disabilities, 8,* 607–626.

Dyer, K., & Peck, C. A. (1987). Current perspectives on social communication curricula for students with autism and severe handicaps. *Education and Treatment of Children, 10,* 338–351.

Dyer, K., Schwartz, I. S., & Luce, S. C. (1984). A supervision program for increasing functional activities for severely handicapped students in a residential setting. *Journal of Applied Behavior Analysis, 17,* 249–259.

Eagle, E. (1967). Prognosis and outcome of community placement of institutionalized retardates. *American Journal of Mental Deficiency, 72,* 232–243.

Edgerton, R., & Bercovici, S. (1976). The clock of competence: Years later. *American Journal of Mental Deficiency, 80,* 485–497.

Egan, P., Luce, S. C., & Hall, R. V. (1988). Use of a concurrent treatment design to analyze the effects of a peer review system in a residential setting. *Behavior Modification, 12,* 35–56.

Egel, A. L. (1981). Reinforcer variation: Implications for motivating developmentally delayed children. *Journal of Applied Behavior Analysis, 14,* 345–351.

Egel, A. L., Richman, G. S., & Koegel, R. L. (1981). Normal peer models and autistic children's learning. *Journal of Applied Behavior Analysis, 14,* 3–12.

Eisenberg, L. (1968). Psychotic disorders in childhood. In R. E. Cooke (Eds.), *The biologic basis of pediatric practice.* New York: McGraw-Hill.

Eyman, R. K., & Call, T. (1977). Maladaptive behavior and community placement of mentally retarded persons. *American Journal of Mental Deficiency, 82,* 137–144.

Favell, J. E., & Greene, J. W. (1981). *How to treat self-injurious behavior.* Austin, TX: Pro-ed.

Favell, J. E., Favell, J. E., & Risley, T. R. (1981). A quality-assurance system for ensuring client rights in mental retardation facilities. In G. T. Hannah, W. P. Christian, & H. B.

Clark (Eds.), *Preservation of client rights: A handbook for practitioners providing therapeutic, educational, and rehabilitative services* (pp. 345–364). New York: Free Press.
Ferster, C. B. (1961). Positive reinforcement and behavioral deficits of autistic children. *Child Development, 32,* 437–456.
Foxx, R. M., & Azrin, N. H. (1972). Restitution: A method of eliminating aggressive-disruptive behavior of retarded and brain-damaged patients. *Behavior Research and Therapy, 10,* 15–27.
Halderman v. Pennhurst, 466 F. Supp. 1295 (E.D. Pa. 1977).
Hall, R. V., & Van Houten, R. (1983). *Managing behavior: Volume I.* Austin, TX: Pro-ed.
Halle, J. W., Marshall, A. M., & Spradlin, J. E. (1979). Time delay: A technique to increase language use and facilitate generalization in retarded children. *Journal of Applied Behavior Analysis, 12,* 431–441.
Hannah, G. T., & Christian, W. P. (1984). Assessing the client's readiness for transition to the community. In W. P. Christian, G. T. Hannah, & T. J. Glahn (Eds.), *Programming effective human services: Strategies for institutional change and client transition* (pp. 139–156). New York: Plenum Press.
Herbert-Jackson, E., O'Brien, M., Porterfield, J., & Risley, T. R. (1977). *The infant center: A complete guide to organizing and managing infant day care.* Baltimore: University Park Press.
Joint Commission on Accreditation of Hospitals. (1978). *Standards for services for developmentally disabled individuals.* Chicago: Joint Commission on Accreditation of Hospitals.
Kaimowitz v. Michigan Department of Mental Health, 42 U.S.L. Week 2063 (Mich. Cir. Ct. Wayne City, July 10, 1973).
Kanner, L. (1943). Autistic disturbances of affective contact. *Nervous Child, 2,* 181–197.
Koegel, R. L. (1982). *How to integrate autistic and other severely handicapped children into a classroom group.* Austin, TX: Pro-ed.
Koegel, R. L., Dunlap, G., & Dyer, K. (1980). Intertrial interval duration and learning in autistic children. *Journal of Applied Behavior Analysis, 13,* 91–99.
Koegel, R. L., & Scheibman, L. (1982). *How to teach autistic and severely handicapped children.* Austin, TX: Pro-ed.
Koegel, R. L., Rincover, A., & Egel, A. (1982). *Educating and understanding autistic children.* San Diego: College-Hill Press.
Koegel, R. L., Schreibman, L., Britten, K. R., Burke, J. C., & O'Neill, R. E. (1982). In A comparison of parent training to direct child treatment. R. L. Koegel, A. Rincover, & A. Egel (Eds.), *Educating and understanding autistic children* (pp. 260–279). San Diego: College-Hill Press.
Koegel, R. L., Dyer, K., & Bell, L. K. (1987). The influence of child-preferred activities on autistic children's social behavior. *Journal of Applied Behavior Analysis, 20,* 243–252.
Lake v. Cameron, 364 F. 2nd 657 (D.C. 1966).
Lakin, K. C., Bruiniks, R. H., & Sigford, B. B. (1981). Early preparation on the community adjustment of mentally retarded people. In R. H. Bruiniks, C. E. Meyers, B. B. Sigford, & K. C. Lakin (Eds.), *Deinstitutionalization and community adjustment of mentally retarded people.* Monograph of the American Association on Mental Deficiency (No. 4), Washington, D.C.
Larsson, D. G., Luce, S. C., & Christian, W. P. (1989). Attaining clinical competence at the May Institute. *Behavior Therapist.* 12(9), 219–220.
Lattimore, J., Jones, M. L., & Calvert, T. L. (1978). *Roadrunner project: Caregiver manual.* Morganton: Western Carolina Center.
Leidholt, P. Lipsker, L. E., Luce, S. C., & Christian, W. P., (1981, May). *A middle management strategy for increasing staff-to-client interaction in a residential treatment setting.* Paper

presented at the annual convention of the Association for Behavior Analysis, Milwaukee.

Lovaas, O. I. (1969). *Behavior modification: Teaching language to psychotic children (film)*. New York: Appleton-Century-Crofts.

Lovaas, O. I. (1981). *Teaching developmentally disabled children: The me book*. Baltimore: University Park Press.

Lovaas, O. I., & Favell, J. E. (1987). Protection for clients undergoing aversive restrictive interventions. *Education and Treatment of Children, 10*, 311–325.

Lovaas, O. I., & Simmons, J. Q. (1969). Manipulation of self-destruction in three retarded children. *Journal of Applied Behavior Analysis, 2*, 143–157.

Lovaas, O. I., Litrownik, A., & Mann, R. (1971). Response latencies to auditory stimuli in children engaged in self-stimulatory behavior. *Behaviour Research and Therapy, 9*, 934–939.

Lovaas, O. I., Koegel, R. L., Simmons, J. Q., & Long, J. S. (1973). Some generalization and follow-up measures on autistic children. *Journal of Applied Behavior Analysis, 6*, 131–166.

Lovaas, O. I., Ackerman, A. B., & Taubman, M. T. (1983). An overview of behavioral treatment of autistic persons. In M. Rosenbaum, C. Franks, & Y. Jaffe (Eds.), *Perspectives on behavior therapy in the 80's*. New York: Springer Publishing.

Luce, S. C. (1979, December). *Reducing autistic behaviors: A review of the literature*. Paper presented at the annual conference of the Association for the Advancement of Behavior Therapy. San Francisco.

Luce, S. C. (1986). Autistic children and adolescents. In F. J. Fuoco, & W. P. Christian (Eds.), *Behavior therapy in residential treatment environments*. New York: Van Nostrand Reinhold Company.

Luce, S. C., & Christian, W. P. (1981). *How to reduce autistic and severely maladaptive behaviors*. Austin, TX: Pro-ed.

Luce, S. C., & Hall, R. V. (1981). Contingent exercise: A mild but powerful procedure used with differential reinforcement to reduce bizarre behavior. *Education and Treatment of Children, 4*, 309–329.

Luce, S. C., Christian, W. P., Lipsker, L. E., & Hall, R. V. (1980). Response cost: A case for specificity. *Behavior Analyst, 4*, 78–80.

Luce, S. C., Delquadri, J., & Hall, R. V. (1980). Contingent exercise: A mild but powerful procedure used to reduce inappropriate verbal and aggressive behavior. *Journal of Applied Behavior Analysis, 13*, 583–594.

Luce, S. C., Anderson, S. R., Thibadeau, S. F., & Lipsker, L. E. (1984). Preparing the client for transition to the community. In W. P. Christian, G. T. Hannah, & T. J. Glahn (Eds.), *Programming effective human services: Strategies for institutional change and client transition* (pp. 157–176). New York: Plenum Press.

Martin, R. (1975). *Legal challenges to behavior modification*. Champaign, IL: Research Press.

McClannahan, L. E., & Krantz, P. J. (1981). Accountability systems for protection of the rights of autistic children and youth. In G. T. Hannah, W. P. Christian, & H. B. Clark (Eds.), *Preservation of client rights: A handbook for practitioners providing therapeutic, educational, and rehabilitative services* (pp. 83–106). New York: Macmillan/Free Press.

Mithaug, D. E. (1981). *How to teach prevocational skills to severely handicapped persons*. Austin, TX: Pro-ed.

Newsom, C. D., & Rincover, A. (1981). Autism. In E. J. Mash & L. G. Terdal (Eds.), *Behavioral assessment of childhood disorders*. New York: Guilford Press.

New York State Association for Retarded Children, Inc. v. Carey & Parisi, 393 F. Supp. 715 (E.D.N.Y. 1975), 357 F. Supp. 752 (E.D.N.Y. 1973).

Nihira, K., Foster, R., Shelhaas, M., & Leland, H. (1974). *The adaptive behavior scale*. Washington, DC: American Association of Mental Deficiency.

Peck, C. A. (1985). Increasing opportunities for social control by children with autism and severe handicaps: Effects on student behavior and perceived classroom climate. *Journal of the Association for the Severely Handicapped, 10*, 183–193.

Phillips, E. L., Fixsen, D. L., Phillips, E. A., & Wolf, M. M. (1979). The teaching family model: A comprehensive approach to residential treatment of youth. In D. Cullinane & M. H. Epstein (Eds.), *Special education for adolescents: Issues and perspectives*. Columbus, OH: Charles E. Merrill.

Polan, C. G., & Spencer, B. C. (1959). A checklist of symptoms of autism of early life. *West Virginia Medical Journal, 55*, 198–204.

Porterfield, J. K., Herbert-Jackson, E., & Risley, T. R. (1976). Contingent observation: An effective and acceptable procedure for reducing disruptive behavior of young children in a group setting. *Journal of Applied Behavior Analysis, 9*, 55–64.

Reid, D. (1983). Trends and issues on training feeding and dressing skills. In J. L. Matson & F. Andrasik (Eds.), *Treatment issues and innovations in mental retardation* (pp. 213–240). New York: Plenum Press.

Reid, D. H., & Whitman, T. L. (1983). Behavioral staff management in institutions: A critical review of effectiveness and acceptability. *Analysis and Intervention in Developmental Disabilities, 3*, 131–149.

Rimland, B. (1964). *Infantile autism*. New York: Appleton-Century-Crofts.

Rincover, A. (1978). Sensory extinction: A procedure for elimination of self-stimulatory behavior in psychotic children. *Journal of Abnormal Child Psychology, 6*, 299–301.

Rincover, A. (1982). *How to use sensory extinction*. Austin, TX: Pro-ed.

Rincover, A., & Koegel, R. L. (1975). Setting and stimulus control in autistic children. *Journal of Applied Behavior Analysis, 8*, 235–246.

Risley, T. R., & Wolf, M. M. (1967). Establishing functional speech in echolalic children. *Behaviour Research and Therapy, 5*, 73–88.

Romanczyk, R., & Lockshin, S. (1981). *How to create a curriculum for autistic and other handicapped children*. Austin, TX: Pro-ed.

Rotholz, D. A., & Luce, S. C. (1983). Alternative strategies for the reduction of self-stimulatory behavior in autistic youth. *Education and Treatment, 6*, 363–377.

Rouse v. Cameron, 373 F. 2nd. 451 (D.C. 1966).

Rutter, M. (1978). Diagnosis and definition. In M. Rutter & E. Schopler (Eds.), *Autism: A reappraisal of concepts and treatment*. New York: Plenum.

Sidman, M. (1960). *Tactics of scientific research*. New York: Basic Books.

Solnick, J. V., Rincover, A., & Peterson, C. (1977). Some determinants of reinforcing and punishing effects of time-out. *Journal of Applied Behavior Analysis, 10*, 415–424.

Sternlicht, M. (1978). Variables affecting foster care placement of institutionalized retarded residents. *Mental Retardation, 16*, 25–27.

Stokes, T. F., & Baer, D. M. (1977). An implicit technology of generalization. *Journal of Applied Behavior Analysis, 10*, 349–367.

Sulzer-Azaroff, B., & Mayer, G. R. (1977). *Applying behavior analysis procedures with children and youth*. New York: Holt, Rinehart & Winston.

Timbers, G. D., Jones, R. J., & Davis, J. L. (1981). Safeguarding the rights of children and youth in group-home settings. In G. T. Hannah, W. P. Christian, & H. B. Clark (Eds.), *Preservation of client rights: A handbook for practitioners providing therapeutic, educational, and rehabilitative services*. New York: Macmillan/Free Press.

Van Houten, R. (1980). Social validation: The evaluation of standards of competency for target behaviors. *Journal of Applied Behavior Analysis, 12*, 581–591.

Welch, S. J., & Pear, J. (1980). Generalization of naming responses to objects in the natural environment as a function of stimulus modality with retarded children. *Journal of Applied Behavior Analysis, 13,* 629–643.

Westaway, A. M., & Apolloni, I. (Eds.). (1978). Becoming independent: A living skills system. Bellevue, WA: Edmark.

Wolf, M. M., Risley, T. R., & Meese, H. (1964). Application of operant conditioning procedures to the behavior problems of an autistic child. *Behaviour Research and Therapy, 1,* 305–312.

Wolfensberger, W. (1972). The principle of normalization in human services. Toronto: National Institute on Mental Retardation.

Wyatt v. Stickney, 344 F. Supp. 373, 344 F. Supp. 387 (M.D. Ala. 1972).

7

Pediatric Pain

Gary A. Walco, Lawrence J. Siegel, Michael J. Dolgin, and James W. Varni

Introduction

Pain in children represents a complex cognitive-developmental phenomenon, involving a number of biobehavioral components that synergistically interact to produce differential levels of pain perception and verbal and nonverbal manifestations (Varni, 1983). Given children's various cognitive-developmental stages, conceptualizations of pain and discomfort must be taken into consideration (Thompson & Varni, 1986). Thus, an accurate understanding of pain perception in children cannot be gleaned from simply applying downward the knowledge of pain perception in adults. Instead, research and clinical practice in pediatric pain assessment and management must develop a separate, if not parallel, database from the adult field which is sensitive to the unique characteristics of children.

Varni (1983) has identified four primary categories of pediatric pain:

Gary A. Walco • Schneider Children's Hospital of Long Island Jewish Medical Center, and Albert Einstein College of Medicine, New Hyde Park, New York 11042. Lawrence J. Siegel • Ferkauf Graduate School of Psychology, Yeshiva University, Bronx, New York 10461. Michael J. Dolgin • Children's Hospital of Los Angeles, and University of Southern California, Los Angeles, California 90089-1061. James W. Varni • Orthopaedic Hospital, and University of Southern California, Los Angeles, California 90089-1061.

Inpatient Behavior Therapy for Children and Adolescents, edited by Vincent B. Van Hasselt and David J. Kolko. Plenum Press, New York, 1992.

(1) pain associated with a disease state (e.g., hemophilia, arthritis, sickle-cell disease); (2) pain associated with an observable physical injury or trauma (e.g., burns, lacerations, fractures); (3) pain not associated with a well-defined or specific disease state or identifiable physical injury (e.g., migraine and tension headaches, recurrent abdominal pain); and (4) pain associated with medical and dental procedures (e.g., lumbar punctures, bone marrow aspirations, surgery, injections, venipuncture, tooth extractions). To exemplify assessment and intervention strategies implemented in inpatient settings, we will focus on three issues: procedural pain and acute iatrogenic distress, postoperative pain, and pain associated with chronic diseases.

PROCEDURAL PAIN AND ACUTE IATROGENIC DISTRESS

Noninvasive medical procedures, such as X rays and physical examinations, can create significant distress in the general pediatric population. Children with serious or chronic illnesses endure a variety of more intrusive procedures, including catheterizations, spinal taps, bone marrow aspirations, endoscopies, etc. For these children, repeated medical procedures are often considered more aversive than the threat of their disease itself, and constitute a primary reason for psychological referral (Kellerman & Katz, 1979; Zeltzer, Kellerman, Ellenberg, Dash, & Rigler, 1980).

Studies of pediatric cancer patients undergoing bone marrow aspirations and spinal taps indicate that in most cases a stable pattern of habituation is not evident (Katz, Kellerman, & Siegel, 1980; Kellerman, Zeltzer, Ellenberg, & Dash, 1983). Some patients develop symptoms of anticipatory distress that may include anxiety, somatic complaints, nausea and vomiting, avoidance, and resistance (Kellerman & Varni, 1982). Owing to the fact that painful medical procedures are acute and generally predictable events, and because the sensory (nociception) and affective (anxiety) components are so intertwined, some investigators have adopted the more inclusive concept of "distress" as the focus of assessment and intervention (e.g., Jay, 1988; Katz *et al.*, 1980).

With regard to any medical procedure, the most fundamental intervention involves prior preparation of the child. Typically, this includes giving the child information regarding what will be done, letting the child handle equipment, practicing the procedure on a doll, introducing the child to medical personnel, and discussing fears and concerns. Such preparation serves multiple functions, including education, desensitization, modeling, reassurance, mastery, and trust. Fernald and Corry (1981) found that empathic preparation that was supportive, child-centered, and that described the sensations, anxieties, and reactions that might occur during an injection produced less crying and better cooperation than a directive preparation where the child was informed of what would occur and was told to be "big, brave, and still." In the empathic preparation, the child was assured that the injection was in no way a punishment, that anxiety was natural, and that crying was permissible. The directive preparation focused on the importance of cooperation and the negative consequences of noncompliance (e.g., prolonging the procedure).

The beneficial effects of preparation can be enhanced by offering children a skill they can actively use. *In vivo* systematic desensitization that combines relaxation training, modeling, and behavioral rehearsal has been successfully employed with adult patients who experience high levels of anxiety associated with injections (e.g., Ferguson, Taylor, & Wermuth, 1978). Although hypnosis, pleasant imagery, participant modeling, and *in vivo* desensitization have been reported as anxiety-reduction strategies in case studies of children with needle phobias, more systematic, data-based studies are needed.

In one such case, Dash (1981) treated severe needle phobia in a 5-year-old cardiac patient during three sessions of *in vivo* participant modeling that involved pairing needles, syringes, and test tubes with the child's most valuable reinforcer, sugarless bubble gum. The needles were exposed gradually as the child unwrapped her gum. As the therapist then began handling the needles and placing them against his own arm, the child gradually modeled this behavior without distress. The child was then hypnotized by use of a rapid induction consisting of eye fixation, deep breathing, and visualization of herself walking down a flight of stairs, through a large door, and entering her favorite place. The therapist also trained the nursing staff to assist the child in utilizing these skills when he was not present. Follow-up 2 and 24 months later indicated no further needle phobias or other problem behaviors. Peterson and Shigetomi (1981) also reported that children who were taught active coping skills in addition to filmed modeling preparation were calmer and more cooperative during tonsillectomies than children who had received either one of the interventions alone.

The issue of individual coping styles and of tailoring behavioral intervention and preparatory information to children's actual preferences and needs is a matter for further investigation (Hubert, Jay, Saltoun, & Hayes, 1988). Smith, Ackerson, and Blotcky (1989) have moved in this direction with children who have cancer and who are undergoing bone marrow aspirations and spinal taps by matching the usual coping style (i.e., repression or sensitization) of these children with behavioral interventions aimed at either distraction or sensory information. Dependent measures included self-reported pain and fear, heart rate, and observed distress. Neither coping style nor behavioral intervention mode demonstrated a superior main effect, although an interaction of matched coping style and treatment was found. Interestingly, children offered an intervention matching their usual coping style (e.g., repressors receiving distraction) exhibited the highest levels of self-reported pain. Also of interest are the data suggesting that children's usual coping behaviors may evolve over time and repeated procedures. Despite the methodological difficulties inherent in this area of research study, the investigation by Smith *et al.* (1989) broke important new ground for future research. For a review of the important theoretical, research, and therapeutic issues related to children's coping styles and stressful medical procedures as well as representative studies in the area, see Peterson (1989).

A number of investigative efforts have demonstrated the effectiveness of behavioral interventions in reducing pain and anxiety in children with cancer who are undergoing painful medical procedures. Conditioned anxiety in response to bone marrow aspirations and lumbar punctures occurs frequently in these patients and contributes to the pain-anxiety–distress cycle. Most investigations have focused on hypnotic techniques (see Dash, 1980). Several case studies (e.g., Ellenberg, Kellerman, Dash, Higgins, & Zeltzer, 1980; Gardner, 1976) have provided in-depth accounts of the utility of hypnosis in reducing the perceived pain and anxiety in children and adolescents who are undergoing these procedures.

Research employing hypnosis with larger groups of pediatric cancer patients shows significant improvements in procedure-related distress over baseline measurements (Hilgard & LeBaron, 1982; Kellerman *et al.*, 1983). Zeltzer and LeBaron (1982) found hypnosis to be superior to nonhypnotic techniques (i.e., supportive counseling). Katz, Kellerman, and Ellenberg (1987) compared hypnosis and nondirected play in a randomized study of 36 children with acute leukemia who were undergoing routine bone marrow aspirations. Self-report ratings of pain and fear, nurses' ratings of distress, and behavioral observations of distress were recorded. When the two interventions were compared, no significant differences were noted on any measure. Both groups reported improvements on self-report measures, with no demonstrable changes in observed distress behavior. Intervention by sex interactions were significant for all dependent measures (i.e., boys benefited more in the nondirected play condition, whereas girls did better with hypnosis). Results were most apparent on self-report measures of pain and fear. The investigators pointed out that this finding warrants future scrutiny because it may reflect the differential utility of active versus passive coping skills with boys and girls. These data also underscore the advantages of multimodal assessment since treatment gains were more evident on subjective (self-report) pain perception indices than on objective (observational) measures. Interventions may have an important impact on the patient's covert experience that may be obscured by an emphasis on achieving dramatic, visible improvements.

Jay, Elliott, Katz, and Siegel (1987) developed a multiple-component cognitive-behavioral treatment package designed to teach effective coping skills and to reduce children's distress during bone marrow aspirations. The rationale for using a multidimensional intervention is to offer patients more than one strategy and to maximize the likelihood of therapeutic benefit. The package is based on the stress inoculation model described by Meichenbaum and Turk (1976) and incorporates filmed modeling, positive incentive, breathing exercises, emotive imagery, and behavioral rehearsal. Dependent measures included self-report, physiological, and observational data. A counterbalanced design with 56 children aged 3 to 14 years with leukemia was used in order to compare the effectiveness of this behavioral package to that of oral sedation (Valium) and a minimal-attention control condition.

Results indicated that the cognitive-behavioral package was significantly more efficacious than the control condition in reducing children's observed distress, self-reported pain, pulse rate, and blood pressure. Data regarding the Valium condition were equivocal, with a reduction in blood pressure being the only significant difference from the other two conditions. There was some evidence suggesting that Valium was useful in reducing anticipatory anxiety, but less helpful during the actual bone marrow aspiration—a logical finding given that no information or coping skills were offered in the Valium condition. An additional advantage of the cognitive-behavioral package was its utility with preschool as well as with older children. Studies of hypnosis or other behavioral techniques generally do not address children under 7 years, despite the fact that these children exhibit significantly higher levels of distress (Jay, Ozolins, Elliott, & Caldwell, 1983).

Parental distress during children's medical procedures must also be considered, especially for young children. The relationship between children's observed distress and parental anxiety has been documented (Jay *et al.*, 1983). Jay and Elliott (1990) have completed a study evaluating a stress inoculation program for parents whose children were undergoing bone marrow aspirations or spinal taps. Parent intervention involved filmed modeling, education, self-statement training, cognitive rehearsal, and relaxation training. Observational, self-report, and physiological data regarding parent and child distress during the procedure were collected and compared to those of a group of parents who merely observed the behavioral intervention their children were receiving during the procedure. Although parents receiving the stress inoculation training reported lower anxiety scores and higher positive self-statement scores, behavioral and physiological variables were not impacted. Future studies of the interaction between parent and child distress and coping behavior will promote our understanding of systems influences in childhood pain and its management (e.g., Blount *et al.*, 1989).

POSTOPERATIVE PAIN

Pain is associated with all surgical procedures that involve children and adults. Although acute pain generally serves as a warning signal that tissue damage is occurring (as in the case of injury or disease process), the acute pain following surgery serves no such adaptive purpose (Chapman & Bonica, 1983). Investigators have only recently begun to systematically examine the nature and incidence of postoperative pain in children. In contrast to the literature addressing this issue with adults, research pertaining to postoperative pain in child populations is sparse (Beyer & Levine, 1987).

The limited data on postoperative pain in children can be attributed to two primary factors. One is the problem associated with the assessment of pain in children, since it is only within the past decade that valid and reliable measures of pain for pediatric populations have been developed (Johnston, 1989; Karoly, 1988; Savedra & Tesler, 1989). The second factor is the pervasive and erroneous beliefs shared by many medical practitioners who work with children. McIlvaine (1989) noted a number of myths concerning pain in children that have served to impede progress in understanding the nature and management of pain following surgical procedures with children. These myths include beliefs that (1) children do not experience pain as intensely as do adults, (2) children are unable to describe or locate their pain, (3) children recover quickly, (4) children may become addicted to narcotics, and (5) narcotics always depress respiratory functions in children.

Assessment of Postoperative Pain

The assessment of postoperative pain in children presents some unique challenges even with children who are capable of providing self-reports of their pain. This is particularly true of the first 24-hour period following surgery when the child is emerging from the effects of anesthesia and lapses in and out of periods of wakefulness. As a result, one often must rely on nonverbal indices of behavior to assess pain intensity. Typically, these indices involve physiological and behavioral manifestations which are thought to reflect pain and discomfort (e.g., groaning, grimacing, restlessness, guarding the operative site, cardiovascular and respiratory functions) (Johnston, 1989; Savedra & Tesler, 1989; Troug & Anand, 1989).

With infants, postoperative pain assessment obviously must rely on nonverbal pain cues. An example of the assessment approach with infants is represented by the work of Attia, Amiel-Tison, and Mayer (1987) who developed the Postoperative Comfort Score. This multidimensional instrument evaluates the infant across 10 behavioral variables: (1) sleep patterns, (2) facial expression, (3) quality of cry, (4) motor activity, (5) excitability, (6) flexion of fingers and toes, (7) sucking behavior, (8) global evaluation of tone, (9) consolability, and (10) responsiveness to people. Using this measure with infants undergoing minor surgical procedures, these authors found a relationship between high scores on the scale (indicating greater pain/discomfort) and higher plasma catecholamine and beta-endorphin levels.

For children who are capable of providing self-reports of pain, the visual analogue scale (VAS) has been found to be useful as a method for evaluating pain intensity following surgical procedures (O'Hara, McGrath, D'Astous, & Vair, 1987; Tree-Trakarn, Pirayavaraporam, & Lertakyamanee, 1987). An advantage of the VAS in these circumstances is that it provides a quick and fairly unobtrusive procedure for assessing the severity of a child's pain.

Siegel (1989) investigated several measures to assess postoperative pain in children 4 to 12 years of age who were undergoing abdominal surgery. All children received the same premedication prior to surgery and the same method of anesthesia induction. In the recovery room, postsurgical pain was measured with the modified version of the Pain/Discomfort Scale reported by Hannallah, Broadman, Belman, Abramowitz, and Epstein (1987). This scale measures five pain indices, including blood pressure, crying, movement, agitation, posture, and pain verbalizations. Following the child's return to the hospital room, self-reported pain was assessed by the VAS and pain behaviors were assessed using the UAB Pain Behavior Scale (Richards, Nepomuceno, Riles, & Suer, 1982). The Pain Behavior Scale was developed to be sensitive to small changes in behavior, to be scored quickly, and to provide good rater reliability. These instruments were administered at four time intervals during the second and third day following surgery. In addition, mothers and nurses completed the VAS at the same time as the child. Parents also completed the State Anxiety Scale (Spielberger, Gorsuch, & Lushene, 1970).

Scores from the Pain/Discomfort Scale indicated that a significant number of children were experiencing moderate levels of pain/discomfort in the recovery room as they were coming off of the general anesthesia. Correlations between the UAB Pain Scale and Child VAS ranged from $r = .43$ to $r = .58$. Moderate to high correlations were found between child and nurse VAS scores. Although mother and child VAS scores were significantly related, the correlations were considerably lower than those of the child and nurse. An explanation of these lower correlations can be found in the relationship between maternal anxiety and the mothers' ratings of their children's pain. Significant positive correlations were obtained between maternal state anxiety scores and scores on the VAS. Interestingly, as the anxiety of the mothers consistently decreased over 3 days in the hospital, their VAS scores were increasingly related to the VAS scores of their child.

Postoperative Pain Management

The objectives of postoperative pain management are twofold and include (1) minimizing discomfort for the psychological well-being of the patient, and (2) facilitating physical recovery. In the latter situation, failure to adequately control the pain following surgery can lead to physiological stress responses (e.g., muscle contractions, muscle tension) and postoperative complications, which thereby impede recovery and discharge from the hospital (Beyer & Bournaki, 1989).

To date, the preponderance of evidence clearly indicates that children, compared to adults, do not receive adequate pain management during the postsurgical period (Schechter, 1989). A number of investigations indicate that given the same type of surgery, and controlling for body weight, children generally are given less therapeutically prescribed dosages of analgesics and less potent types of medication than are adult patients, even when significant levels of postoperative pain are identified by medical personnel (Beyer, DeGood, Ashley, & Russell, 1983; Burokas, 1985; Bush, Holmbeck, Cockrell, 1989; Mather & Mackie, 1983; Schechter, Allen, & Hanson, 1986). These findings have been replicated with children and adults who have undergone minor elective surgeries (e.g., hernia repair) as well as more serious major surgical procedures (e.g., open-heart surgery). It has been suggested by these investigators that the consistent findings of inadequate pain management in children following surgery may be attributed in large part to the myths noted earlier.

Currently, the primary method for postoperative pain management in children is analgesic medication delivered by means of nerve blocks, local anesthetic infusions, or patient-controlled analgesia (Shannon & Berde, 1989). It is standard practice for the physician to write a prescription order on a p.r.n. (as needed) basis. This dosing regimen is based on the assumption that children can adequately verbalize their pain experience and/or that medical personnel can adequately assess the occurrence and nature of the child's pain experience. As a result, it becomes the responsibility of nurses and physicians to determine when and how much medication the child needs for pain management. However, the studies discussed earlier indicating the undermedication of children on a p.r.n. basis call this method into serious question. As Bush *et al.* (1989) noted with regard to postoperative pain treatment, "p.r.n. pain prescription in children essentially guarantees very low drug delivery" (p. 46).

A recent advance in postoperative pain management is the use of patient-controlled analgesia (PCA). PCA involves the use of a microprocessor-operated pump that connects to an indwelling intravenous catheter that permits the patient to self-administer small, frequent boluses of an analgesic by pressing a button. After each administration of the medication, an automatic lockout device is activated so that the patient cannot repeat a dose before a specified time (Berde, 1989). Although this method has been used most frequently with adults, PCA has shown considerable promise as an effective and safe treatment for postoperative pain in children as young as 6 years (Dodd, Wang, & Rauk, 1988; Gaukroger, Tomkins, & van der Walt, 1989; Rodgers, Webb, Stergios, & Newman, 1988). From a psychological perspective, a major advantage of PCA is the high degree of control over postoperative pain that this technique provides to the child. Research has demonstrated that a sense of control over painful events may affect an individual's experience of pain and the ability to cope with the pain (Siegel & Smith, 1989).

There have been few empirical investigations of nonpharmacological approaches to postoperative pain management in children. For example, the efficacy of techniques, such as relaxation training and cognitive-behavioral approaches, have yet to be examined as adjunctive methods for the treatment of pain in children following surgery. Although several studies have investigated the use of transcutaneous electrical nerve stimulation (TENS) as a method of postoperative pain relief in children, findings to date are inconclusive (Carman & Roach, 1988).

PAIN ASSOCIATED WITH CHRONIC DISEASES

Acute procedural pain and postoperative pain are finite events. The discomfort has a known onset and lasts until the procedure is over or the healing process is complete. In contrast, pain associated with chronic illness is typically either recurrent or chronic and is often unpredictable with respect to occurrence or intensity. Thus, acute anxiety related to pain is less significant, and children and their families must learn to adapt to the ongoing difficulties associated with pain and chronic illness. As a result, assessment issues are quite different, and interventions focus more on coping with pain rather than eradicating it. A discussion of comprehensive pain assessment and factors related to coping with pain in pediatric chronic illness is well beyond the scope of this chapter (for a review, see Walco & Varni, 1991); thus, advances in cognitive-behavioral intervention strategies will be highlighted.

The primary cognitive-biobehavioral treatment techniques utilized in the management of pediatric chronic and recurrent pain have been categorized by Varni (1983) into two categories: (1) *pain perception regulation* modalities through such self-regulatory techniques as progressive muscle relaxation, meditative breathing, and guided imagery, and (2) *pain behavior regulation,* which identifies and modifies socioenvironmental factors that influence pain expression and rehabilitation. In the following sections, we will describe the utilization and clinical research findings of cognitive-biobehavioral assessment and management techniques for three pediatric chronic diseases: hemophilia, juvenile rheumatoid arthritis, and sickle-cell disease.

Hemophilia

Whereas recurrent acute pain in the hemophiliac is associated with a specific bleeding episode, chronic musculoskeletal pain as a result of hemophilic arthropathy (similar to osteoarthritis and caused by repeated hemorrhages into the joint areas) represents a sustained condition over an extended period of time. Thus, pain perception in the hemophiliac truly represents a complex psychophysiological event, complicated by the existence of both recurrent bleeding pain and chronic arthritic pain, requiring differential treatment strategies. More specifically, acute pain of hemorrhage provides a functional signal indicating the necessity of intravenous infusion of factor replacement which temporarily replaces the missing clotting factor, converts the clotting status to normal, and allows a functional blood clot to form. Arthritic pain, on the other hand, represents a potentially debilitating chronic condition which may result in impaired life functioning and analgesic dependence (Varni & Gilbert, 1982). Consequently, the development of an effective alternative to analgesic dependency is the reduction of perceived chronic arthritic pain secondary to hemophilic arthropathy that does not interfere with the essential functional signal of acute recurrent bleeding pain; this has been the goal of the behavioral medicine approach to hemophilia pain management (Varni, 1981a).

Varni and his associates (Varni, 1981a,b; Varni & Gilbert, 1982; Varni, Gilbert, & Dietrich, 1981) conducted a series of studies that examined chronic arthritic pain management in both child and adult hemophiliacs. Instruction in the self-regulation of arthritic pain perception consists of three sequential phases. First the child is taught a 25-step progressive muscle-relaxation sequence involving the alternative tensing and relaxing of major muscle groups (see Varni, 1983). Then the child is taught meditative breathing exercises, consisting of medium deep breaths inhaled through the nose and slowly exhaled through the mouth. While exhaling, the child is instructed to say the word "relax" silently and to initially describe aloud and subsequently visualize the word "relax" in warm colors, as if written in colored chalk on a blackboard. Finally, the child is instructed in the use of guided-imagery techniques (i.e., pleasant, distracting scenes selected by the child). Initially, children are instructed to imagine themselves actually in the scene, not simply observing themselves there. The scene is evoked by a detailed multisensory description by the therapist and subsequently described aloud by the child. Once the scene is clearly visualized, the therapist instructs the child to experiment with other, different scenes to maintain interest and variety. The child is asked to practice these techniques on a regular basis in the home, and to return for sessions with the therapist to maintain the techniques and for encouragement and problem-solving. Data have demonstrated the successful utilization of these techniques with both child and adult patients in controlling chronic musculoskeletal pain secondary to hemophilic arthropathy.

Juvenile Rheumatoid Arthritis

In children with chronic musculoskeletal pain, the prototype for inflammatory chronic athropathy is juvenile rheumatoid arthritis (Varni & Jay, 1984). Typically, this disease manifests itself before 16 years of age, with peak onset in the age groups 1 to 3 and 8 to 12 years. In general, girls are affected twice as often as boys. Although the precise mechanisms of joint pain in juvenile rheumatoid arthritis are not fully understood, it is clear that the effects of this pain are substantial. From a clinical standpoint, pain is thus seen as the major mediating factor in one's ability to cope with the disease (Lovell & Walco, 1989).

In a study of cognitive-biobehavioral interventions for pain associated with juvenile rheumatoid arthritis (Walco, Varni, & Ilowite, in press), children between the ages of 5 and 16 years were seen for a total of eight sessions in which they were taught progressive muscle relaxation, meditative breathing, and guided imagery in an attempt to moderate joint pain and increase adaptive functioning. In addition, parents were seen for two sessions during which pain behavior regulation was discussed.

Central to this study was the use of the Pediatric Pain Questionnaire (PPQ) (Varni & Thompson, 1985), which was employed for initial assessment and to evaluate both immediate as well as long-term effects of the intervention. Modeled after the McGill Pain Questionnaire (Melzack, 1975), the PPQ includes visual analogue scales to assess pain intensity, pain descriptors related to the sensory, affective, and evaluative aspects of pain, and a number of questions focused on emotional concomitants and impact of pain. The reliability, validity, and clinical utility of the PPQ in children and adolescents with juvenile rheumatoid arthritis have been shown (Varni, Thompson, & Hanson, 1987).

Although the general intervention paradigm was similar to that described above for patients with hemophilia, the specific contents of images and means of inducing relaxation varied to some degree depending on the age and interests of the particular child. It is here that data gathered on the PPQ were so essential to the implementation of specific interventions. For example, in addition to self-regulatory techniques that were used to distract children from their pain were images aimed at "undoing" the pain. If among the verbal descriptors the child used "hot" to describe pain, then images involving cooling were used. Similarly, if "squeezing" was chosen as a descriptor, the child was asked to elaborate on a metaphor for this pain (e.g., "My knee feels like it is in a vise"), and then this metaphor would be applied to an image involving a reversal of the pain process (e.g., the vise opening).

Data from the body outlines, in which young children use specific colors to identify relative levels of pain intensity, were also utilized to generate images. For example, a child may have chosen red to represent the most intense level of pain and used it to color in a specific joint. Once relaxed, the child was asked to picture that area of the body and to visualize it painted red. Images were then invoked in which the red area continually shrinks, with healthy pain-free tissue replacing those that had previously been painful.

The findings indicate that there is tremendous short-term benefit from such strategies. Indeed, virtually all subjects dramatically reduced their level of subjective pain. Audio tapes were provided for rehearsal at home, and instructions to practice the techniques on a regular basis were given. Although descriptive data indicate that generalization from clinic sessions to strategies employed at home occurred, not all subjects spontaneously used these skills outside of the clinical setting.

Within the PPQ, there are also questions focusing on behavioral sequelae of the child's pain, psychosocial factors which may mediate the pain, and outcomes related to the child's pain. These data were incorporated into discussions with parents on pain behavior regulation. Essentially, this is an operant paradigm aimed at increasing "well behaviors" while minimizing "pain behaviors." Using specific issues and examples previously provided by the child or parent appears to facilitate parents' comprehension of these issues and the modification of stimuli that may be eliciting or reinforcing maladaptive pain behaviors. Analyses of 6- and 12-month follow-up data indicate improved adaptive daily functioning (e.g., physical activities).

Sickle-Cell Disease

The need for careful assessment of pain associated with sickle-cell disease is very important since little is known about its specific causes and course. Reversible microvascular occlusion at the arteriolar or capillary level affecting bone or bone marrow circulation causes the characteristic painful "crisis" (painful episode) which is the hallmark of sickle-cell disease. Although a variety of biochemical (Karayalcin, Lanzkowsky, & Kazi, 1981; Lawrence & Fabry, 1986) or hematologic (Warth & Rucknagel, 1984) variables are altered during acute painful episodes, most are nonspecific and thus are not diagnostic for this event.

The frequency and severity of pain that is due to vaso-occlusive episodes varies greatly both across and within individuals. Data indicate that the average pediatric sickle-cell disease patient experiences one to two severe episodes per year (Shapiro, 1989). The variation is great, however, in that some patients may experience no pain in a year, whereas others experience pain more than once a week. Furthermore, within a given individual, there may be extended pain-free periods followed by a number of vaso-occlusive episodes over a relatively short period of time.

There are few reliable hematologic parameters by which the severity of a vaso-occlusive episode may be gauged. Thus, unlike the pain associated with acute bleeds in hemophilia or joint flare-ups in arthritis in which there are objective indices of medical factors related to pain, in sickle-cell disease one is limited to subjective reports of the patient and behavioral observations as a means of evaluating the intensity of pain that is due to vaso-occlusion.

A study has been conducted utilizing the PPQ to assess sickle-cell pain (Walco & Dampier, 1990). Thirty-five subjects between the ages of 5 and 15 years were evaluated in the outpatient clinic. Results indicated that the relative infrequency of vaso-occlusive episodes apparently limited the number of opportunities parents had to evaluate their child's pain; thus, retrospective accounts of pain intensity were poor. Significant relationships between physician estimates of disease severity, restrictions in activity, impact on daily functioning, and reported levels of present pain were consistently shown. It was clear that pain adjectives, colors (for younger children), and body outlines could be used meaningfully to describe pain.

As a second aspect of the investigation, the present pain visual analogue scale (VAS) and pain adjective checklist were used on a daily basis with patients admitted to the hospital for uncomplicated painful episodes. Findings indicated that the VAS was quite useful in this situation; patients were able to express different levels of discomfort throughout the course of their hospitalization and VAS ratings correlated with dosage of analgesic (an independent criterion since the house physician was not privy to VAS ratings). In addition, patients utilized the adjective checklist in a meaningful way throughout the hospitalization. It was noted that a large number of pain descriptors were selected at the beginning of the hospital stay, and were steadily dropped as days passed. This trend was especially obvious for the affective and evaluative pain descriptors. Finally, body outlines proved to be worthwhile as patients labeled specific pain sites and, to a large extent, differentiated relative levels of pain intensity among the sites.

These assessment data are essential in planning both pharmacological as well as psychological treatment strategies. Currently, studies are under way in which optimal analgesic regimens are being matched to individual patients' reported pain experiences. In addition, attempts are being made to identify those patients who may benefit most from learning self-regulatory techniques as well as those who may require behavioral programs aimed at enhancing daily functioning.

By and large, sickle-cell crises may be conceptualized as recurrent, acute, painful episodes. Thus, the average patient appears to maintain a relatively normal life-style which is interrupted periodically by vaso-occlusive episodes. At these times, rest and immobilization are encouraged, and analgesic treatments range from aspirin or acetaminophen

(Tylenol) for less severe episodes to parenterally administered (intramuscular or intravenous) narcotics given during hospitalizations (Cole, Sprinkle, Smith, & Buchanon, 1986; Scott, 1982). In the latter situations, a fixed dosing schedule adjusting for dosage of analgesic is much preferred to either p.r.n. or variable-schedule dosing. Fixed dosing facilitates the maintenance of therapeutic levels of the analgesic, thereby reducing the severe peaks and valleys experienced as the drug is metabolized. This facet, in tandem with the fact that the patient receives the analgesic without having to ask for it, reduces the tendency of constantly attending to one's level of discomfort. In addition, recent data indicate that in adolescents with sickle-cell disease, patient-controlled analgesia is an efficient means of delivering therapeutic doses of narcotic analgesics (Schechter, Berrien, & Katz, 1988).

Zeltzer, Dash, and Holland (1979) described two cases in which self-regulatory techniques were shown to be of benefit to adolescent and young adult patients who were experiencing painful episodes. Hypnosis was induced through the use of eye fixation and progressive muscle relaxation techniques. Images were used in which the patients placed themselves in a favorite place, engaged in an enjoyable activity, and were free of pain or concern. Subsequent images focused on body warmth and vasodilation (a reversal of the vaso-occlusive state); thermal biofeedback was employed to monitor changes in peripheral temperature. Instructions were given to use these techniques at the perceived onset of a sickle-cell crisis. Reductions in the frequency and intensity of pain crises, the need for heavy analgesia, the frequency of emergency room visits, and the frequency and length of hospitalizations were shown.

Similar techniques and results were obtained in a larger study conducted with 15 adults between 22 and 35 years of age (Thomas, Koshy, Patterson, Dorn, & Thomas, 1984). Finally, in an investigation with eight patients between the ages of 10 and 20 years, Cozzi, Tryon, and Sedlacek (1987) demonstrated the immediate short-term effectiveness of biofeedback training (e.g., frontalis muscle tension, digital temperature, frequency of headache as a crisis symptom, analgesic use, perceived pain intensity), but no significant effect on emergency room or inpatient utilization. Clearly, more systematic research is needed concerning the efficacy of both pharmacological and nonpharmacological interventions for recurrent pain in sickle-cell disease.

Sickle-Cell Disease and Chronic Pain

The key assumption underlying an acute pain model of intervention is that the pain is principally peripheral in its origin (Crue, 1985). Implicit here is the notion that once the condition resolves, the pain will dissipate and the patient will return to a normal routine. Also implicit is the fact that psychological factors play a relatively small part in the patient's pain experience; thus, these issues are often ignored. For most pediatric and adolescent sickle-cell disease patients, the acute pain model is valid (Walco & Dampier, 1987). There is a minority, however, for whom psychological and social issues play a major role in affecting their pain experience; thus, these issues should not be ignored. Typically, these patients are adolescents whose life-style is marked by maladaptive coping patterns, poor psychological adjustment, inadequate family and social support, and school absenteeism and failure. Clearly, to ignore these factors and continue hospitalizing such patients for pain only contributes to the cycle of dependency on the medical system and withdrawal from prosocial activities.

Although it seems that these psychological factors parallel those found in adults with chronic pain syndromes, devising appropriate assessment and treatment strategies is difficult. For example, when such a patient presents in the emergency room complaining of severe pain, medical professionals are faced with the truly impossible task of determining the extent to which that pain is due to vaso-occlusion or to psychosocial factors. In actuality, such a strict dichotomization cannot be made and is rarely productive. However, for many professionals, this distinction exists and carries the incorrect implication that the former is "real" pain, while the latter is "all in the patient's head." As a result, antagonistic relationships develop between patients and caregivers which often lead to manipulation and malingering. Furthermore, because treatment of pain follows from assessment, medical professionals are faced with another conflict. As mentioned above, if pathophysiologic factors are emphasized while psychological and social issues are ignored, the maladaptive pattern is reinforced. On the other hand, if one assumes that the pain is purely psychological, there is a strong likelihood of undertreating a severe vaso-occlusive episode.

Walco and his colleagues (Varni, Walco, & Wilcox, 1990; Walco & Dampier, 1987) contended that in order to treat such patients adequately, biomedical, psychological, and social factors must be addressed. Behaviorally based interventions, usually in the form of behavioral contracts, have been employed, including protocols specifying the frequency and duration of hospitalizations (for uncomplicated painful episodes), inpatient analgesic dosing schedules, frequency of emergency room visits, and availability of narcotics for outpatient use. Each of these variables are modified over time to successively approximate norms for matched peers, and all medical personnel are provided with these protocols so that responses are standardized and few relevant decisions are made on a subjective basis.

These behavioral contracts have been successful in curbing inappropriate health care utilization. Also, the frequency and intensity of manipulative or malingering behavior has decreased. Quality of life outside of the hospital, however, does not improve dramatically until other interventions are introduced to specifically address psychological maladjustment. Our clinical work here has included facilitating reentry to school, building social skills, working to improve the family system, and, in some cases, psychopharmacological interventions. Currently, a controlled study is in progress in which these variables, and possible related interventions, are being examined systematically.

SUMMARY

Psychologists workiing on inpatient medical units have been making substantial contributions to the assessment and management of pain in children. It is rarely the case that this is done in isolation, and so a close interdisciplinary tie with medical professionals is essential. The advantages for physicians are clear in that by reducing pain and acute distress, patient management is much easier. It is also a great opportunity for psychologists, since the hospital serves as a relatively well-controlled environment for research protocols that are aimed at refining assessment and intervention strategies. Finally, such interdisciplinary endeavors are ultimately most beneficial to patients because their comprehensive medical and psychosocial needs may be met.

REFERENCES

Attia, J., Amiel-Tison, C., & Mayer, M. N. (1987). Measurement of postoperative pain and narcotic administration in infants using a new clinical scoring system. *Anesthesiology, 67*, 532.

Berde, C. B. (1989). Pediatric postoperative pain management. *Pediatric Clinics of North America, 36*, 921–940.

Beyer, J. E., & Bournaki, M. (1989). Assessment and management of postoperative pain in children. *Pediatrician, 16*, 30–38.

Beyer, J. E., & Levine, C. R. (1987). Issues and advances in pain control in children. *Nursing Clinics of North America, 22*, 661–676.

Beyer, J. E., DeGood, D. E., Ashley, L. C., & Russell, G. A. (1983). Patterns of postoperative analgesic use with adults and children following cardiac surgery. *Pain, 17*, 71–81.

Blount, R. L., Corbin, S. M., Sturges, J. W., Wolfe, V. V., Prater, J. M., & James, L. D.

(1989). The relationship between adults and child coping and distress during BMA/LP procedures: A sequential analysis. *Behavior Therapy, 20*, 586–601.

Burokas, L. D. (1985). Factors affecting nurses' decisions to medicate pediatric patients after surgery. *Heart and Lung, 14*, 373–379.

Bush, J. P., Holmbeck, G. N., & Cockrell, J. L. (1989). Patterns of PRN analgesic drug administration in children following elective surgery. *Journal of Pediatric Psychology, 14*, 433–448.

Carman, D., & Roach, J. W. (1988). Transcutaneous electrical nerve stimulation for the relief of postoperative pain in children. *Spine, 13*, 109–110.

Chapman, C. R., & Bonica, J. J. (1983). *Acute pain. Current concepts*. Kalamazoo, MI: Upjohn.

Cole, T. B., Sprinkle, R. H., Smith, S. J., & Buchanon, G. R. (1986). Intravenous narcotic therapy for children with severe sickle cell pain crisis. *American Journal of Diseases of Children, 140*, 1255–1259.

Cozzi, L., Tryon, W. W., & Sedlacek, K. (1987). The effectiveness of biofeedback-assisted relaxation in modifying sickle cell crisis. *Biofeedback and Self-Regulation, 12*, 51–61.

Crue, B. L. (1985). Multidisciplinary pain treatment programs: Current status. *Clinical Journal of Pain, 1*, 31–38.

Dash, J. (1980). Hypnosis for symptom amelioration. In J. Kellerman (Ed.), *Psychological aspects of childhood cancer* (pp. 215–230). Springfield, IL: Charles C Thomas.

Dash, J. (1981). Rapid hypno-behavioral treatment of a needle phobia in a five-year-old cardiac patient. *Journal of Pediatric Psychology, 6*, 34–42.

Dodd, E., Wang, J. M., & Rauk, R. L. (1988). Patient-controlled analgesia for post-surgical pediatric patients, ages 6–16 years. *Anesthesiology, 68*, 372.

Ellenberg, L., Kellerman, J., Dash, J., Higgins, G., & Zeltzer, L. (1980). Use of hypnosis for multiple symptoms in an adolescent girl with leukemia. *Journal of Adolescent Health Care, 1*, 132–137.

Ferguson, J. M., Taylor, C. B., & Wermuth, B. (1978). A rapid behavioral treatment of needle phobias. *Journal of Nervous and Mental Disease, 166*, 194–298.

Fernald, D. C., & Corry, J. J. (1981). Empathic versus directive preparation of children for needles. *Children's Health Care, 10*, 44–47.

Gardner, G. G. (1976). Childhood death and human dignity: Hypnotherapy for David. *International Journal of Clinical and Experimental Hypnosis, 24*, 122–139.

Gaukroger, P. B., Tomkins, D. P., & van der Walt, J. H. (1989). Patient-controlled analgesia in children. *Anesthesia and Intensive Care, 17*, 264–268.

Hannallah, R. S., Broadman, L. M., Belman, A. B., Abramowitz, M. D., & Epstein, B. S. (1987). Control of post-orchidopexy pain in pediatric outpatients: Comparison of two regional techniques. *Anesthesiology, 66*, 832–834.

Hilgard, J. R., & LeBaron, S. (1982). Relief of anxiety and pain in children and adolescents with cancer: Quantitative measures and clinical observations. *International Journal of Clinical and Experimental Hypnosis, 32*, 417–442.

Hubert, N., Jay, S. M., Saltoun, M., & Hayes, M. (1988). Approach-avoidance and distress in children undergoing preparation for painful medical procedures. *Journal of Child Clinical Psychology, 17*, 194–202.

Jay, S. M. (1988). Invasive medical procedures: Management of pain and discomfort. In D. Routh (Ed.), *Handbook of pediatric psychology* (pp. 401–425). New York: Guilford Press.

Jay, S. M., & Elliott, C. H. (1990). A stress inoculation program for parents of children undergoing painful medical procedures. *Journal of Consullting and Clinical Psychology, 58*, 799–804.

Jay, S. M., Ozolins, M., Elliott, C. H, & Caldwell, S. (1983). Assessment of children's distress during painful medical procedures. *Health Psychology, 2,* 133–147.
Jay, S. M., Elliott, C. H., Katz, E. R., & Siegel, S. E. (1987). Cognitive-behavioral and pharmacologic interventions for children undergoing painful medical procedures. *Journal of Consulting and Clinical Psychology, 55,* 860–865.
Johnston, C. C. (1989). Pain assessment and management in infants. *Pediatrician, 16,* 16–23.
Karoly, P. (1988). Pain assessment in children: I. Concepts and measurement strategies. In P. Karoly (Ed.), *Handbook of child health assessment: Biopsychosocial perspectives* (pp. 357–386). New York: Wiley.
Karayalcin, G., Lanzkowsky, P., & Kazi, A. B. (1981). Serum alpha-hydroxybutyrate dehydrogenase levels in children with sickle cell disease. *American Journal of Pediatric Hematology/Oncology, 3,* 169–171.
Katz, E. R., Kellerman, J., & Ellenberg, L. (1987). Hypnosis in the reduction of acute pain and distress in children with leukemia. *Journal of Pediatric Psychology, 12,* 379–393.
Katz, E. R., Kellerman, J., & Siegel, S. E. (1980). Behavioral distress in children with cancer undergoing medical procedures: Developmental considerations. *Journal of Consulting and Clinical Psychology, 48,* 356–365.
Kellerman, J., & Katz, E. R. (1979). *Psychological referrals in pediatric hematology-oncology.* Unpublished manuscript.
Kellerman, J., & Varni, J. W. (1982). Pediatric hematology-oncology. In D. C. Russo & J. W. Varni (Eds.), *Behavioral pediatrics: Research and practice* (pp. 67–100). New York: Plenum Press.
Kellerman, J., Zeltzer, L., Ellenberg, L., & Dash, J. (1983). Adolescents with cancer: Hypnosis for the reduction of acute pain and anxiety associated with medical procedures. *Journal of Adolescent Health Care, 4,* 85–90.
Lawrence, C., & Fabry, M. E. (1986). Erythocyte sedimentation rate during steady state and painful crisis in sickle cell anemia. *American Journal of Medicine, 81,* 801–809.
Lovell, D. J., & Walco, G. A. (1989). Pain associated with juvenile rheumatoid arthritis. *Pediatric Clinics of North America, 36,* 1015–1027.
Mather, L., & Mackie, J. (1983). The incidence of postoperative pain in children. *Pain, 15,* 271–282.
McIlvaine, W. B. (1989). Perioperative pain management in children: A review. *Journal of Pain and Symptom Management, 4,* 215–229.
Meichenbaum, D., & Turk, D. (1976). The cognitive-behavioral management of anxiety, anger, and pain. In P. O. Davidson (Ed.), *The behavioral management of anxiety, depression, and pain* (pp. 1–34). New York: Brunner/Mazel.
Melzack, R. (1975). The McGill Pain Questionnaire: Major properties and scoring methods. *Pain, 1,* 277–299.
O'Hara, M., McGrath, P. J., D'Astous, J., & Vaip, C. A. (1987). Oral morphine versus injected meperidine (Demerol) for pain relief in children after orthopedic surgery. *Journal of Pediatric Orthopedics, 1,* 78–82.
Peterson, L. (1989). Coping by children undergoing stressful medical procedures: Some conceptual, methodological, and therapeutic issues. *Journal of Consulting and Clinical Psychology, 57,* 380–387.
Peterson, L., & Shigetomi, C. (1981). The use of coping techniques to minimize anxiety in hospitalized children. *Behavior Therapy, 12,* 1–14.
Richards, J. S., Nepomuceno, C., Riles, M., & Suer, Z. (1982). Assessing pain and behavior: The UAB Pain Behavior Scale. *Pain, 14,* 393–398.
Rodgers, B. M., Webb, C. J., Stergios, D., & Newman, B. M. (1988). Patient-controlled analgesia in pediatric surgery. *Journal of Pediatric Surgery, 23,* 259–262.

Savedra, M. C., & Tesler, M. D. (1989). Assessing children's and adolescents' pain. *Pediatrician, 16,* 24–29.
Schechter, N. L. (1989). The undertreatment of pain in children: An overview. *Pediatric Clinics of North America, 36,* 781–794.
Schechter, N. L., Allen, D. A., & Hanson, M. A. (1986). Status of pediatric pain control: A comparison of hospital analgesic usage in children and adults. *Pediatrics, 77,* 11–15.
Schechter, N. L., Berrien, F. B., & Katz, S. M. (1988). The use of patient controlled analgesia in adolescents with sickle cell pain crisis. *Journal of Pain and Symptom Management, 3,* 1–5.
Scott, R. B. (1982). The management of pain in children with sickle cell disease. In R. B. Scott (Ed.), *Advances in the pathophysiology, diagnosis, and treatment of sickle cell disease* (pp. 47–58). New York: Alan R. Liss.
Shannon, M., & Berde, C. B. (1989). Pharmacologic management of pain in children and adolescents. *Pediatric Clinics of North America, 36,* 855–871.
Shapiro, B. S. (1989). The management of pain in sickle cell disease. *Pediatric Clinics of North America, 36,* 1029–1045.
Siegel, L. J. (1989, October). *Postoperative pain in children: Incidence and patterns of management.* Paper presented at the American Pain Society, Phoenix, Arizona.
Siegell, L. J., & Smith, K. E. (1989). Children's strategies for coping with pain. *Pediatrician, 16,* 110–118.
Smith, K. E., Ackerson, J. D., & Blotcky, A. D. (1989). Reducing distress during invasive medical procedures: Relating behavioral interventions to preferred coping style in pediatric cancer patients. *Journal of Pediatric Psychology, 14,* 405–419.
Spielberger, C. D., Gorsuch, R. L., & Lushene, R. (1970). *The State-Trait Anxiety Inventory Manual.* Palo Alto, CA: Consulting Psychologists Press.
Thomas, J. E., Koshy, M., Patterson, L., Dorn, L., & Thomas, K. (1984). Management of pain in sickle cell disease using biofeedback therapy: A preliminary study. *Biofeedback and Self-Regulation, 9,* 413–420.
Thompson, K. L., & Varni, J. W. (1986). A developmental cognitive-biobehavioral approach to pediatric pain assessment. *Pain, 25,* 282–296.
Tree-Trakarn, T., Pirayavaraporn, S., & Lertakyamanee, J. (1987). Topical analgesia for relief of post-circumcision pain. *Anesthesiology, 67,* 395–399.
Troug, R., & Anand, K. J. S. (1989). Management in pain in the postoperative neonate. *Clinics of Perinatology, 16,* 61–78.
Varni, J. W. (1981a). Behavioral medicine in hemophilia arthritic pain management. *Archives of Physical Medicine and Rehabilitation, 62,* 183–187.
Varni, J. W. (1981b). Self-regulation techniques in the management of chronic arthritic pain in hemophilia. *Behavior Therapy, 12,* 185–194.
Varni, J. W. (1983). *Clinical behavioral pediatrics: An interdisciplinary biobehavioral approach.* New York: Pergamon Press.
Varni, J. W., & Gilbert, A. (1982). Self-regulation of chronic arthritic pain and long-term analgesic dependence in a hemophiliac. *Rheumatology and Rehabilitation, 22,* 171–174.
Varni, J. W., & Jay, S. M. (1984). Biobehavioral factors in juvenile rheumatoid arthritis: Implications for research and practice. *Clinical Psychology Review, 4,* 543–560.
Varni, J. W., & Thompson, K. L. (1985). *The Varni/Thompson Pediatric Pain Questionnaire.* Unpublished manuscript.
Varni, J. W., Gilbert, A., & Dietrich, S. L. (1981). Behavioral medicine in pain and analgesia management for the hemophilic child with factor VIII inhibitor. *Pain, 11,* 121–126.
Varni, J. W., Thompson, K. L., & Hanson, V. (1987). The Varni/Thompson Pediatric Pain

Questionnaire: I. Chronic musculoskeletal pain in juvenile rheumatoid arthritis. *Pain, 28,* 27–38.
Varni, J. W., Walco, G. A., & Wilcox, K. T. (1990). Cognitive-biobehavioral assessment and treatment of pediatric pain. In A. M. Gross & R. S. Drabman (Eds.), *Handbook of clinical behavioral pediatrics* (pp. 83–109). New York: Plenum Press.
Walco, G. A., & Dampier, C. D. (1987). Chronic pain in adolescent patients. *Journal of Pediatric Psychology, 12,* 215–225.
Walco, G. A., & Dampier, C. D. (1990). Pain in children and adolescents with sickle cell disease: A descriptive study. *Journal of Pediatric Psychology, 15,* 643–658.
Walco, G. A., & Varni, J. W. (1991). Cognitive-behavioral interventions for children with chronic illnesses. In P. C. Kendall (Ed.), *Child and adolescent therapy: Cognitive-behavioral procedures* (pp. 209–244). New York: Guilford Press.
Walco, G. A., Varni, J. W., & Ilowite, N. T. (in press). Cognitive-behavioral interventions for pain in children with juvenile rheumatoid arthritis. *Pediatrics.*
Warth, J. A., & Rucknagel, D. L. (1984). Density ultra centrifugation of sickle cells during and after pain crisis: Increased dense erythrocytes in crisis. *Blood, 64,* 507–515.
Zeltzer, L., & LeBaron, S. (1982). Hypnosis and non-hypnotic techniques for reduction of pain and anxiety during painful procedures in children and adolescents with cancer. *Journal of Pediatrics, 101,* 1032–1035.
Zeltzer, L., Kellerman, J., Ellenberg, L., Dash, J., & Rigler, D. (1980). Psychological effects of illness in adolescence: II. Impact of illness in adolescents: Crucial issues and coping styles. *Journal of Pediatrics, 97,* 132–138.
Zeltzer, L. K., Dash, J., & Holland, J. P. (1979). Hypnotically induced pain control in sickle cell anemia. *Pediatrics, 64,* 533–536.

8

Conduct Disorder

David J. Kolko

Introduction

The antisocial and aggressive acts that constitute the conduct disorder (CD) syndrome share a number of characteristics. First, many of the behaviors (e.g., fighting, stealing, cruelty, property destruction) that are so pervasive among clinic populations also occur in the general population. Second, a child's involvement in aggressive behaviors is generally stable across time. Third, the adverse impact of a child's antisocial behavior is often felt more by the child's parents, siblings, teachers, and peers. Yet, even though CD children themselves may evince little concern for their behavior, their involvement in troublesome activities may restrict opportunities for receiving desired peer relationships and social supports. These conditions may be salient correlates and/or precipitants of escalating involvement in delinquency, illicit drug use, exposure to harsh parental consequences and violent behavior, and family conflict and dissolution. Not surprisingly, the cost of intervention to society is substantial and, given existing clinical approaches, may be met with only minimal success. Thus, the disorder is both prevalent and associated with diverse forms of impairment (see Offord, Boyle, & Racine,

---

David J. Kolko • Western Psychiatric Institute and Clinic, University of Pittsburgh School of Medicine, 3811 O'Hara Street, Pittsburgh, Pennsylvania 15213.

Inpatient Behavior Therapy for Children and Adolescents, edited by Vincent B. Van Hasselt and David J. Kolko. Plenum Press, New York, 1992.

1991). The clinical aspects of this disorder that convey this prognosis merit further discussion.

CLINICAL DESCRIPTION OF THE DISORDER

The diagnostic criteria for CD have been modified consistently through the years. The most recent symptoms are based on the revised *Diagnostic and Statistical Manual of Mental Disorders* (DSM-III-R) (American Psychiatric Association, 1987). Essentially, the diagnosis is given to children who exhibit a persistent pattern (i.e., for a period of at least 6 months) of conduct that violates age-appropriate social norms and the rights of others. The child's troublesome acts are likely to be exhibited in multiple settings. No single behavior or set of primary symptoms is required for diagnostic classification. Instead, the child merely needs to exhibit at least 3 of 13 individual symptoms. Of course, aggression against both peers and adults that persists despite parental punishment and other sanctions is a primary component. The other symptoms reflect offenses of varying degrees of severity against property (e.g., stealing, destruction, fire setting) and people (e.g., assault, rape), as well as noncriminal status offenses (e.g., lying, running away, truancy). Thus, the disorder involves antisocial activities that generally include physical aggression and other highly provocative behaviors.

Three subtypes of CD are included in the DSM-III-R; namely, the solitary aggressive type, the group type, and the undifferentiated type. The solitary aggressive type, which is similar to the Undersocialized Aggressive type included in the DSM-III (American Psychiatric Association, 1980), is characterized by persistent physical aggression exhibited by the individual alone. In contrast, the group type, which corresponds to the Socialized Nonaggressive type in the DSM-III, involves the display of diverse conduct problems in a group context wherein there exists some loyalty to group members. Finally, the undifferentiated type represents a category with clinical features that preclude classification into either of the two previous types.

The specification of CD subtypes in the DSM-III provided recognition of the breadth, severity, and complexity of its associated features, such as severe defiance of authority, disruptive behaviors, drug use, academic underachievement, depression, impulsivity, and overactivity, as well as limited frustration tolerance, empathy, or guilt (see Kolko, 1989). Other aspects of this disorder reflect deficits in interpersonal, cognitive/problem-solving, academic, and self-control skills.

These include limited conversational skills (Hansen, St. Lawrence, & Christoff, 1988), social skill in response to provocation (Dodge, McClaskey, & Feldman, 1985), and positive affective repertoires displayed towards peers (Panella & Henggeler, 1986). Apart from displaying limited problem-solving skills (see Camp & Ray, 1984), aggressive children have been found to maintain excessive attributions of hostility or blame (Fondacaro & Heller, 1990; Lochman, 1987), highlighting a social information-processing style that is prone to perceptual distortions of others. CD children may have co-diagnoses of clinical concern in their own right, such as attention-deficit/hyperactivity disorder and major depressive disorder. Indeed, subtypes with varied patterns of comorbidity are common in this population (see Hinshaw, 1987; Werry, Reeves, & Elkind, 1987).

Among inpatient populations, CD manifests itself in a range of provocative behaviors and at levels that often raise serious concerns about the safety of the children themselves and others. For example, it is not unusual for such children to inflict serious injuries upon their child victims and to show histories of homicidal threats, self-abuse, and severe mood lability. Recent assessments highlight the breadth of antisocial acts among inpatient CD children that reflect both aggressive and hostile response patterns (Kazdin & Esveldt-Dawson, 1986; Kazdin, Rodgers, Colbus, & Siegel, 1987). The commission of both overt and covert antisocial acts in this population is of significant clinical concern, a combination that seems to portend a poor prognosis (Loeber & Schmaling, 1985). Many of these behaviors are cross-situational and of long-standing duration, persisting across time despite exposure to outpatient interventions (e.g., medications, behavior modification). Not uncommonly, these children evince alternative patterns of chronic involvement in antisocial behavior (Loeber, 1985). Corroboration of this pattern of adjustment comes from a study of child inpatients that found that CD children functioned more poorly at home and at school over the course of a 2-year follow-up than did non-CD children (Kazdin, 1989). However, both CD and non-CD children evinced significant improvements over the course of hospitalization.

Parental and family dysfunction also are well documented among hospitalized CD children. Parents may suffer from their own psychiatric disorders, including depression and substance abuse (Jary & Stewart, 1985), and/or exhibit diverse deficits in child management abilities in such areas as monitoring and discipline (Patterson, 1986; Patterson & Bank, 1986). This overall picture can be exacerbated by marital conflict in an often volatile home environment where inconsistency, coercion, and both physical punishment and family violence are all too frequently used for control purposes (Patterson, Dishion, & Bank, 1984). The degree of conflict among family members is even apparent in clinic meetings or during informal transitional times. A common outcome of this type of severely disturbed and disorganized family situation is out-of-home placement.

Behavioral and Psychiatric Assessment

Numerous assessment strategies for evaluation of the characteristics and correlates of this disorder have been reviewed by Kazdin (1987a) and McMahon (1987), with some sources emphasizing inpatient assessment of aggression and antisocial behavior (Feindler & Ecton, 1986; Goldstein & Keller, 1987). In accord with the broad clinical features and correlates described earlier, present conceptualizations of CD have greatly expanded the context of assessment to include several domains and dimensions. Relevant examples of representative measures for assessment and evaluation of CD from the child, parent, family, and social system/community domains are shown in Table 1.

These measures illustrate characteristics and correlates of CD that provide a comprehensive evaluation of the child and the family. Understandably, a multimodal framework is required in order to best operationalize and then integrate the clinical information gleaned from all these sources. To this end, clinical interviews with the child and parents are conducted to document the child's and parents' psychiatric dysfunction and related clinical concerns (e.g., presenting complaints, past psychiatric history, contact with mental health services), as is generally characteristic of inpatient treatment with any childhood disorder. This diagnostic formulation should be supplemented with data from a family social history (e.g., developmental progress, family events, medical problems, family resources), academic evaluation, and several standardized self-report instruments that evaluate the child's repertoire of both deviant and prosocial behaviors.

Despite its limited resources and inherent artificiality, the inpatient unit permits opportunities for behavioral assessment of child behavior and family interactions that supplement these other measures. The child can be observed during school to assess classroom conduct, academic performance, and peer relations (e.g., Abikoff, Martin, & Gittelman, 1985; Horn, Conners, Wells, & Shaw, 1986), and during general unit settings, such as meals, free-play, and recreational activities, to examine self-care, motor, conversational/social, anger-control and self-control,

Table 1. Measures for Assessment of Individual Domains Associated with Conduct Disorder

Domain/measure	Reference
Child	
Diagnostic profile	
Kiddie-SADS	Chambers, Puig-Antich, Hirsch, Paez, Ambrosini, & Davies, 1985
Psychopathology	
Child Behavior Checklist	Achenbach & Edelbrock, 1983
Teacher Report Form	Edelbrock & Achenbach, 1984
Antisocial behavior/agression	
Interview for Antisocial Behavior	Kazdin & Esveldt-Dawson, 1986
Children's Hostility Inventory	Kazdin, Rodgers, Colbus, & Siegel, 1987
Covert Problem Behavior Scale	Stouthamer-Loeber & Loeber, 1989
Self-Report of Delinquency	Elliot, Huizinga, & Morse, 1985
Ratings of antisocial behavior	Curtiss, Rosenthal, Marohn, Ostrov, Offer, & Trujillo, 1983
Observations of aggression	Feindler, Ecton, Kingsley, & Dubey, 1986
Anger potential	
Children's Inventory of Anger	Finch & Eastman, 1983
Anger ratings in simulations	Kolko, Dorsett, & Milan, 1981
Temperament	
Dimensions of Temperament Scale-R	Windle & Lerner, 1984
Emotionality-Activity-Sociability-Impulsivity Temperament Scale	Plomin, 1983
Social competence	
Matson Evaluation of Social Skills of Youngsters	Matson, Rotatori, & Helsel, 1983
Interpersonal style	
Children's Action Tendency Scale	Deluty, 1979
Peer relations	
Peer Nominations	Coie, Dodge, & Coppotelli, 1982
Loneliness Scale for Children	Asher & Wheeler, 1985
Problem-solving ability	
Open Middle Test—Revised	Pellegrini, 1985
Social-information processing style	
Dyadic interaction ratings	Lochman, 1987

(*continued*)

Table 1. (Continued)

Domain/measure	Reference
Parent	
Psychopathology	
Schedule of Affective Disorders and Schizophrenia—Lifetime	Endicott & Spitzer, 1978
Schedule of Affective Disorders and Schizophrenia—Children	Johnson, Magrao, & Stern, 1986
Marital discord	
Dyadic Adjustment Scale	Spanier, 1976
Child management ability	
Structured Observation System	Budd, Riner, & Brockman, 1983
Family	
Verbal/physical conflict resolution	
Conflict Tactics Scales	Straus, 1979
Family Interaction Coding System	Reid, 1978
Family/home environment	
Family Environment Scale	Moos, Insel, & Humphrey, 1974
Home Environment Questionnaire	Laing & Sines, 1982
Parent–child relationships	
Children's Report of Parenting Behavior Inventory	Crook, Raskin, & Eliot, 1981
Life experiences	
Children's Life Events Inventory	Chandler, 1984
Extrafamily Relationships/Resources	
Community/family relations	
Community Interaction Checklist	Dumas & Wahler, 1983
Social/economic support	
Socioeconomic profile	Dumas & Wahler, 1983
Social Network Support	Salzinger, Kaplan, & Artemyeff, 1983

and organizational skills. More general measures of psychopathology that tap clusters of symptoms documented during clinical interviews can also be obtained on a daily basis using the Child Behavior Rating Form (CBRF) (Kolko, 1988), along with a profile representing the frequency of times-out, number of points earned and lost in any unit-wide token or point system, and involvement in prosocial, "bonus" behaviors. Of course, assessment may be enhanced through the use of standardized, analogue, role-play measures of social competence (Dodge *et al.*, 1985) and retrospective problem-solving reviews of critical incidents documented by staff that complement observations of the child's actual unit performances.

The ability to structure situations and to manipulate stimulus conditions (e.g., play, work tasks, compliance) based on information derived from existing measures of home behavior (e.g., Chamberlain & Reid, 1987) can facilitate inpatient assessment of family interaction. For example, commonly used clinic-based tasks and measures can be simplified to examine the parent's role and efficacy during child management situations, the child's responsiveness to each parent, and each participant's overall behavioral repertoire (Budd, Riner, & Brockman, 1983; Dishion, Gardner, Patterson, Reid, Spyrou, & Thibodeaux, 1984; Forehand & McMahon, 1981). Additionally, the processes by which coercion escalates (e.g., positive or negative reinforcement of child deviant behavior) may be carefully documented for diagnostic purposes and later reviewed to assess progress during treatment. The role of siblings may be pursued when functional analysis details suggest either differential responsiveness by the children or to the children by the parents.

COGNITIVE-BEHAVIORAL TREATMENTS

Conceptual Model of Aggression

Several complementary behavioral approaches to treatment appear warranted during inpatient hospitalization, many of which may be applied on an outpatient basis (Dumas, 1989; Frankel & Simmons, 1985; Kazdin, 1985, 1987a,b; Kolko, 1989; Scruggs, Mastropieri, Cook, & Escobar, 1986). Because of the complexity and residential nature of the inpatient environment, a clear understanding of the role of aggression and both the policy and procedures governing its regulation and control is a therapeutic prerequisite.

A model has been proposed for managing aggressive adults in an inpatient setting that addresses these considerations (Maier, Stava, Morrow, Van Rybroek, & Bauman, 1987). Apart from examining different phases associated with the process of aggression, the model describes factors that perpetuate the cycle, provides descriptions of patients' seclusion experiences and staff perspectives on aggression, and indicates the differences between verbal and physical aggression. A notable component in the model is the postulation of a hierarchy of therapeutic responses to different forms of aggression and at different points in the process (e.g., ambulatory restraints, special "me-time," verbal control, seclusion). Several treatment/management issues that impact on the consistency with which these strategies are implemented must be addressed, such as effective leadership, adequate staffing patterns, concerns for the rights of patients and the use of medication. These general considerations are particularly important in managing highly aggressive child inpatients.

Contingency Management

One of the most basic interventions designed to provide a consistent set of expectations covering a broad range of behaviors and to facilitate general child management is integrated through the use of contingency management. Based on the assumption that antisocial behavior and the environment in which it is expressed are functionally related, explicit consequences are arranged for strengthening desired and weakening undesired behaviors (Stumphauzer, 1973).

Token Economy. The token economy (or point system), in particular, is a comprehensive system for motivating patients to engage in or refrain from appropriate and inappropriate behaviors, respectively (Ayllon & Azrin, 1968; Kazdin, 1982). The rationale, operations, resources, and outcome evidence associated with this approach have been well detailed elsewhere (Kazdin, 1977), as well as specific applications with antisocial youth (Karacki & Levinson, 1970). Briefly, the token economy describes the relationship between individual behaviors and their immediate consequences. Children earn tokens or other symbols (e.g., points, checks, stars) contingent upon exhibiting positive behaviors which are later exchanged for more preferred, backup reinforcers. These backup reinforcers can include tangible items (e.g., toys, self-care products), social time (e.g., talking with staff), activity privileges (e.g., air hockey time), and edible items (e.g., snacks). Among the prerequisites for a successful token economy are the following: (1) objective and clear definitions of all behaviors/expectations, (2) a convenient and reliable medium for registering or monitoring token performances, (3) a diverse range of presumably effective backup reinforcers, (4) explicit arrangements between each behavior and its intended consequence, and (5) exchange rates indicating the costs of backup reinforcers.

A few issues may be considered to enhance the implementation and impact of token systems. First, children may benefit from prompts to engage in any additional desired behaviors which were not exhibited and a review of the number of tokens earned in each individual activity. Second, the frequency with which children receive backup reinforcers and the range of available reinforcers should be tailored to the specific population. Reinforcers for some children may need to be delivered frequently at first (e.g., on a daily basis), whereas others may be able to be delayed for longer time periods. Third, the reasons for a child's apparent unresponsiveness to the system should be carefully examined. Potential reasons include unusual reinforcer preferences, the child already possessing many of the reinforcers in the system, and the absence of a well-developed repertoire for making use of the reinforcer. Many of these suggestions might be addressed using a levels system in which different levels of performance and types of reinforcers are balanced. Accordingly, children who meet certain expectations at the most basic level proceed to a higher level with more diverse expectations and reinforcers. Such systems provide some degree of individualization in the context of a unit-wide program (see Gable & Strain, 1981).

Time-out and Seclusion. Although still controversial, time-out and seclusion in residential settings are regarded as generally beneficial in promptly reducing the level of serious antisocial behavior and in protecting remaining children in the area (Foxx, 1982; Gair, Bullard, & Corwin, 1984; Soloff, 1987). Different forms of time-out from positive reinforcement can be implemented following aggressive behavior, including brief momentary time-out within a setting, isolation in a separate setting, or seclusion in a room with the door locked (Romoff, 1987). In many settings, the form of time-out is contingent upon the type and severity of the infraction. For example, mild noncompliance or provocation may be managed using a one-minute, corner time-out, whereas assault or involvement in a fight may be more effectively handled using seclusion. Isolation has also been used effectively to reduce more mild forms of disruption and misbehavior (Tyler & Brown, 1967).

Apart from determining its location, several components and parameters may be considered in using time-out (Forehand & McMahon, 1981; Foxx, 1982; Wilson & Lyman, 1982). A few specific procedures are suggested: (1) provide a warning for certain behaviors; (2) state a reason for time-out; (3) minimize use of physical methods to enforce the procedure by using backup contingencies for compliance; (4) limit the duration of time-out (generally $<$ 20 min) and impose it in a convenient place; (5) provide a clear indication as to the conclusion of time-out; and (6) discuss prosocial alternatives following the procedure during a short debriefing period. In addition, the imposition of additional fines for needing to take a time-out or seclusion may enhance the impact of this procedure. Additional decisions should be made to determine whether a child is released contingent upon being calm for a specific period of time, whether time-out should be used intermittently during the later stages of hospitalization, and whether exclusionary time-out or isolation should be used for more serious behaviors. A clear illustration of the procedural components of time-out is found in Foxx (1982).

Instructions and Commands. The staff of an inpatient setting constantly present instructions to initiate or terminate behavior. Because noncompliance with instructions is not only common among psychiatrically disturbed children but also a potential precursor to antisocial behavior, special attention must be paid to the manner in which commands are delivered. Technical aspects of appropriate instructions and reprimands have been described (Forehand & McMahon, 1981; Van Houten, Nau, MacKenzie-Keating, Sameoto, & Colavecchia, 1982) and include the use of simple, clear, and singular commands, eye contact and firm tone of voice, close physical proximity, and frequent praise. Administration of appropriate instructions in a relatively positive manner may enhance compliance and, ultimately, reduce the need to consequate any ensuing deviant behavior. Moreover, carefully executed reprimands may elicit more desired behavior among nontargeted children (Van Houten *et al.*, 1982), whereas general methods for improving compliance may be associated with reductions in nontargeted deviant behavior (Parrish, Cataldo, Kolko, Neef, & Egel, 1986).

Child Skills Training

The increasing role of skills training or psychoeducational programming in inpatient settings is designed, in part, to address the limited generalization and maintenance that often follows exposure to contingency management programs (see Lochman, 1990). Direct training also provides more focused opportunities to expand the prosocial repertoire of the CD child. Three related approaches whose training emphasis lies predominantly in the social, cognitive, and affective domains will be highlighted here.

General Social and Conversational Skills. As noted earlier, youths exhibiting aggressive behavior have been found to exhibit deficiencies in prosocial skill (Freedman, Rosenthal, Donahoe, Schlundt, & McFall,

1978; Hansen *et al.*, 1988). To remediate these deficits, aggressive inpatients have been exposed to training techniques (e.g., instructions, modeling, behavioral rehearsal or role-playing, performance feedback, social/tangible reinforcement) designed to teach discrete social and anger-control skills on an individual basis (e.g., Bornstein, Bellack, & Hersen, 1980; Kolko, Dorsett, & Milan, 1981). Treatment may be associated with improvements in social interaction and reductions in aggressivity (Goldstein & Glick, 1987; Ladd, 1985; Schneider & Byrne, 1987).

As applied on an inpatient unit, a group format for skills training provides exposure to multiple models and opportunities for interaction, closely approximates the child's actual peer system or network, and is likely to be efficient and cost-effective (Rose & LeCroy, 1985). Group applications with CD patients in residential settings (Hansen, St. Lawrence, & Christoff, 1989; Jamison, Lambert, & McCloud, 1987; Kolko, Loar, & Sturnick, 1990) and with adolescent male offenders (Long & Sherer, 1985) have reported at least one improvement in a targeted skill (e.g., eye contact) or an associated psychological attribute likely to mediate one's social interactions (locus of control). However, only two of these studies reported consistent gains in individual skills and improved social competence during hospitalization (Hansen *et al.*, 1989; Kolko *et al.*, 1990).

Incorporation of recent improvements in procedure, curriculum, and methodology could bolster program impact during hospitalization. To assure that the content and skills selected for training are based on the deficiencies of the targeted population, an effort should be made to socially validate the skills selected for training (Hansen *et al.*, 1988; Kolko *et al.*, 1990). Procedures that individualize the targets of training by developing idiosyncratic skill sequences and mastery criteria have been found helpful before initiating instruction (Schneider & Byrne, 1987). Of course, numerous skill targets that can be observed during hospitalization appear relevant for aggressive children, including helping others, sharing, providing positive support, being empathic, and expressing affection (Dubow, Huesmann, & Eron, 1987; Goldstein & Glick, 1987).

Group programs may also benefit from the use of specialized audiovisual materials, including interactional games and skits, cooperative role-play tasks, program workbooks and worksheets, and modeling films (Bierman & Furman, 1984; Hardwick, Pounds, & Brown, 1985; Rose & LeCroy, 1985). By attending to the appeal and reinforcing value of the curriculum, these materials may facilitate group cohesion, motivation and task involvement, participation, and overall mastery of program concepts. For example, board games that have been used to teach verbal social skills to adult psychiatric inpatients (Foxx, McMorrow, Bittle, & Fenlon, 1987) are among the many curricula that have been developed for teaching social skills. In addition, the inclusion of problem scenarios directed toward various key "significant others" (e.g., parents, teachers, peers) and use of multiple role-play partners may enhance the realism and functional significance of training (Dubow *et al.*, 1987; Goldstein & Glick, 1987).

Guidelines for inpatient instruction also emerge from recent training applications. Attention should be paid to increasing the child's involvement in and satisfaction with peer relationships, in addition to mastery of behavioral skill objectives. Suggested program components include involvement in cooperative peer group experiences that provide explicit opportunities for peer interaction (Bierman & Furman, 1984) and the use of prohibitions and consequences for misbehavior (Bierman, Miller, & Stabb, 1987). The combination of these procedures may be needed to enhance both behavioral performances and peer sociometric status, and may maximize the benefit of participation in cooperative peer interactions (see Bierman & Schwartz, 1986).

Generalization and maintenance of performance should be addressed from the inception of training, especially in view of the artificial nature and temporary stay of an inpatient setting. In the study by Kolko *et al.* (1990), teachers and randomly selected staff members ("Secret Agents") monitored participants' interactions following training and reinforced correct use of the skill learned that day. This *in vivo* enhancement procedure was designed to promote skill use in more naturalistic settings (e.g., classroom, meals, free-play). Inpatient settings permit multiple opportunities for reinforcement of extratherapy behavior and for brief "tutorials" that review and correct the failure to engage in prosocial skills. Programs that integrate diverse skills, these and other training techniques, and related procedural considerations in the context of scripted session outlines have been disseminated (Goldstein & Glick, 1987; Goldstein & Keller, 1987).

Problem-Solving Skills. Difficulties in the use of cognitive-mediational strategies to regulate behavior have been documented among impulsive and aggressive children (Camp & Bash, 1981; Kendall & Braswell, 1985; Lochman, 1987; Lochman & Lampron, 1986; Spivack & Shure, 1974). Initial applications of problem-solving training conducted in classrooms and directed toward children who are at risk for social adjustment (Spivack, Platt, & Shure, 1976; Spivack & Shure, 1974, 1982) and school mental health problems (Weissberg, 1985) provide a therapeutic approach suitable for inpatient populations. These group-based programs offer a range of didactic training manuals, teacher and therapist guidelines, worksheets, and supplementary materials. In general, training consists of modeling specific responses to individual tasks, soliciting and evaluating potential solutions, and then providing practice exercises to promote use of the skill. Among the many skills taught are the following: (1) problem definition, (2) goal statement, (3) impulse delay, (4) generation of alternatives, (5) consideration of consequences, and (6) implementation. Training may result in improvements in problem-solving performance and, to some extent, general child adjustment.

Aggressive or patient populations have been encouraged to apply cognitive mediational skills to novel interpersonal situations using repeated practice and therapist feedback. For example, the Think Aloud program (see Camp & Ray, 1984) incorporates both self-regulatory skills (e.g., using verbalization to inhibit behavior, understanding cause and effect) and techniques designed to foster spontaneous use of the skills (e.g., overt followed by covert verbalization, multiple contexts). The lessons emphasize the use of various cognitive, academic, and social problems (e.g., mazes, puzzles, conflicts) that are increased in complexity and the degree of required verbal control over nonverbal behavior. The initial program (Camp & Bash, 1981) has been updated in the form of a comprehensive curriculum for regular classrooms (Camp & Bash, 1985) that, with a few modifications, would be applicable to group-based inpatient treatment. Problem-solving can also be supplemented by related strategies, such as training in social-perspective taking, observation of modeling videotapes, the making of personalized problem-solving videotapes, and the use of behavioral goal setting (Lochman, Burch, Curry, & Lampron, 1984; Lochman & Curry, 1986), and may be enhanced if intervention is of sufficient duration (Lochman, 1985). In one study, outpatient CD children met in groups over a 20-week period while parents attended similar group meetings in which they were exposed to program concepts and principles and were encouraged to apply these principles to the home (Yu, Harris, Solovitz, & Franklin, 1986). These applications have reported reductions in aggression and behavioral dysfunction, and/or improved prosocial orientation or social competence, although long-term follow-up results reflect moderate improvements (Lochman, 1988).

The integration of many of these program components with psychiatrically hospitalized children has been reported in noteworthy studies by Kazdin (Kazdin, Bass, Siegel, & Thomas, 1989; Kazdin, Esveldt-Dawson, French, & Unis, 1987a,b). Apart from extending this approach to inpatients, these studies are significant due to their inclusion of comparison conditions (nondirective relationship therapy, treatment-contact control), collection of 1-year follow-up data, use of multidimensional parent and teacher rating scales, and documentation of treatment integrity. For example, in the Kazdin *et al.* 1987a study, children received a structured individual skills training program that provided exposure to academic tasks and games followed by real-life social situations, a response cost component involving a loss of chips to discourage noncompliance and program errors, and individualized homework assignments. Compared to the two comparison conditions, trained children showed significant reductions in aggressive and externalizing behaviors and increases in prosocial behaviors both at home and in school, which were maintained at follow-up.

In the second study (Kazdin *et al.*, 1989), problem-solving skills training was supplemented with an *in vivo* practice component directed toward encouraging the children's use of their skills in extratherapy contexts. Relative to an extended version of problem-solving skills training alone, the combined condition was associated with greater changes in child performance at posttraining but not at follow-up. Both problem-solving conditions were superior to a relationship therapy condition. The fact that many children from all three groups still remained outside the normative range for prosocial behavior invites further elaborations of this approach with inpatients, such as more intensive treatment, the addition of home-based programming, school consultation, and booster sessions. With further attention being paid to observational assessment methods (Ladd, 1985), the clinical relevance of training in problem-solving skills may be more fully promoted.

Self-Control and Combined Social-Cognitive Skills. Given their complementary nature, social and cognitive skills training approaches have been combined in order to target several response domains that may enhance overall impact, a level of therapeutic intensity that is likely to be achieved on an inpatient unit. Thus, the integration of group training in problem-solving and progressive muscle relaxation with focused practice (Nardone, Tryon, & O'Connor, 1986) and other self-control procedures (e.g., self-instructions, positive assertion, self-evaluation) may aid in controlling aggression (Feindler, Ecton, Kingsley, & Dubey, 1986). Training in problem-solving and prosocial skills has also targeted aggressive schoolchildren (Dubow *et al.*, 1987) and adolescents in residential treatment (Baum, Clark, McCarthy, Sandler, & Carpenter, 1986). For example, Baum *et al.* (1986) provided training in social skills and imagery/self-instructions, cue-controlled relaxation, along with booster sessions, homework review, and specialized incentives to improve therapeutic outcome. After training in coping/problem-solving skills and exposure to other procedures (modeling, response cost, reinforcement for correct performances), children in day treatment have shown improved self-control and prosocial behavior and reported greater social competence, although the maintenance of treatment effects appeared somewhat limited (Kendall, Reber, McLeer, Epps, & Ronan, 1990).

One recently disseminated curriculum for residential youth is noteworthy for its selection of program elements that individually have been found to influence aggression or prosocial behavior (Goldstein & Glick, 1987). Accordingly, the program consists of structured learning in prosocial skills, anger control training, and moral education as a means of improving the aggressive adolescent's social, affective, and cognitive repertoires, respectively. A recent extension of this effort includes material covering communication training, contracting, and contingent management (Goldstein & Keller, 1987). Given their novelty, such comprehensive and multimodal programs would seem to be applicable on an inpatient basis, but require further evaluation in order to document their relative utility and cost-effectiveness.

Parent, Marital, and Family Skills Training

The long history of teaching behavioral principles and procedures to parents in an attempt to improve their childrens' adjustment takes on special significance when working with psychiatrically disturbed children (see Griest & Wells, 1983). In addition to suffering from their own behavioral and emotional problems, parents often utilize physically punitive child-rearing techniques that encourage the expression of aggression as a problem-solving or conflict-resolution strategy, avoid positive disciplinary methods, and possess few resources likely to facilitate treatment (Patterson, 1982). Not surprisingly, the instigation of aggressive or coercive parent–child interactions often eventuates in reciprocally aversive, intense, and escalating sequences of antisocial behavior. Consequently, therapeutic services directed towards parents and/or families are likely to be both comprehensive and intensive (see Miller & Prinz, 1990).

In terms of recommended program components, parents should first be familiarized with the terms and techniques associated with social learning theory (Patterson, 1975, 1976) before receiving intensive training in the contingent application of behavioral methods. For example, Patterson, Reid, Jones, and Conger (1975) required parents to review program materials, observe and record deviant child behavior in the home, and then apply behavioral techniques (e.g., positive reinforcement, time-out, response-cost). It is often advisable to train parents initially to use clear instructions, warnings, and positive attention, among other basic procedures, in order to improve the child's generalized compliance (Forehand & McMahon, 1981). To facilitate inpatient application, parents may be given opportunities to observe *in vivo* application of consequences by staff members and then be encouraged to practice the skills with siblings at home, to observe their children in different hospital settings (perhaps behind a one-way mirror), and to implement new techniques during unstructured visits and family meetings. The clinical utility of this general approach with the families of aggressive and antisocial children has been well documented (Fleischman, 1982; Fleischman & Szykula, 1981; Patterson & Fleischman, 1979).

In accord with these components, one recent application consisted of parent training conducted during short-term hospitalization which provided instruction in several management tasks, such as positive reinforcement, contracting, and time-out, in combination with child-directed problem-solving (Kazdin *et al.*, 1987b). The individualized treatment, which was subsequently completed on an outpatient basis, led to reductions in deviant behavior and improvements in social competence at home and in school which were maintained at 1-year follow-up.

Variations of the parent's basic training package are often needed to facilitate the involvement of parents of hospitalized CD children. One option is the use of group training methods that integrate exposure to modeling videotapes and therapist-led discussion (Webster-Stratton, 1984, 1985; Weinrott, Bauske, & Patterson, 1979). In addition to their cost-effectiveness, inpatient groups offer parents opportunities to share common problems and experiences, receive group feedback, and obtain social suppport. This particular curriculum seems especially well-suited to parents who require training in several basic monitoring and disciplinary skills. An alternative includes self-administration of parent training videotapes that depict the application of individual skills to various interactions (Webster-Stratton, Hollinsworth, & Kolpacoff, 1989). This videotape "library" allows parents to take the training program home or to schedule training at any time that is convenient for them. To supplement training, written materials and worksheets that can be reviewed at home under less stressful conditions may be used to facilitate parents' understanding of frequently foreign technical procedures (Barkley, 1987; Dangel & Polster, 1988; Fleischman, Horne, & Arthur, 1983), a strategy that may minimize common obstacles (e.g., reluctance, limited time/money) to continued participation in didactic training sessions.

Additional procedures that embellish the targets and content of treatment may be needed to maximize the utility of parent training programs. For parents with psychiatric disturbances, notably, maternal depression, formal evaluation and treatment may be needed in order to enhance the parent's general effectiveness and motivation (see Dumas, 1989). Treatment designed to alleviate severe marital discord or spousal violence by improving the couple's cohesion or supportiveness may actually precede training in child management skills (Griest & Forehand, 1982). Several brief training programs have emphasized positive forms of communication, marital problem-solving and conflict-resolution, and self-control skills with good results (Dadds, Sanders, Behrens, & James, 1987; Dadds, Schwartz, & Sanders, 1987; Kelley, Embrey, & Baer, 1979; Sanders, 1982; Sanders & Glynn, 1981; Wells, Griest, & Forehand, 1980). For example, the use of "partner support training" (e.g., providing immediate responses to problems, communication and problem-solving skills) with maritally discordant couples is likely to enhance outcome following standard Parent Management Training (PMT) (Dadds, *et al.*, 1987). Generalization of behavior to novel settings and follow-up maintenance may be promoted if parents are taught to use planned activities with their children (Dadds, Sanders, & James, 1987).

Other methods are directed toward improving parental adjustment and functioning, and, ultimately, the generalized effectiveness of parent training (Wahler, 1980). To address parents' tendencies to overstate the negative behavior of their children, efforts can be made to improve the accuracy of their perceptions by providing mothers with redefinitions of their summary reports of coercive child behaviors (Wahler, Sansbury, Benders, & Bryant, 1985). This form of attributional retraining is consistent with the more general approach of altering parents' communication patterns pertaining to interactions with their children during parent training (Wahler, Sansbury, Benders, Bryant, & Bond, 1988) and functional family therapy (Alexander & Parson, 1982).

Improvements in parents' social support and the quality of their extrafamily relationships likewise may be beneficial (Dumas & Whaler, 1983; Wahler, 1980), though intervention methods have not yet emerged. Possibilities for parents of hospitalized children include establishing friendships during group training programs, incorporating extended family members during specific training sessions, and providing parents with special "nights out" during designated hospital visiting hours. It also may prove clinically beneficial to advocate on behalf of the family when negotiating financial arrangements, cross-system or agency contacts, and the introduction of novel child treatments. Several of these targets have been incorporated successfully into parent training programs (Griest *et al.*, 1982).

CASE HISTORY

Background

H. was an 11.6-year-old, black female who was placed in respite care the week prior to admission because of several episodes of running away from her current foster family. She had a long history of conduct problems, including fighting, lying, truancy, impulsivity, stealing, noncompliance, and school underachievement. The primary reasons for referral included increasing unmanageability in foster care, throwing lighted matches, attempts to set furniture on fire, and running away. In addition, the foster mother awoke one night and found H. standing at the foot of her bed holding two butcher knives. She had also become increasingly threatening/aggressive and sexually provocative.

H. attended the fifth grade of a regular elementary school. For the past 3 years, she had resided with her foster parents and their five children, ages 6 to 16 years. She was also in the custody of the local Children and Youth Services agency. Foster placement was initiated after the child proved unmanageable under her biological mother's care. H. was reported to have been physically and sexually abused by her biological father who was serving a jail sentence for theft.

Assessment

Psychiatric assessment upon admission revealed an Axis I diagnosis of CD: undersocialized aggressive, with no diagnoses on Axes II or III. A Child Behavior Checklist (CBCL) completed by her foster mother yielded the following significant T-scores: Delinquent (82), Aggressive (72), Cruel (70), Hyperactive (77), Sex Problems (82), and Schizoid/Obsessive (70). Her Wechsler Intelligence (WISC-R) subscale scores were 77 Verbal, 92 Performance, and 83 Full Scale. On the Peabody Individual Achievement Test (PIAT), she received a reading recognition score of 8.9 and a reading comprehension score of 8.1. There was no history of psychosis, neurological deficits, seizures, metabolic or endocrine encephalopathies, or severe medical illness. She was admitted on no medication.

Conditions and Outcome

Unit observations during a 2-week baseline condition confirmed H.'s frequent and often volatile acts of physical aggression directed toward staff and peers, as well as noncompliance. She was also observed making threats of aggression on several occasions. In accord with unit protocol, aggression precipitated a 10-point loss and a 10-minute, locked seclusion, whereas continued noncompliance resulted in a sequence of consequences (i.e., initial 2-point loss, open seclusion, locked seclusion). To reflect these outcomes, the total number of seclusions because of physical aggression and general noncompliance were recorded (see Figure 1). Beginning with the third week, seclusions for threats of aggression were recorded. During the first and second weeks of hospitalization (Baseline), H. had four and nine seclusions for aggression, respectively (M = 6.5). She punched staff members on several occasions, with two incidents resulting in physical injuries. Release from seclusion was often followed by out-of-control behaviors that eventuated in provocation or further aggression. The aggres-

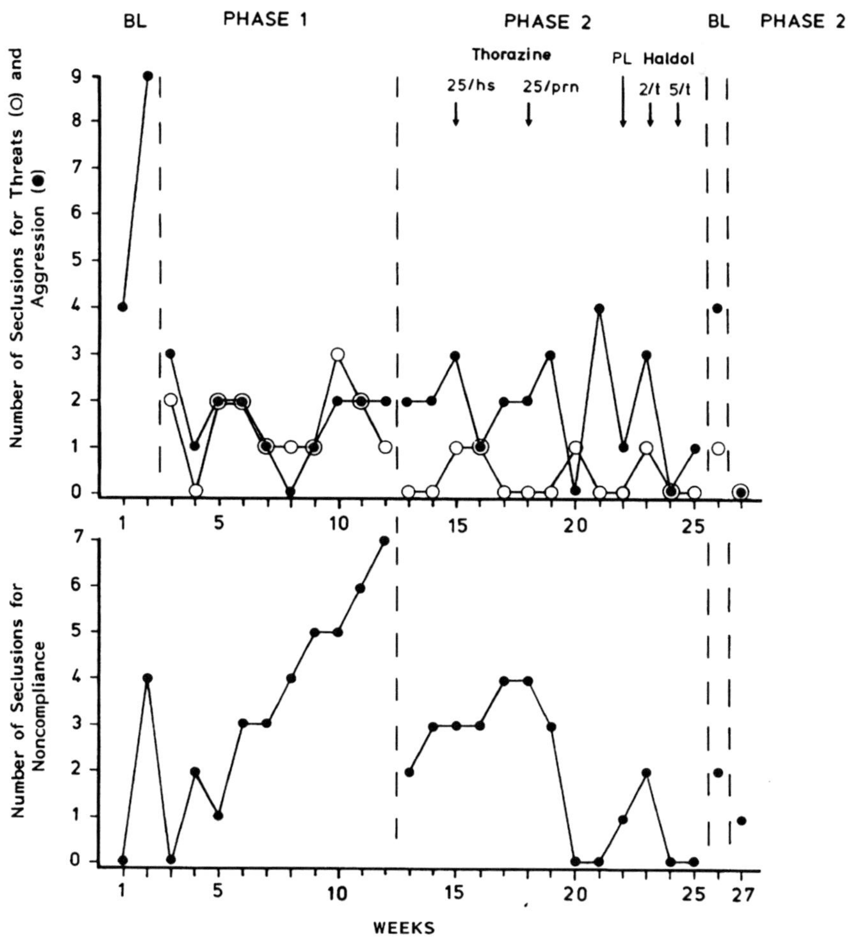

Figure 1. Weekly frequency of seclusions for aggression, threats, and noncompliance across the different phases of inpatient treatment.

sion was often preceded by loud and hostile threatening statements which generally reflected her unwillingness to comply with unit rules, explicit staff requests, or staff-administered consequences for deviant behavior.

In light of these functional analysis details, initial intervention (Phase 1) consisted of a 2-Hour Threat Contingency/Problem-Solving "Talk Down" condition. Thus, as shown in Figure 1, seclusions for threats were initiated in this condition. Accordingly, each episode of threatening behavior resulted in a 1-hour locked seclusion, whereas aggression resulted in a 2-hour seclusion. Following seclusion, a problem-solving debriefing was implemented in which she reviewed with a staff member the details of the incident (e.g., what happened, what she did, and what staff did) and specific alternative solutions (e.g., what did she really want; how could she really get this). Differential reinforcement of other behavior (DRO) using praise was also used to strengthen her problem-solving and other prosocial behaviors. Introduction of this condition resulted in a dramatic and generally stable reduction in seclusions for aggression ($M = 1.5$). Seclusions for threats also occurred intermittently ($M = 1.5$); however, seclusions for noncompliance showed a consistent increase throughout this condition ($M = 3.3$).

Therefore, Phase 2 consisted of a general DRO contingency in which H. received a preferred reinforcer (e.g., bag of assorted edibles, toy, art supply) for demonstrating good compliance and controls, and being seclusion-free during each of four, 4-hour periods. Ratings of these two behaviors were made each period. In addition, all locked seclusions were reduced in duration to 1-hour for the first 3 weeks of the condition before being reduced to 30-minutes. A bonus contingency was also added whereby she earned 1:1 time with staff if she remained seclusion-free for the entire day, an outcome that occurred for 75% of the days in this phase. As shown in Figure 1, the number of seclusions for noncompliance were reduced considerably during the first 2 weeks of this condition ($M = 1.9$). H. had no seclusions for threats of aggression, but she continued to have intermittent seclusions for aggression.

To explore the incremental benefit of medication, Thorazine (25 mg/HS) was added (weeks 15–17) and then administered on an as-needed basis (weeks 18–21) before being discontinued. Next, a brief, double-blind, Haldol/placebo trial was initiated with placebo (week 22) being followed by Haldol (2 mg/TID, weeks 23; 5 mg/TID, weeks 24–25). The number of seclusions for aggression and threats continued to remain comparably low during all of these medication conditions, especially the Haldol/placebo trial. Of course it is difficult to determine whether the eventual reduction in seclusions for noncompliance was aided by the introduction of Thorazine.

Discontinuation of the DRO/30-minute seclusion contingency program was attempted (week 26) to examine the relative impact of intervention, but it resulted in an immediate increase in the number of seclusions for both aggression and noncompliance. Resumption of this behavioral procedure in her final week of hospitalization was associated with the return to a near zero rate in all seclusions.

Conclusions

Although such findings do not emerge from a well-controlled experimental design, they nonetheless suggest the clinical utility of integrating operant consequences for antecedent behaviors (threats that precede physical aggression), focused problem-solving skills training (debriefing, generating alternatives), and subsequent DRO procedures that target seclusions in general (tangible/social reinforcement for no seclusions) in controlling serious aggression and noncompliance. Continued improvement was achieved when the length of seclusion was generally reduced to a routine duration, which may have been abetted by the development of greater self-control over threatening behavior. Numerous procedures were combined in order to target various aspects of H.'s antisocial behaviors. The case also suggests that behavioral and pharmacological interventions may provide complementary approaches to the control of physically aggressive and provocative behavior.

PROBLEM AREAS

Contingency Management

Based on samples of staff–patient interactions, staff implementation of specific contingencies may be inconsistent (Kolko, McCanna, & Donaldson, 1989), largely on account of stressful or chaotic circumstances or general disorganization. To maximize their participation, all staff should participate in in-service training programs and then demonstrate criterion mastery of all principles and procedures before being monitored on a regular basis (see Milne, 1985). Because of the CD child's intimidating repertoires, the appropriateness of staff responses to child behavior once training has been completed should then be periodically monitored. With aggressive and hostile children, in particular, staff members often find themselves perpetuating a similar cycle of increased coercion and punitiveness that may obstruct therapeutic progress.

An additional obstacle to behavioral consistency is the diffusion of responsibility inherent in the use of multiple change agents who interact with individual children both briefly and at different times. On a large unit, for example, there is a tendency to imitate certain staff members who may or may not perform completely and/or to experience difficulty communicating important details regarding changes in contingencies. Relatedly, the integrity of specific procedures varies as a function of the frequency with which the procedure is needed and/or used. That is, staff may begin to misapply or fail to apply a procedure once it has proven helpful with a given child. This may reflect the tendency to rapidly shift attention to a child's remaining deviant behaviors that have not responded to intervention.

Child Skills Training

One of the more obvious limitations of skills training during an inpatient stay is the unavailability of nondeviant peers to reinforce appropriate behavior. Although children may acquire prosocial skills, high levels of antisocial and defiant behavior may interfere with sincere attempts to practice these skills. It is not uncommon for children to show mastery of skill concepts and engage in adaptive role-plays in a training session only to engage in impulsive and antisocial acts once they return to the unit. Thus, it may be necessary to have the children return to small but well-controlled group situations in which there is a high density of reinforcing activities and staff members (see Bierman *et al.*, 1987; Kolko *et al.*, 1990).

The artificial and restricted environment of an inpatient unit also carries therapeutic limitations. First, many of the settings or situations in which CD children evince their behavior problems are not found in the hospital, thereby precluding *in vivo* practice, although practical methods for promoting generalization have been reported (Kazdin *et al.*, 1989). Similarly, certain deviant behaviors that often occur under conditions of reduced monitoring in the community (e.g., firesetting, drug use, truancy, curfew violations) are obviously prevented during hospitalization. The difficulty in training children to engage in alternative behaviors upon exposure to the cues or precipitants inherent in these settings presents a challenge that requires considerable creativity in developing meaningful simulations of these situations.

A final issue pertains to the children's individual motives or goals. The majority of skills-based programs assume that training will alter the motivation to behave appropriately once the child is exposed to program concepts. However, few programs provide explicit attention to procedures or information that will alter the child's preferences for self-serving or antisocial behaviors. That is, children are trained to engage in prosocial behaviors or to think constructively about alternative options in solving a problem such that various outcomes or effects are considered (e.g., hitting may result in harm, whereas asking nicely may result in compliance). However, further attention is needed to the mechanism by which one can alter a child's preference for deviant behavior in the direction of expecting benefits from prosocial behaviors and believing in the worthiness of goals that promote or value self-enhancement and social-system enhancement. The work of Arbuthnot and Gordon (1986) and Goldstein and Glick (1987) is supportive of this direction. Perhaps incorporation of these techniques will expedite treatment and shorten what are otherwise the often delayed effects of skills training programs.

Parent, Marital, and Family Skills Training

Because families with severely dysfunctional children are often extremely disorganized and dysfunctional themselves, they exhibit various risk factors and therapeutic obstacles that complicate parental involvement (e.g., parental psychopathology, family dysfunction, significant role confusion, limited family resources and social supports, frequent crises). Indeed, the adverse clinical impacts of many of these contextual or ecological characteristics make them worthwhile therapeutic targets in their own right (see Dumas, 1989; Lochman, 1990). It is not surprising, for example, that these variables impede attendance, in-session compliance and mastery of program concepts, home practice of individual techniques, and *in vivo* application once the child has returned home. Disturbed parents may require their own psychiatric treatment while the child is hospitalized which then may postpone parent training or family therapy until after the child is discharged. Likewise, other aspects of the family's limited socioeconomic resources may constrain a child's opportunities for peer socialization and involvement in out-of-home activities, or parent's participation in outpatient treatment.

The desire to promote a child's return home and the motivation to negotiate or reciprocate during sessions are perhaps the most basic significant prerequisites to treatment which many parents may fail to satisfy. In many cases, the discord between hospitalized children and their parents has become so extensive that the parents are no longer interested in caring for and in maintaining custody of the child. The dissolution of some families during hospitalization, then, is not always antagonistic to the child's overall welfare, though it obviously curtails participation in certain therapeutic activities and, in all likelihood, disrupts other treatments in which these parties might be involved.

Discharge Planning and Community Outreach

Providing attention devoted to improving parental and family functioning is one of the ways to promote a child's home and community adjustment. This objective is greatly abetted to the extent that the child's return to the home and school environment has been well planned and reviewed. This often involves discussing treatment plans and procedures with parents, making arrangements for weekend visits, reviewing successful treatment procedures with the child's community teacher to promote generalization, establishing a liaison and effective working relationship with the child's community therapist, and clarifying the criteria for using hospitalization in the future. All too often, however, these tasks are delegated to a member of the treatment team just prior to discharge. Clearly, efforts to facilitate the child's efficient return home, as with other therapeutic considerations, should be addressed soon after admission (Rancurrelo, 1987).

SUMMARY

Hospitalized CD children and their parents have multiple psychological and psychiatric problems, few personal and social resources, and histories of limited response to prior outpatient interventions. At the same time, inpatient treatment is often short and unable to accommodate the staff and time resources required to conduct labor-intensive behavioral training efforts. Despite these impediments, admission is often needed to initiate treatments so that children are exposed to operant consequences for deviant behavior and interventions that train cognitive, affective, and social skills, and parents are involved in both child- and family-focused interventions. Indeed, certain data suggest long-term improvements in the adjustment of hospitalized CD children, though fewer gains have been found for these children relative to non-CD children (Kazdin, 1989; see Pfeiffer & Strzelecki, 1990). Of course, these integrated services must be continued in the form of follow-up treatment to maximize gains. To this end, close contact and monitoring of family stability should be maintained so that imminent crises can be addressed and revisions in home programming made in the context of booster sessions. The addition of pharmacological treatments is also likely to enhance long-term outcome (see Campbell, Green, & Deutsch, 1985; Leventhal, 1984; Stewart, Myers, Burket, & Lyles, 1990; Tupin, 1987).

At present, there is cautious optimism about the utility of inpatient behavioral treatment of CD children in light of limited data regarding generalization across time and settings. This provides a significant challenge to the proponents of cognitive-behavioral approaches who must begin to integrate psychological methods with alternative therapeutic approaches while establishing a mechanism by which families can receive continuity of care throughout the developmental and family-system changes associated with this chronic disorder.

REFERENCES

Abikoff, H., Martin, D., & Gittelman, R. (1985). Social interaction observation code. *Psychopharmacology Bulletin, 21,* 869–873.

Achenbach, T. M., & Edelbrock, C. S. (1983). *Manual for the Child Behavior Checklist and Revised Child Behavior Profile.* Burlington: University of Vermont, Department of Psychiatry.

Alexander, J. F., & Parson, B. V. (1982). *Functional family therapy.* Monterey, CA: Brooks/Cole.

American Psychiatric Association. (1980). *Diagnostic and statistical manual of mental disorders* (3rd ed.). Washington, DC: Author.

American Psychiatric Association. (1987). *Diagnostic and statistical manual of mental disorders (3rd ed., rev.).* Washington, DC: Author.

Arbuthnot, J., & Gordon, D. A. (1986). Behavioral and cognitive effects of a moral reasoning development intervention for high-risk behavior-disordered adolescents. *Journal of Consulting and Clinical Psychology, 54,* 208–216.

Asher, S. R., & Wheeler, V. A. (1985). Children's loneliness: A comparison of rejected and neglected peer status. *Journal of Consulting and Clinical Psychology, 53,* 500–505.

Ayllon, T., & Azrin, N. H. (1968). *The token economy: A motivational system for therapy and rehabilitation.* New York: Appleton-Century-Crofts.

Barkley, R. A. (1987). *Defiant children: A clinician's manual for parent training.* New York: Guilford Press.

Baum, J. G., Clark, H. B., McCarthy, W., Sandler, J., & Carpenter, R. (1986). An analysis of the acquisition and generalization of social skills in troubled youths: Combining social skills training, cognitive self-talk, and relaxation procedures. *Child and Family Behavior Therapy, 8,* 1–27.

Bierman, K. L., & Furman, W. (1984). The effects of social skills training and peer involvement on the social adjustment of preadolescents. *Child Development, 55,* 151–162.

Bierman, K. L., & Schwartz, L. A. (1986, August). *Selecting social intervention techniques for aggressive rejected children.* Paper presented at the annual meeting of the American Psychological Association, Washington, DC.

Bierman, K. L., Miller, C. L., & Stabb, S. D. (1987). Improving the social behavior and peer acceptance of rejected boys: Effects of social skill training with instructions and prohibitions. *Journal of Consulting and Clinical Psychology, 55,* 194–200.

Bornstein, M., Bellack, A. S., & Hersen, M. (1980). Social skills training for highly aggressive children: Treatment in an inpatient setting. *Behavior Modification, 4,* 173–186.

Budd, K. S., Riner, L. S., & Brockman, M. P. (1983). A structured observation system for clinical evaluation of parent training. *Behavioral Assessment, 5,* 373–393.

Camp, B. W., & Bash, M. A. S. (1981). *Think aloud: Increasing social and cognitive skills—A problem solving program for children* (Primary level). Champaign, IL: Research Press.
Camp, B. W., & Bash, M. A. S. (1985). *Think aloud: Increasing social and cognitive skills—A problem solving program for children*. Champaign, IL: Research Press.
Camp, B. W., & Ray, R. S. (1984). Aggression. In A. W. Meyers & W. E. Craighead (Eds.), *Cognitive behavior therapy with children* (pp. 315–350). New York: Plenum Press.
Campbell, M., Green, W. H., & Deutsch, S. I. (1985). *Child and adolescent psychopharmacology*. Beverly Hills, CA: Sage Publications.
Chamberlain, P., & Reid, J. B. (1987). Parent observation and report of child symptoms. *Behavioral Assessment, 9*, 97–109.
Chambers, W. J., Puig-Antich, J., Hirsch, M., Paez, P., Ambrosini, P. J., Tabrizi, M. A., & Davies, M. (1985). The assessment of affective disorders in children and adolescents by semistructured interview: Test-retest reliability of the Schedule for Affective Disorders and Schizophrenia for school-age children, present episode version. *Archives of General Psychiatry, 42*, 696–702.
Chandler, L. A. (1984). *The Children's Life Events Inventory: Its use in clinical assessment*. Unpublished manuscript, University of Pittsburgh.
Coie, J. D., Dodge, K. A., & Coppotelli, H. A. (1982). Dimensions and types of social status: A cross-age perspective. *Developmental Psychology, 18*, 557–569.
Crook, T., Raskin, A., & Eliot, J. (1981). Parent–child relationships and adult depression. *Child Development, 52*, 950–957.
Curtiss, G., Rosenthal, R. H., Marohn, R. C., Ostrov, E., Offer, D. J., & Trujillo, J. (1983). Measuring delinquent behavior in inpatient treatment settings: Revision and validation of the Adolescent Antisocial Behavior Checklist. *Journal of the American Academy of Child Psychiatry, 22*, 459–466.
Dadds, M. R., Sanders, M. R., Behrens, B. C., & James, J. E. (1987). Marital discord and child behavior problems: A description of family interactions during treatment. *Journal of Clinical Child Psychology, 16*, 192–203.
Dadds, M. R., Sanders, M. R., & James, J. E. (1987). The generalization of treatment effects in parent training with multidistressed parents. *Behavioural Psychotherapy, 15*, 289–313.
Dadds, M. R., Schwartz, S., & Sanders, M. R. (1987). Marital discord and treatment outcome in behavioral treatment of child conduct disorders. *Journal of Consulting and Clinical Psychology, 55*, 396–403.
Dangel, R. F., & Polster, R. A. (1988). *Teaching child management skills*. New York: Pergamon Press.
Deluty, R. H. (1979). Children's Action Tendency Scale: A self-report measure of aggressiveness, assertiveness, and submissiveness in children. *Journal of Consulting and Clinical Psychology, 47*, 1061–1071.
Dishion, T. J., Gardner, K., Patterson, G., Reid, J., Spyrou, S., & Thibodeaux, S. (1984). *The Family Process Code: A multidimensional system for observing family interactions* (Oregon Social Learning Center Technical Report). (Available from Oregon Social Learning Center, 207 E. 5th Ave., Suite 202, Eugene, OR, 97401.)
Dodge, K. A., McClaskey, C. L., & Feldman, E. (1985). Situational approach to the assessment of social competence in children. *Journal of Consulting and Clinical Psychology, 53*, 344–355.
Dubow, E. F., Huesmann, L. R., & Eron, L. D. (1987). Mitigating aggression and promoting prosocial behavior in aggressive elementary school boys. *Behavioral Residential Treatment, 25*, 527–531.

Dumas, J. E. (1989). Treating antisocial behavior in children: Child and family approaches. *Clinical Psychology Review, 9*, 197–222.
Dumas, J. E., & Wahler, R. C. (1983). Predictors of treatment outcome in parent training: Mother insularity and socioeconomic disadvantage. *Behavioral Assessment, 5*, 301–313.
Edelbrock, C., & Achenbach, T. M. (1984). The teacher version of the Child Behavior Profile: I. Boys aged 6–11. *Journal of Consulting and Clinical Psychology, 52*, 207–217.
Elliot, D. S., Huizinga, D., & Morse, B. J. (1985). *Dynamics of deviant behavior: A national survey* (progress report). Boulder, CO: Behavioral Research Institute.
Endicott, J., & Spitzer, R. L. (1978). A diagnostic interview: The Schedule of Affective Disorders and Schizophrenia. *Archives of General Psychiatry, 35*, 837–844.
Feindler, E. L., & Ecton, R. B.(1986). *Adolescent anger control: Cognitive-behavioral techniques.* New York: Pergamon Press.
Feindler, E. L., Ecton, R. B., Kingsley, D., & Dubey, D. R. (1986). Group anger-control training for institutionalized psychiatric male adolescents. *Behavior Therapy, 17*, 109–123.
Finch, A. J., & Eastman, E. S. (1983). A multimethod approach to measuring anger in children. *Journal of Psychology, 115*, 55–60.
Fleischman, M. J. (1982). Social learning interventions for aggressive children: From the laboratory to the real world. *Behavior Therapist, 5*, 55–58.
Fleischman, M. J., & Szykula, S. A. (1981). A community setting replication of a social learning treatment for aggressive children. *Behavior Therapy, 12*, 115–122.
Fleischman, M. J., Horne, A. M., & Arthur, J. L. (1983). *Troubled families: A treatment program.* Champaign, IL: Research Press.
Fondacaro, M. R., & Heller, K. (1990). Attributional style in aggressive adolescent boys. *Journal of Abnormal Child Psychology, 18*, 75–89.
Forehand, R., & McMahon, R. J. (1981). *Helping the noncompliant child: A clinician's guide to parent training.* New York: Guilford Press.
Foxx, R. M. (1982). *Decreasing behaviors of severely retarded and autistic persons.* Champaign, IL: Research Press.
Foxx, R. M., McMorrow, M. J., Bittle, R. G., & Fenlon, S. J. (1987). Teaching social skills to psychiatric inpatients. *Behavior Research Therapy, 23*, 531–537.
Frankel, F., & Simmons, J. Q. (1985). Behavioral treatment approaches to pathological unsocialized physical aggression in young children. *Journal of Child Psychology and Psychiatry, 26*, 525–551.
Freedman, B. J., Rosenthal, L., Donahoe, C. P., Schlundt, D. G., & McFall, R. M. (1978). A social-behavioral analysis of skills deficits in delinquent and nondelinquent adolescent boys. *Journal of Consulting and Clinical Psychology, 46*, 1448–1462.
Gable, R., & Strain, P. (1981). Individualizing a token reinforcement system for the treatment of children's behavior disorders. *Behavioral Disorders, 7*, 39–45.
Gair, D. S., Bullard, D. M., & Corwin, J. M. (1984). Guidelines for children and adolescents. In K. Tardiff (Ed.), *The psychiatric uses of seclusion and restraint* (pp. 69–85). Washington, DC: American Psychiatric Press.
Goldstein, A. P., & Glick, B. (1987). *Aggression replacement training: A comprehensive intervention for aggressive youth.* Champaign, IL: Research Press.
Goldstein, A. P., & Keller, H. (1987). *Aggressive behavior: Assessment and intervention.* New York: Pergamon Press.
Griest, D. L., & Forehand, R. (1982). "How can I get any parent training done with all these other problems going on?": The role of family variables in child behavior therapy. *Child and Family Behavior Therapy, 4*, 73–80.

Griest, D. L., & Wells, K. C. (1983). Behavioral family therapy with conduct disorders in children. *Behavior Therapy, 14,* 37–53.
Griest, D. L., Forehand, R., Rogers, T., Breiner, J., Furey, W., & Williams, C. A. (1982). Effects of parent enhancement therapy on the treatment outcome and generalization of a parent training program. *Behaviour Research and Therapy, 20,* 429–436.
Hansen, D. J., St. Lawrence, J. S., & Christoff, K. A. (1988). Conversational skills of inpatient conduct-disordered youths: Social validation of component behaviors and implications for skills training. *Behavior Modification, 12,* 424–444.
Hansen, D. J., St. Lawrence, J. S., & Christoff, K. A. (1989). Group conversational-skills training with inpatient children and adolescents: Social validation, generalization, and maintenance. *Behavior Modification, 13,* 4–31.
Hardwick, P. J., Pounds, A. B., & Brown, M. (1985). Preventive adolescent psychiatry: Practical problems in running social skills groups for the younger adolescent. *Journal of Adolescence, 8,* 357–367.
Hinshaw, S. P. (1987). On the distinction between attentional deficits/hyperactivity and conduct problems/aggression in child psychopathology. *Psychological Bulletin, 101,* 443–463.
Horn, W. F., Conners, C. K., Wells, K. C., & Shaw, D. (1986). Use of the Abikoff Classroom Observation Coding System on a children's inpatient unit. *Journal of Psychopathology and Behavioral Assessment, 8,* 9–23.
Jamison, R. N., Lambert, E. W., & McCloud, D. J. (1987). Social skills training with hospitalized adolescents: An evaluative experiment. *Adolescence, 21,* 55–65.
Jary, M. L., & Stewart, M. A. (1985). Psychiatric disorder in the parents of adopted children with aggressive conduct disorder. *Neuropsychobiology, 13,* 7–11.
Johnson, M. H., Magrao, P. A., & Stern, S. L. (1986). Use of the SADS-C as a diagnostic and symptom severity measure. *Journal of Consulting and Clinical Psychology, 54,* 546–551.
Karacki, L., & Levinson, R. B. (1970). A token economy in a correctional institution for youthful offenders. *Howard Journal of Penology and Crime Prevention, 13,* 20–30.
Kazdin, A. E. (1977). *The token economy: A review and evaluation.* New York: Plenum Press.
Kazdin, A. E. (1982). The token economy: A decade later. *Journal of Applied Behavior Analysis, 15,* 431–445.
Kazdin, A. E. (1985). *Treatment of antisocial behavior in children and adolescents.* Homewood, IL: Dorsey Press.
Kazdin, A. E. (1987a). *Conduct disorders in childhood and adolescence.* Beverly Hills, CA: Sage Publications.
Kazdin, A. E. (1987b). Treatment of antisocial behavior in children: Current status and future directions. *Psychological Bulletin, 102,* 187–203.
Kazdin, A. E. (1989). Hospitalization of antisocial children: Clinical course, follow-up status, and predictors of outcome. *Advances in Behaviour Research and Therapy, 11,* 1–67.
Kazdin, A. E., & Esveldt-Dawson, K. (1986). The Interview for Antisocial Behavior: Psychometric characteristics and concurrent validity with child psychiatric inpatients. *Journal of Psychopathology and Behavioral Assessment, 8,* 289–303.
Kazdin, A. E., Esveldt-Dawson, K., French, N. H., & Unis, A. S. (1987a). Effects of parent management training and problem-solving skills training combined in the treatment of antisocial child behavior. *Journal of the American Academy of Child and Adolescent Psychiatry, 26,* 416–424.
Kazdin, A. E., Esveldt-Dawson, K., French, N. H., & Unis, A. S. (1987b). Problem-solving skills training and relationship therapy in the treatment of antisocial child behavior. *Journal of Consulting and Clinical Psychology, 55,* 76–85.

Kazdin, A. E., Rodgers, A., Colbus, D., & Siegel, T. (1987). Children's Hostility Inventory: Measurement of aggression and hostility in psychiatric inpatient children. *Journal of Clinical Child Psychology, 16*, 320–328.

Kazdin, A. E., Bass, D., Siegel, T., & Thomas, C. (1989). Cognitive-behavioral therapy and relationship therapy in the treatment of children referred for antisocial behavior. *Journal of Consulting and Clinical Psychology, 57*, 522–535.

Kelley, M. L., Embrey, L. H., & Baer, D. M. (1979). Skills for child management and family support: Training parents for maintenance. *Behavior Modification, 3*, 373–396.

Kendall, P. C., & Braswell, L. (1985). *Cognitive-behavioral therapy for impulsive children*. New York: Guilford Press.

Kendall, P. C., Reber, M., McLeer, S., Epps, J., & Ronan, K. R. (1990). Cognitive-behavioral treatment of conduct-disordered children. *Cognitive Therapy and Research, 14*, 279–297.

Kolko, D. J. (1988). Fire setting and pyromania. In C. Last & M. Hersen (Eds.), *Handbook of child psychiatric diagnosis* (pp. 443–459). New York: Wiley.

Kolko, D. J. (1989). Conduct disorder. In M. Hersen (Ed.), *Innovations in child behavior therapy* (pp. 324–352). New York: Springer.

Kolko, D. J., Dorsett, P. G., & Milan, M. A. (1981). A total-assessment approach in the evaluation of social skills training: The effectiveness of an anger-control program for adolescent psychiatric patients. *Behavioral Assessment, 3*, 383–401.

Kolko, D. J., McCanna, M., & Donaldson, L. (1989). Sequential assessment of staff administration of contingency management procedures on a child psychiatric unit. *Behavior Modification, 13*, 216–244.

Kolko, D. J., Loar, L. L., & Sturnick, D. (1990). Inpatient social-cognitive skills training for conduct disordered and attention deficit disordered children. *Journal of Child Psychology and Psychiatry, 31*, 737–748.

Ladd, G. W. (1985). Documenting the effects of social skill training with children: Process and outcome assessment. In B. Schneider, K. H. Rubin, & J. E. Ledingham (Eds.), *Children's peer relations: Issues in assessment and intervention* (pp. 243–269). New York: Springer-Verlag.

Laing, J. A., & Sines, J. O. (1982). The Home Environment Questionnaire: An instrument for assessing several behaviorally relevant dimensions of children's environments. *Journal of Pediatric Psychology, 7*, 425–449.

Leventhal, B. L. (1984). The neuropharmacology of violent and aggressive behavior in children and adolescents. In C. R. Keith (Ed.), *The aggressive adolescent* (pp. 299–358). New York: Free Press.

Lochman, J. E. (1985). Effects of different treatment lengths in cognitive behavioral interventions with aggressive boys. *Child Psychiatry and Human Development, 16*, 45–56.

Lochman, J. E. (1987). Self- and peer perceptions and attributional biases of aggressive and nonaggressive boys in dyadic interactions. *Journal of Consulting and Clinical Psychology, 55*, 404–410.

Lochman, J. E. (1988, August). Cognitive-behavioral intervention with aggressive boys: Three-year follow-up effects. In F. D. Armstrong (Chair), *Disruptive behavior disorders in children*. Paper presented at the annual meeting of the American Psychological Association, Atlanta, GA.

Lochman, J. E. (1990). Modification of childhood aggression. In M. Hersen, R. M. Eisler, & P. M. Miller (Eds.), *Progress in behavior modification* (pp. 47–85). Newbury Park, CA: Sage.

Lochman, J. E., & Curry, J. F. (1986). Effects of social problem-solving training and self-instruction training with aggressive boys. *Journal of Clinical Child Psychology, 15*, 159–164.

Lochman, J. E., & Lampron, L. B. (1986). Situational social problem-solving skills and self-esteem of aggressive and nonaggressive boys. *Journal of Abnormal Child Psychology, 14,* 605–617.

Lochman, J. E., Burch, P. R., Curry, J. F., & Lampron, L. B. (1984). Treatment and generalization effects of cognitive-behavioral and goal-setting interventions with aggressive boys. *Journal of Consulting and Clinical Psychology, 52,* 915–916.

Loeber, R. (1985). Patterns and development of antisocial child behavior. *Annals of Child Development, 2,* 77–116.

Loeber, R., & Schmaling, K. B. (1985). The utility of differentiating between mixed and pure forms of antisocial child behavior. *Journal of Abnormal Child Psychology, 13,* 315–336.

Long, S. J., & Sherer, M. (1985). Social skills training with juvenile offenders. *Child and Family Behavior Therapy, 6,* 1–11.

Maier, G. J., Stava, L. J., Morrow, B. R., Van Rybroek, G. J., & Bauman, K. G. (1987). A model for understanding and managing cycles of aggression among psychiatric inpatients. *Hospital and Community Psychiatry, 35,* 520–524.

Matson, J. L., Rotatori, A. F., & Helsel, W. J. (1983). Development of a rating scale to measure social skills in children: The Matson Evaluation of Social Skills of Youngsters (MESSY). *Behaviour Research and Therapy, 21,* 335–340.

McMahon, R. J. (1987). Some current issues in the behavioral assessment of conduct disordered children and their families. *Behavioral Assessment, 9,* 235–252.

Miller, G. E., & Prinz, R. J. (1990). Enhancement of social learning family interventions for childhood conduct disorder. *Psychological Bulletin, 108,* 291–307.

Milne, D. (1985). A review of the in-service training of nurses in behavior therapy. *Behavioural Psychotherapy, 13,* 120–131.

Moos, R. H., Insel, P. M., & Humphrey, B. (1974). *Family, work and group environment scales.* Palo Alto: Consulting Psychologists Press.

Nardone, M. J., Tryon, W. W., & O'Connor, K. (1986). The effectiveness and generalization of a cognitive-behavioral group treatment to reduce impulsive/aggressive behavior for boys in a residential setting. *Behavioral Residential Treatment, 1,* 93–103.

Offord, D. R., Boyle, M. C., & Racine, Y. A. (1991). The epidemiology of antisocial behavior in childhood and adolescence. In D. J. Pepler & K. H. Rubin (Eds.). *The development and treatment of childhood aggression* (pp. 31–54). Hillsdale, NJ: Lawrence Erlbaum.

Panella, D., & Henggeler, S. W. (1986). Peer interactions of conduct-disordered, anxious-withdrawn, and well-adjusted black adolescents. *Journal of Abnormal Child Psychology, 14,* 1–12.

Parrish, J. P., Cataldo, M. F., Kolko, D. J., Neef, N. A., & Egel, A. L. (1986). Experimental analysis of response covariation among compliant and inappropriate behaviors. *Journal of Applied Behavior Analysis, 19,* 241–254.

Patterson, G. R. (1975). *Families.* Champaign, IL: Research Press.

Patterson, G. R. (1976). *Living with children: New methods for parents and teachers* (3rd ed.). Champaign, IL: Research Press.

Patterson, G. R. (1982). *Coercive family process.* Eugene, OR: Castalia.

Patterson, G. R. (1986). Performance models for antisocial boys. *American Psychologist, 41,* 432–444.

Patterson, G. R., & Bank, L. (1986). Bootstrapping your way in the nomological thicket. *Behavioral Assessment, 8,* 49–73.

Patterson, G. R., & Fleischman, M. (1979). Maintenance of treatment effects: Some considerations concerning family systems and follow-up data. *Behavior Therapy, 10,* 168–185.

Patterson, G. R., Reid, J. B., Jones, R. R., & Conger, R. E. (1975). *A social learning approach to family intervention* (Vol. 1). Eugene, OR: Castalia.
Patterson, G. R., Dishion, T. J., & Bank, L. (1984). Family interaction: A process model of deviancy training. *Aggressive Behavior, 10*, 253–267.
Pellegrini, D. S. (1985). Social cognition and competence in middle childhood. *Child Development, 56*, 253–264.
Pfeiffer, S. I., & Strzelecki, S. C. (1990). Inpatient psychiatric treatment of children and adolescents: A review of outcome studies. *Journal of the American Academy of Child and Adolescent Psychiatry, 29*, 847–853.
Plomin, R. (1983). Childhood temperament. In B. B. Lahey & A. E. Kazdin (Eds.), *Advances in clinical child psychology* (Vol. 6, pp. 45–92). New York: Plenum Press.
Rancurello, M. (1987). Special aspects of the care of the severely disturbed child and use of psychiatric inpatient services. In R. L. Cohen & M. K. Duncan (Eds.), *Basic handbook of training in child and adolescent psychiatry* (pp. 105–116). Springfield, IL: Charles C. Thomas.
Reid, J. B. (1978). *A social learning approach to family intervention. Volume 2: Observation in home settings.* Eugene, OR: Castalia.
Romoff, V. (1987). Management and control of violent patients at the Western Psychiatric Institute and Clinic. In L. H. Roth (Ed.), *Clinical treatment of the violent person* (pp. 235–260). New York: Guilford Press.
Rose, S. D., & LeCroy, C. W. (1985). Improving children's social competence: A multimodal behavioral group approach. In D. Upper & S. M. Ross (Eds.), *Handbook of behavioral group therapy* (pp. 25–62). New York: Plenum Press.
Salzinger, S., Kaplan, S., & Artemyeff, C. (1983). Mothers' personal social networks and child maltreatment. *Journal of Abnormal Psychology, 92*, 68–76.
Sanders, M. R. (1982). The generalization of parent responding to community settings: The effects of instructions, plus feedback, and self management training. *Behavioural Psychotherapy, 10*, 273–287.
Sanders, M. R., & Glynn, T. (1981). Training parents in behavioural self management: An analysis of generalization and maintenance. *Journal of Applied Behavior Analysis, 14*, 223–247.
Schneider, B. H., & Byrne, B. M. (1987). Individualizing social skills training for behavior-disordered children. *Journal of Consulting and Clinical Psychology, 55*, 444–445.
Scruggs, T. E., Mastropieri, M. A., Cook, S. B., & Escobar, C. (1986). Early intervention for children with conduct disorders: A quantitative synthesis of single-subject research. *Behavioral Disorders, 11*, 260–271.
Soloff, P. H. (1987). Physical controls: The use of seclusion and restraint in modern psychiatric practice. In L. H. Roth (Ed.), *Clinical treatment of the violent person* (pp. 119–137). New York: Guilford Press.
Spanier, G. B. (1976). Measuring dyadic adjustment: New scales for assessing the quality of marriage and similar dyads. *Journal of Marriage and the Family, 38*, 15–28.
Spivack, G., & Shure, M. B. (1974). *Social adjustment of young children: A cognitive approach to solving real-life problems.* San Francisco: Jossey-Bass.
Spivack, G., & Shure, M. B. (1982). The cognition of social adjustment: Interpersonal cognitive problem solving thinking. In B. B. Lahey & A. E. Kazdin (Eds.), *Advances in clinical child psychology* (Vol. 5, pp. 323–372). New York: Plenum Press.
Spivack, G., Platt, J. J., & Shure, M. B. (1976). *The problem-solving approach to adjustment.* San Francisco: Jossey-Bass.
Stewart, J. T., Myers, W. C., Burket, R. C., & Lyles, W. B. (1990). A review of the phar-

macotherapy of aggression in children and adolescents. *Journal of the American Academy of Child and Adolescent Psychiatry, 29*, 269–277.

Stouthamer-Loeber, M., & Loeber, R. (1989, February). Toward a better definition of dishonesty and concealing antisocial behavior patterns in boys. In D. J. Kolko (Chair), *"Covert" child antisocial behaviors: Patterns and developmental context*. Symposium presented at the first annual meeting of the Society for Research in Child and Adolescent Psychopathology, Miami, FL.

Straus, M. A. (1979). Measuring intrafamily conflict and violence: The Conflict Tactics (CT) Scales. *Journal of Marriage and the Family, 41*, 75–88.

Stumphauzer, J. S. (Ed.). (1973). *Behavior therapy with delinquents*. Springfield, IL: Charles C. Thomas.

Tupin, J. P. (1987). Psychopharmacology and aggression. In L. H. Roth (Ed.), *Clinical treatment of the violent person* (pp. 79–95). New York: Guilford Press.

Tyler, V. O., & Brown, G. D. (1967). The use of swift, brief isolation as a group control device for institutionalized delinquents. *Behaviour Research and Therapy, 5*, 1–9.

Van Houten, R., Nau, P. A., MacKenzie-Keating, S. E., Sameoto, D., & Colavecchia, B. (1982). An analysis of some variables influencing the effectiveness of reprimands. *Journal of Applied Behavior Analysis, 15*, 65–83.

Wahler, R. G. (1980). The insular mother: Her problems in parent-child treatment. *Journal of Applied Behavior Analysis, 13*, 207–219.

Wahler, R. G., Sansbury, L. L., Benders, I., & Bryant, S. (1985). *Discriminative restructuring of the insular mother's ecosystem: A means of enhancing her problem solving capabilities*. Paper presented at the annual meeting of the Association for Advancement of Behavior Therapy, Houston.

Wahler, R. G., Sansbury, L. L., Benders, I., Bryant, S., & Bond, D. (1988). *Communication patterns in parent training interventions: A system for coding speaker and listener interactions*. Unpublished manuscript.

Webster-Stratton, C. (1984). Randomized trial of two parent-training programs for families with conduct-disordered children. *Journal of Consulting and Clinical Psychology, 52*, 666–678.

Webster-Stratton, C. (1985). The effects of father involvement in parent training for conduct problem children. *Journal of Child Psychiatry and Psychology, 26*, 801–810.

Webster-Stratton, C., Hollinsworth, T., & Kolpacoff, M. (1989). The long-term effectiveness and clinical significance of three cost-effective training programs for families with conduct-problem children. *Journal of Consulting and Clinical Psychology, 57*, 550–553.

Weinrott, M. R., Bauske, B. W., & Patterson, G. R. (1979). Systematic replication of a social learning approach to parent training. In P. Sjoden, S. Bates, & W. S. Dockens (Eds.), *Trends in behavior therapy* (pp. 331–351). New York: Academic Press.

Weissberg, R. P. (1985). Designing effective social problem-solving programs for the classroom. In B. H. Schneider, K. H. Rubin, & J. E. Ledingham (Eds.), *Children's peer relations: Issues in assessment and intervention* (pp. 225–242). New York: Springer-Verlag.

Wells, K. C., Griest, D. L., & Forehand, R. (1980). The use of a self-control package to enhance the temporal generality of a parent training program. *Behaviour Research and Therapy, 18*, 347–354.

Werry, J. S., Reeves, J. C., & Elkind, G. S. (1987). Attention deficit, conduct, oppositional, and anxiety disorders in children: A review of research on differentiating characteristics. *Journal of American Academy of Child and Adolescent Psychiatry, 26*, 133–143.

Wilson, D. R., & Lyman, R. D. (1982). Time-out in the treatment of childhood behavior problems: Implementation and research issues. *Child and Family Behavior Therapy, 4*, 5–20.

Windle, M., & Lerner, R. M. (1984). *Revised Dimensions of Temperament Survey* (DOTS-R). Unpublished scale.

Yu, P., Harris, G. E., Solovitz, B. L., & Franklin, J. L. (1986). A social problem-solving intervention for children at high risk for later psychopathology. *Journal of Clinical Child Psychology, 15,* 30–40.

9

Attention-Deficit Hyperactivity Disorder

MARK D. RAPPORT, CAROLY S. PATAKI, AND GABRIELLE A. CARLSON

INTRODUCTION

The hospitalization and treatment of children on child psychiatry inpatient units has evolved from its previous primary tasks of containment and custodial care to a more sophisticated level. Currently, there is an emphasis on the exploration of conflicts and their origins while attempting to reconstruct dysfunctions of personality and rehabilitate the child to the environment (Nurcombe, 1989). And, more recently, the child inpatient unit has become a highly specialized setting in which comprehensive diagnostic evaluation, stabilization, and brief intervention can be conducted (Jemerin & Philips, 1988). Factors responsible for these changes (e.g., the metamorphosis of the inpatient population, the costs and reimbursement associated with hospitalization, and the community resources available) (Jemerin & Philips, 1988), and their impact on the administration (Geraty, 1989), treatment (Harper, 1989; Nurcombe, 1989;

MARK D. RAPPORT • Department of Psychology, University of Hawaii, Honolulu, Hawaii 96822. CAROLY S. PATAKI AND GABRIELLE A. CARLSON • Department of Psychiatry and Behavioral Science, State University of New York at Stony Brook, Stony Brook, New York 11794–8790.

Inpatient Behavior Therapy for Children and Adolescents, edited by Vincent B. Van Hasselt and David J. Kolko. Plenum Press, New York, 1992.

Woolston, 1989), and research (Riddle, 1989) that are associated with psychiatric hospitalization have been detailed recently in a special section of the *Journal of the American Academy of Child and Adolescent Psychiatry* (Volume 28, No. 1, 1989). These factors bear directly on the topic of this chapter because they dictate the (1) type of children admitted, (2) the length, course, and goals of hospital stay, and (3) the range, potency, and delivery of therapeutic modalities that are administered.

Under usual circumstances, children suspected of having attention-deficit hyperactivity disorder (ADHD) are referred by the parent and/or the school to the family's physician, a mental health center, or a psychiatric/psychological outpatient clinic for evaluation. Treatment typically begins in a unimodal fashion and extends to a multimodal approach depending on the child's unique difficulties, the chronicity/severity of problems exhibited, the existing environment support(s), the availability of community resources, and the extent of parent/school involvement. Needless to say, the overwhelming majority of children with ADHD are neither referred to nor seen on child psychiatry inpatient units. Does the relatively small percentage of children with ADHD referred for and provided inpatient care represent, then, merely the outer portion on a severity curve for symptomatology, or are they a qualitatively different population of children? Although the breadth and complexity of this question are beyond the scope of this chapter, the empirical evidence available, albeit scant, suggests that there may be a bimodal distribution of outcome in children with ADHD (Mannuzza, Klein, Bonagura, Konig, & Shenker, 1988). Those children who continue to experience dysfunction of sufficient magnitude to qualify for a formal diagnosis at follow-up may be at risk in adulthood for the triad of ADHD, antisocial personality disorder, and substance abuse (Gittelman, Mannuzza, Shenker, & Bonagura, 1985). Children who evidence more severe manifestations of ADHD symptomatology and who are co-morbid for other disorders of childhood may thus represent not only a more deviant but a distinct population of children compared to those seen in outpatient settings.

This chapter will focus initially on providing a clinical description of children with ADHD who are admitted to and treated on child psychiatry inpatient units. The manner in which behavioral and psychiatric assessment is utilized with respect to diagnosis, implementing and monitoring treatment, and discharge planning will be discussed subsequently. Owing to the physical structure of inpatient units, the diverse populations served, and the multifaceted requirements associated with hospital care, the section on treatment will focus on describing a recently developed behavioral Inpatient Management Program (IMP)

(Rapport, Kelly, & Carlson, 1989) and its heuristic value in treating children and monitoring patient progress. A detailed case study then will be presented to illustrate the differential and combined effects of psychotherapeutic and psychopharmacological interventions on a child's ability to function on a child psychiatry inpatient unit. The interplay between these two therapeutic modalities and the manner in which their effects differ as a function of situation, structure, task, and temporal parameters on an inpatient unit will be highlighted. The remaining section will discuss problem areas associated with inpatient care of children with ADHD.

CLINICAL DESCRIPTION OF THE DISORDER

The evolution from DSM-III (American Psychiatric Association, 1980) to DSM-III-R (American Psychiatric Association, 1987) was more mercuric than had been the case with earlier evolutions of psychiatric nomenclature, with a resulting change in the name of attention deficit disorder (with or without hyperactivity) to its current moniker, Attention-Deficit Hyperactivity Disorder (ADHD). The reemergence of "hyperactivity" in the name of the disorder *suggests* to some that both excessive gross motor activity and attentional dysfunction in their various manifestations are necessary and sufficient to define the disorder. Aside from the name change, the way in which a diagnosis is derived also has been altered considerably. Diagnostic criteria are arranged in "descending order of discriminating power based on DSM-III-R field trials" rather than by core clinical areas of inattention, impulsivity, and hyperactivity. This represents a conceptual shift from a monothetic (i.e., a diagnosis made only in children exhibiting behaviors characteristic of each of the three primary core areas of the disorder) to a polythetic phenotypic category schema; that is, one in which no single characteristic is essential or sufficient for group membership, and members having the greatest number of shared characteristics or clinical features are grouped together. Some researchers disagree with the conceptual shift. However, these concerns are beyond the scope of the present chapter and have been discussed elsewhere (see reviews by Carlson & Rapport, 1989).

Current Diagnostic Criteria and Essential Features of the Disorder

The current DSM-III-R diagnostic criteria for Attention-Deficit Hyperactivity Disorder (ADHD) are presented in Table 1. They require a

Table 1. Diagnostic Criteria for Attention-Deficit Hyperactivity Disorder

Note: Consider a criterion met only if the behavior is considerably more frequent than that of most people of the same mental age.

A. A disturbance of at least 6 months during which at least eight of the following are present:
   1. Often fidgets with hands or feet or squirms in seat (in adolescents, may be limited to subjective feelings of restlessness).
   2. Has difficulty remaining seated when required to do so.
   3. Is easily distracted by extraneous stimuli.
   4. Has difficulty awaiting turn in games or group situations.
   5. Often blurts out answers to questions before they have been completed.
   6. Has difficulty following through on instructions from others (not due to oppositional behavior or failure of comprehension) for example, fails to finish chores.
   7. Has difficulty sustaining attention in tasks or play activities.
   8. Often shifts from one uncompleted activity to another.
   9. Has difficulty playing quietly.
   10. Often talks excessively.
   11. Often interrupts or intrudes on others (e.g., butts into other children's games).
   12. Often does not seem to listen to what is being said to him or her.
   13. Often loses things necessary for tasks or activities at school or at home (e.g., toys, pencils, books, assignments).
   14. Often engages in physically dangerous activities without considering possible consequences (not for the purpose of thrill-seeking), for example runs into street without looking.

   Note: The above items are listed in descending order of discriminating power based on data from a national field trial of the DSM-III-R criteria for Disruptive Behavior Disorders.

B. Onset before the age of seven.

C. Does not meet the criteria for a Pervasive Developmental Disorder.

Criteria for severity of Attention-Deficit Hyperactivity Disorder:

Mild: Few, if any, symptoms in excess of those required to make the diagnosis *and* only minimal or no impairment in school and social functioning.

Moderate: Symptoms or functional impairment intermediate between "mild" and "severe."

Severe: Many symptoms in excess of those required to make the diagnosis *and* significant and pervasive impairment in functioning at home and school and with peers.

Note: From the *Diagnostic and Statistical Manual of Mental Disorders* (3rd ed., rev. by the American Psychiatric Association, 1987, Washington, DC. Copyright 1987 by the American Psychiatric Association. Adapted by permission.

child to exhibit any 8 of the 14 symptoms or behaviors listed under the "A" criterion (see Table 1). The essential features of the disorder continue to include developmentally inappropriate levels of inattention, impulsiveness, and hyperactivity (similar to DSM-III criteria) to varying degrees, with additional emphasis placed on the developmental or age-specific nature associated with the clinical picture. For example, the predominant feature "excessive gross motor activity" found typically in very young children with the disorder may adumbrate many of the clinical manifestations of inattention and impulsiveness in early years. In contrast, older children with the disorder tend to evidence excessive gross motor activity as fidgetiness and restlessness; it is their attentional difficulties and impulsiveness that become the predominant features attended to during middle childhood, prepubescent, and adolescent years. This becomes apparent because of the increasing emphasis on and more difficult cognitive demands associated with academic performance in successive years, as well as the proclivity for social activities and peer acceptance to play a more significant role in everyday functioning.

Attempts to identify the "core components" of the disorder (i.e., inattention, impulsiveness, and hyperactivity) by means of laboratory (clinic-based) and field studies have produced inconsistent, often equivocal, and largely discouraging results. With regard to the clinic-based studies, the enigma appears to lie in (1) defining and measuring such broad constructs as attention and impulsiveness; (2) the faulty assumption that laboratory measures that assess behavioral domains, such as attention (e.g,. the Continuous Performance Test [CPT]), learning (e.g., Paired Associates Learning [PAL]), impulsiveness (e.g., Matching Familiar Figures Test [MFFT]), and gross motor activity (e.g., wrist actometers, grid crossings, seat cushions) can be used interchangeably and compared with one another without regard to their psychometric properties, inherent properties, or external validity; (3) the failure to use and/or the inconsistent use of appropriate diagnostic criteria in classifying children which results in a preponderance of "mixed" groups of children in the literature; and (4) the failure to identify a single feature of the disorder or unique response to treatment that could be considered pathognomonic of ADHD. This last issue takes on special importance because of the relatively high degree of covariation in symptomatology and behavioral dysfunction associated with various disorders of childhood.

Field studies have been plagued with similar difficulties. There are serious concerns, for example, regarding the (1) psychometric properties and structure of the most popularly used parent and teacher rating scales (e.g., nonindependent factors, factor contamination); (2) typically poor agreement obtained between rating sources (parent and teacher); (3) lack of established relationship (external validity) of most scales with direct observations of children's behavior; and (4) a recent and increasing trend to "diagnose by rating scale" without appropriate clinical interview of child and parent, comprehensive history taking, adequate testing/evaluation, and observation.

On a more realistic basis, however, it may be naive to expect that a complex disorder of brain, behavior, and development will respond to simplistic attempts at diagnosis made with teacher rating scales or laboratory instruments. This viewpoint takes on additional significance if factors hypothesized to be associated with ADHD are related to an underlying central defect in self-regulation (Douglas, 1988), an imbalance between or dysregulation of the behavioral inhibition and reward systems that underlie learning (Quay, 1988), or deficiencies in functional and/or structural control mechanisms related to efficient allocation of control over one's own behavior (Sergeant, 1988). Each of these current theoretical positions would posit that the myriad of behavioral and cognitive sequelae associated with ADHD should pervade disparate areas of children's behavior and performance across different modalities (e.g., visual, perceptual-motor, auditory), situations, and settings. A host of other factors would also be expected to differentially affect the ADHD child's behavior or susceptibility to these factors (see reviews by Douglas, 1988; Quay, 1988; Sergeant, 1988).

Secondary Features of the Disorder

Aside from the primary clinical descriptors provided in the DSM-III-R, a variety of associated symptoms or behaviors are reported frequently in children with ADHD. Many of these symptoms or patterns of behavior are reported early in the developmental course of the disorder, and thus may represent less prominent features of the disorder. These include: lability of mood, temper tantrums, low frustration tolerance, social disinhibition, cognitive impairment with associated learning disability, and perceptual motor difficulties. Other aspects of disturbance or behavioral difficulties may be secondary to or direct and indirect consequences of ADHD. For example, disturbed peer and interpersonal relationships, academic underachievement, school failure, decreased self-esteem, depressed mood, conduct problems, and aggression are frequently reported in children with ADHD.

Coexisting Disorders

Many disorders are found to coexist with ADHD; however, relatively little is known regarding specific prevalence estimates in children. As might be expected, the disorders that tend to coexist most commonly with ADHD are those of an externalizing nature: Conduct Disorders (CD) and Oppositional Defiant Disorder (ODD). These are listed under the subclass "Disruptive Behavior Disorders" in the DSM-III-R and described (along with ADHD) as "socially disruptive" and often more distressing to others than to the individuals with the disorders. The relatively high degree of covariation in symptomatology among these disorders has resulted in significant controversy and debate (see Hinshaw, 1987; Lahey *et al.*, 1988; Loney, 1988; Milich, Widiger, & Landau, 1987; Quay, 1986; Taylor, Schachar, Thorley, & Wieselberg, 1986; Werry, Reeves, & Elkind, 1987; Werry, Elkind & Reeves, 1987). This has led many to question whether they are simply different aspects or presentations of a similar underlying psychopathological condition. There is little or no evidence, for example, that Oppositional Defiant Disorder meets even minimal criteria for categorization as a formal "disorder," and it is difficult to imagine a child with ADHD not exhibiting many if not most of the symptoms described under ODD criteria. The debate regarding the independence of conduct disorder from ADHD continues, with existing evidence in favor of independent disorders but with a relatively high rate of co-occurrence (Hinshaw, 1987; Loney, 1988; Trites & Laprade, 1983).

Other disorders or conditions that coexist or overlap symptomatically with ADHD are listed in Table 2, with assignment corresponding to Axis I (i.e., clinical syndromes and adjustment reactions), Axis II (developmental disorders), or Axis III (physical disorders and conditions) categorization. The clinical manifestations of many of these disorders and physical conditions often present with one or more features that are seen in children with ADHD. For example, attentional difficulties are frequently present in children with Tourette's syndrome, disorders involving mood and anxiety, as well as in early onset schizophrenia and a variety of adjustment reactions (see Axis I disorders in Table 2). Attentional disturbance is also relatively common in the developmental disorders listed under Axis II and in a variety of physical conditions listed under Axis III (e.g., those involving ingestion of toxic substances and infectious diseases). Consequently, the onset and developmental course of disturbance (e.g., early versus late, acute versus chronic), antecedent/postcedent and contributing factors, clinical presentation (e.g., episodic versus continuous), and appearance of expected and unex-

Table 2. Disorders That Can Co-occur with or Mimic Attention-Deficit Hyperactivity Disorder

Axis I: Clinical syndromes (and adjustment reactions)	Axis II: Developmental disorders
Oppositional defiant disorder	Mental retardation
Conduct disorder	Pervasive developmental disorder
Anxiety disorders	Specific developmental disorders
Separation anxiety	Academic skills disorders
Avoidant disorder	Language and speech disorders
Overanxious disorder	Motor skills disorders
Phobic disorders	
Posttraumatic stress disorder	Axis III: Physical disorders/conditions
Tic disorders	Toxic (e.g., lead, side effects of drugs)
Tourette's disorder	Traumatic (e.g., subdural effusions)
Chronic tic disorder	Infectious (e.g., meningitis, encephalitis)
Transient tic disorder	Idiopathic (e.g., Reye's syndrome)
Elimination disorders	Neoplastic (e.g., brain tumors)
Functional encopresis	Nutritional (e.g., vitamin deficiencies)
Functional enuresis	Collagen vascular, autoimmune, allergic
Schizophrenia—Childhood onset	Congenital and hereditary (e.g., Tourette's disorder)
Mood disorders	Endocrine (e.g., hyper/hypothyroidism, diabetes)
Bipolar disorder (cyclothymia)	Vascular (e.g., subdural hematoma)
Depressive disorder (dysthymia)	Metabolic (e.g., cerebral hypoxia)
Adjustment disorder	Multiple causes (vision, hearing, epilepsy)
with anxious mood	
with depressed mood	
with disturbance of conduct	
with mixed features of emotion and conduct	

pected coexisting features of a particular disorder must be examined closely. The broad categories of physical disorders and conditions listed in Table 2 under Axis III were derived from Strayhorn (1987) and are not intended to be inclusive. Although uncommon, they represent conditions that may predispose to or mimic some aspects of ADHD in children and should be considered or listed on Axis III to the degree that they are relevant to understanding and managing a case (see Strayhorn, 1987, for a detailed review).

Although reliable estimates are unavailable at present, it would be reasonable to suspect (owing to admission criteria) a higher rate of coexisting disorders on child psychiatry inpatient units compared to outpatient facilities, including children with ADHD. Of 107 consecutive children admitted to child psychiatry (10 bed) inpatient service at the State University of New York (SUNY) Medical School at Stony Brook, University Hospital, approximately 49% percent carried a discharge diagnosis of Attention Deficit Disorder with Hyperactivity (ADDH) or Attention-Deficit Hyperactivity Disorder (ADHD). Of these, 39% and 16% of the children met DSM-III or DSM-III-R criteria for a second or third clinical (Axis I) disorder, respectively, based on comprehensive evaluation and assessment (see following section on Behavioral and Psychiatric Assessment). At least 20% met diagnostic criteria for a coexisting developmental (Axis II) disorder, and 2% to 3% for a coexisting physical disorder or condition (Axis III) that was believed to contribute to the child's condition. In other words, only 14% of all children with ADHD admitted to this inpatient service over a 2½-year period carried a single diagnosis at discharge. (Note that percentage estimates vary depending on which variables are used in determining learning disability diagnoses. For example, the 14% of ADHD children cited above with no coexisting diagnosis would decrease to approximately 2% if DSM-III-R (Axis II) criteria were applied for academic skill disorders. The 14% estimate was calculated based on the more stringent, New York state criteria for learning disability.) The overall rate of coexistence in other inpatient facilities is probably similar. However, the frequencies of specific coexisting diagnostic cases would be expected to vary considerably according to such variables as geographic region and population served.

Psychosocial Stressors

Aside from meeting criteria for dual or multiple diagnoses, the number and severity of psychosocial stressors affecting a child and his or her family are likely to be higher in children with ADHD admitted for inpatient care compared to those seen in outpatient facilities. Frequently, one or more stressors of an acute nature (i.e., less than 6 months) occur just prior to admission and exacerbate a child's clinical condition (i.e., the proverbial straw that broke the camel's back), whereas multiple stressors of an enduring or chronic nature are identified routinely during review of family history. The distinction between identifiable acute and chronic stressors should be noted owing to their potential implications for (1) diagnostic evaluation and treatment planning (i.e., for both the child and his or her family), (2) helping the child to cope/adjust during the course of hospitalization, (3) obtaining/establishing necessary community/social supports, and (4) planning a suitable disposition for the child. There is also evidence, albeit scant, that enduring stressors may increase the likelihood of developing other mental disorders in adulthood as well as influencing outcome. The categorization of stressors by primary types along with representative examples is depicted in Table 3, derived principally from the DSM-III-R. No attempt is made, however, to delineate whether a specific stressor is relevant to an entire family or to the child in question.

Many of the children seen on inpatient services may be considered "functional orphans" (Jemerin & Philips, 1988) in that they have never experienced or been exposed to adequate parenting. Others have been

Table 3. Primary Types of Psychosocial Stressors Reported in Families of Children with Attention-Deficit Hyperactivity Disorder Seen on Inpatient Services

Primary type	Examples
Conjugal	Marital discord, separation, single parenting, abusive spouse, chronic parental discord.
Parenting	Inadequate parenting skills, inadequate discipline and/or monitoring of a child, inadequate provision of external resources or opportunities for appropriate interactional patterns to develop.
Other interpersonal	Poor or disturbed peer relationships, aggressive behavior.
Occupational	Learning disability, impaired cognitive functioning, inability to function in school, school placement, school failure/retention, associated academic skills disorder, loss of job or change in classroom placement.
Living circumstances	Change in residence, threats to personal safety, abusive parenting, other nonrelated adults present in familial environment, multiple foster home placements, frequent changes in the living arrangements at home, frequent changes in the number and types of individuals living at home.
Family factors	Hostile, intrusive, abusive parents, physical and/or mental illness in members of family, lack of parental guidance, inconsistent parental control, complex or inconsistent parental custody and/or visitation rights, foster family placement, loss of nuclear family members, family dysfunction, persistent and harsh parental discipline, physical, sexual, and/or psychological abuse by parent, alcoholism/substance abuse in family.
Other	Minimum of no support by family, lack of established community support network or services, low socioeconomic conditions (income, education, residence in high-crime area), difficulty with legal authorities, no transportation.

severely abused and/or neglected. Relatively few come from intact families. Many if not most come from situations in which one or more of the family members themselves are seriously affected psychiatrically and in dire need of multiple support, community, and placement services.

Children with ADHD who are admitted for inpatient care thus appear to represent the extreme portion of the distribution curve with respect to psychopathology and severity of symptomatology and an entirely distinct subset of children who are faced with an inordinate amount of environmental stressors. As a group, they evidence multiple and chronic behavioral difficulties that are primarily of an externalizing nature, as well as learning difficulties that affect disparate areas of functioning. Most are co-morbid for a second clinical disorder and meet criteria for one or more academic skill disorders. A much smaller percentage have a coexisting physical condition that contributes to their clinical presentation (e.g., poorly controlled seizure disorders or organic brain syndromes of other etiologies). Nearly all of the families of inpatient children with ADHD appear to have multiple psychosocial stressors of both an acute and chronic nature, with severity ranging from moderate to extreme. Their problems are therefore of both an endogenous (psychiatric) and exogenous (psychosocial) nature, with a resulting pattern of interaction that exacerbates both components and is almost always transsituational.

BEHAVIORAL AND PSYCHIATRIC ASSESSMENT

The assessment of children prior to and following admission to a child psychiatry inpatient unit is a complex, multifaceted endeavor that involves a formidable effort by a highly skilled, multidisciplinary team. A comprehensive evaluation begins with standardized parent and teacher questionnaires and rating scales which are sent out and returned prior to the initial intake session (except in cases that involve an emergency admission). The information elicited generally includes ratings pertaining to DSM-III-R diagnosis, broad- and narrow-band descriptions of child psychopathology, such as parent and teacher forms of the Child Behavior Checklist (Achenbach, 1978; Edelbrock & Achenbach, 1984; McConaughy, Achenbach, & Gent, 1988), and ratings pertinent to specific aspects of child psychopathology, such as the IOWA Conners (Loney & Milich, 1982), the Teacher Self-Control Rating Scale (Humphrey, 1982), and the ADD-H: Comprehensive Teacher's Rating Scale (Ullmann, Sleator, & Sprague, 1985). The benefits of obtaining standardized ratings and descriptions of a child's behavior from multiple informants across settings are critical given the fact that not only do children exhibit different behaviors across settings, but informants may be subjectively focused on only certain aspects of behaviors (for an extensive description, see Barkley, 1984). Relevant information regarding a family's socioeconomic status, past and present psychosocial stressors, current living arrangements, as well as information relevant to understanding a child's medical, educational, and developmental history is obtained and reviewed.

A semistructured psychiatric interview is conducted with the parent (or guardian), the child, and later with both the child and parent present during the initial screening. This interview is conducted by an experienced child psychiatrist with active participation by members critical to the functioning of the multidisciplinary team (e.g., the unit social worker, clinical nurse specialist, psychiatry fellows and/or residents). A variety of specialized self-completed (child) and parent-completed ratings are also obtained during the initial screening (e.g., anxiety scales, depression inventories). A decision regarding appropriateness for hospital admission is made thereafter, depending on multiple and complex factors relative to the child's present functioning, safety, risk, and alternative community resources available.

Following admission to the unit, a variety of psychiatric and behavioral measures are administered. A formal, structured psychiatric interview (Kiddie-SADS-E) (Orvaschel, Puig-Antich, Chambers, Tabrizi, & Johnson, 1982) is completed separately for both the parent and child within 2 weeks following admission. The child and parents are seen individually by the inpatient team, consisting of the medical director of the unit, the resident(s), and primary nursing staff for a second, comprehensive psychiatric assessment, and a resident completes a standard physical examination. Standardized nursing ratings relevant to developmental history, medical history, adaptive functioning, and child psychopathology are obtained. Specialty rating scales are administered to both the patient and relevant family members, as well as completed by nursing staff members depending on presenting symptomatology and suspected areas of dysfunction (e.g., depression, anxiety, hyperactivity rating scales). A battery of standardized ratings is obtained during a child's initial week of hospitalization (baseline week) and weekly thereafter from multiple informants using a variety of broad (e.g., In-Patient Global Rating Scale [IGRS]; Conners, 1985) and narrow-band scales across the different microsettings (e.g., staff ratings of behavior displayed on the unit versus teacher ratings of behavior exhibited in the classroom) and temporal parameters (e.g., observations of behavior exhibited during the day versus evening shift) inherent to an inpatient service.

Depending on the child's problems and availability of recent data, initial psychological and educational assessment is completed within the first several weeks of hospitalization. A comprehensive psychoeducational battery (e.g., WISC-R, Kaufmann K-TEA, Bender Gestalt, tests of learning ability) is administered to each child by a certified school psychologist to provide a homogeneous measure of intellectual functioning and academic achievement, followed by appropriate specialty tests when indicated (e.g., to assess language, visual/auditory processing, specific dimensions of personality, highly specific aspects of reading comprehension, or computational abilities pertaining to mathematics). Educational testing to assess specific competencies, mastery of information, and level of current functioning is completed by the unit's special education teachers.

A computerized assessment battery is administered prior to initiation of formal treatment to assess different aspects of attention, cognitive style, short-term memory, ability to learn directly and indirectly taught information, and long-term recall. Some aspects of the battery are used subsequently to provide information regarding the effects of pharmacological treatments on attentional and cognitive functioning.

The complexity of the medical evaluation is determined by the presenting problems of the child. On admission, all patients receive a routine blood screen which includes an electrolyte panel, complete blood count (CBC), thyroid and liver function tests. A baseline electrocardiogram (EKG), electroencephalogram (EEG), as well as an audiologic screen is obtained. Computerized tomography (CT) scan and/or magnetic resonance imaging (MRI) scan are obtained when indicated (e.g., when there has been a recent change in the patient's mental status, or when a structural brain abnormality must be ruled out). Neurologic consultation and other subspecialty consultations are obtained when specific medical questions arise.

Both formal and informal observations of behavior are used continually as an integral part of assessment by various professional staff members throughout a child's hospital stay. Formal observations (ratings of behavior, somatic complaints, etc.) are presented during weekly psychiatry rounds and case discussions (verbal reports of informal observations) by multidisciplinary team members (see Inpatient Management Program in the following section). Initially, this information is used primarily for diagnostic purposes and treatment planning; later, it is utilized to assess and evaluate behavior change with regard to discharge planning and disposition.

Behavioral and psychiatric assessment on inpatient services has evolved from a practice that relied traditionally on subjective reporting of symptomatology and clinical improvement to a dynamic and interminable process that emphasizes objective evaluation with regard to both diagnosis and treatment outcome. The results of these changes will be consequential for clinical care and hospital system service delivery. Further, they wiill be of inherent heuristic value for child psychiatry as a rapidly developing field of scientific inquiry.

BEHAVIORAL TREATMENT

A combined treatment approach is typically used with children with ADHD who are admitted to inpatient services because of the nature, chronicity, breadth, and severity of their dysfunction. Except in highly unusual cases, a variety of standard behavioral and medical interventions have been tried either alone or in combination on an outpatient basis prior to admission. The results of past interventions are carefully reviewed by the clinical treatmment team to maximize hospital-based treatment initiatives and minimize length of hospital stay.

Unless clinically contraindicated, active treatments applied to children at the time of admission are discontinued during the initial week or two of hospitalization to allow for an accurate diagnostic evaluation and assessment of functioning. During this time, behavioral observations, standardized rating scales, and those specific to the child's difficulties are completed weekly by the child's primary and co-primary nursing team members, as well as by the unit's special education teachers. As mentioned, baseline data are also obtained regarding the child's attention, memory function, learning, and problem-solving abilities. Collectively, this information is used to assess the patient's functioning and response to various treatment interventions throughout the course of hospitalization.

Many inpatient services have found that it is neither cost-effective nor practical to establish an individual comprehensive behavioral program for each child that affects most aspects of his or her behavior throughout the day. Rather, unit-wide behavioral programs have been preferred. The inter- and intraday inconsistencies inherent in individualized programs are unavoidable due to factors ranging from daily changes in staff scheduling/shortages, significant differences in staff training/experience at any given time, and between- and across-shift communication regarding changes in treatment parameters, to programmatic issues involving scheduling of daily activities, subjective determination regarding participation therein, and the short-term nature of inpatient hospitalization. Consequently, several inpatient services are electing to develop and implement a highly structured, systems style/data-based approach to facilitate the daily management and clinical care of children. The In-Patient Management Program (IMP) (Rapport *et al.*, 1989) used on the child psychiatry inpatient unit at SUNY Medical School at Stony Brook, University Hospital utilizes this type of system. A brief description of a few of the program's components is provided below. It is noteworthy that, although this program serves as a basis for the behavioral and milieu treatment of all children admitted for inpatient care, it is always supplemented by specific and individually titrated treatments including but not limited to pharmacotherapy, explicit behavioral interventions targeted at certain types of presenting problems or types of psychopathology, parent training, family therapy, educational intervention, and development of liaisons with community support systems.

The Inpatient Management Program: An Overview

The Inpatient Management Program (IMP) was designed to provide a highly structured therapeutic milieu for children within the pediatric age range (6 to 12 years) who are primarily of borderline or above intelligence, and who are admitted for inpatient psychiatric care. The primary goals of the IMP are (1) to facilitate the completion of a comprehensive diagnostic evaluation by the multidisciplinary team; (2) to provide a positive and therapeutic setting in which children with various types and degrees of psychopathology can be stabilized and learn more adapttive means of interacting with their environment; (3) to provide a standardized means of assessing a child's behavior and the relative efficacy of treatment(s); and (4) to promote the generalizability of treatment gains upon discharge for aftercare follow-up.

Structure of the Inpatient Management Program

The IMP is structured so that children are provided continual feedback via consequences throughout the day. The importance of establishing this type of structured social ecology is critical to the successful functioning of a child psychiatry inpatient unit for several reasons. It provides children with a high degree of certainty, predictability, and stability. Consequently, it serves initially to reduce the anxiety and apprehension that many children experience upon being admitted to a hospital. The structure of the unit also facilitates the treatment team's ability to engage in diagnostic decision making by reducing environmental stressors and their influence on children's behavior, and by stabilizing the environment to an extent that nonenvironmentally related dysfunction, if present, can be detected more readily.

A third reason for introducing this level of structure involves the treatment process itself. Many children admitted to a child psychiatry inpatient unit, for example, require a variety of treatment interventions to properly address their current level of dysfunction. Although the therapeutic effects associated with the milieu are an integral component of a child's treatment, the structure, consistency, and stability inherent to the unit enable the treatment team to determine to what degree additional interventions are required and the relative success of these interventions beyond the effects of the milieu alone.

Finally, the structure of the IMP serves as an ongoing instructional model and learning process for children. Upon awakening, children are expected to behave in a responsible manner and to engage in age-appropriate personal care and control over themselves throughout the day. Expectations range from relatively simple, personal hygiene habits, such as brushing one's teeth, putting away laundry, making one's bed, and using appropriate manners, to accepting responsibility for one's behavior and its consequential effects on the environment.

The Inpatient Management Program Unit Point System

The IMP point system was designed specifically for inpatient care. Certain elements were based on empirical research findings whereby positive and enduring therapeutic changes have occurred as a result of using specific procedures. Other aspects of the system were a result of the senior author's professional experiences in designing therapeutic systems for use in public schools, mental health centers, inpatient units, residential facilities, and familial environments.

The system was designed to be broadly applicable but highly practical given the diversity of children and differing types and severity of psychopathology encountered on inpatient services. Whenever possible, naturally occurring environmental consequences are relied upon (e.g., staying-up later if personal nightly hygiene is completed on time, engaging in a greater number of weekend activities, or spending more quality time with one's parents based upon the child's ability to control himself or herself during the week). The traditional use of primary reinforcers (e.g., food), or secondary reinforcers, such as stereotyped verbal praise and token stores replete with toys and goodies, has been abandoned entirely. These have been replaced primarily with opportunities to engage in various activities on and off the unit throughout the day and evening. This increases children's participation in socialization experiences with adults and peers and concomitantly enables staff members to assess, teach, and monitor individual behavior as well as interpersonal and social skill deficits.

Organization and Use of the Inpatient Management Point System

The IMP point system is composed of two primary components: *daily living points* and *personal goal points*. Daily living points are based on broadly applicable behavioral criteria and are assigned to all children in a unified fashion throughout the day, from the time they awaken until they are asleep at night (see below). Personal goal points are individualized to reflect and promote gains in specific areas of dysfunction as designated by the unit treatment team.

Daily Living Points. The daily living points are assigned for behaviors that children are expected to engage in on a daily basis, such as brushing their teeth, dressing themselves, applying appropriate grooming, preparing for meals, general health care, attending school, participating in unit and therapeutic activities, and behaving responsibly and appropriately with staff members and peers.

A fixed number of daily living points are awarded to children by staff members upon completion of specific responsibilities and at designated time intervals throughout the day based on the child's behavior. These responsibilities are recorded on a daily living point sheet which, accompanied by a daily goal point sheet and cumulative weekly point sheet, are attached to the outside of each child's bedroom door to enable review by staff and children throughout the day. Point assignment is verbalized to each child individually at the time of recording with appropriate explanation provided as required. Because point assignment is nonnegotiable, staff–child interactions focus primarily on problem-solving and providing encouragement and constructive suggestions to the child for behavioral improvement.

The criteria for successful completion of a task or activity are agreed upon by the unit's treatment team and remain in effect for all children unless clinically contraindicated. In the latter cases, criteria for successful task completion are determined by the treatment team during its weekly meeting to ensure that a consistent therapeutic approach is employed by all staff members. During time frames in which children attend school or certain other structured activities (e.g., therapeutic groups, mealtime), the criteria for and breakdown of point assignment are posted in the setting. For example, a large block of daily living points are designated and available for assignment by classroom teachers during the morning and afternoon school sessions. These blocks include smaller numbers of points that are awarded for diverse behaviors ranging from completion of academic assignments to exhibiting appropriate self-help skills.

Daily living points may also be subtracted at anytime during the day if a child engages in or exhibits certain types of inappropriate behavior. These behaviors and associated point loss values are established by the unit treatment team and remain in effect as formal policy. As might be expected, higher point losses are associated with physically dangerous behaviors (e.g., physical aggression, destruction of property) and require no verbal warning. Lower point deductions are routinely preceded by a warning and are applied as consequences for inappropriate behaviors that have less serious potential consequences to the child or others in the immediate environment (e.g., failing to follow verbal instructions). Specific procedures, appropriate entry codes, and relevant point values that may be lost for inappropriate behavior are detailed in the IMP manual.

In summary, point values are awarded and subtracted to reflect a child's behavior throughout the day. This provides continual feedback to the child in addition to written documentation of his or her behavior and its short-term (daily) and long-term (weekend) consequences. The system is structured and based largely on response-cost principles that are considered by some to be more analogous to real-life situations in which, depending on one's behavior, may be followed by either positive or negative events (Rapport, 1988).

Personal Goal Points. A set number of personal goal points may also be earned daily (and accumulated weekly), but are awarded at designated times (e.g., ranging from every few minutes to a few times daily) and for specific behaviors throughout the day as determined by the treatment team. For example, some children are awarded personal goal points for demonstrating newly acquired social skills or increased compliance to verbal requests. Others are awarded points for exhibiting improved interpersonal relationships, participating in a specific therapeutic intervention, or initiating self-control techniques with minimal or no staff involvement. The criteria for and awarding of daily living points are identical for all children on the unit throughout their hospital stay (unless changed formally by the unit treatment team). Specific goals (and points awarded) that individual children work on are reviewed continually and altered to promote therapeutic change. These changes may involve successive approximations to a singular treatment goal that involves multiple phases, or accomplishment of multiple goals worked on concurrently.

Daily and Weekly Accumulated Points. Daily living points are used throughout the day to help children gain control over themselves and because many children are initially unable to work for longer term goal attainment. An established number of points, for example, are required for participation in various activities on and off the unit during the day, for use of the activities room at designated times (instead of playing quietly by oneself with a more restricted range of materials), and for special privileges, such as engaging in computer games or staying up later in the evening. Thus, the more successful a child's day, the more activities he or she is able to participate in on and off the unit.

Therapeutic activities and certain other scheduled events (e.g., community meetings) do not require points. Rather, attendance is mandatory (unless clinically contraindicated), and part of the child's daily living points are assigned for appropriate participation during these regularly scheduled time intervals.

Although daily living points are used by each child throughout the day, they are added back in at the day's end to a weekly point accumulation sheet posted on each child's door. This sheet depicts each child's accumulated daily living points and personal goal points throughout the week and serves to bridge the gap between attainment of short- and long-term goals. A "new week" begins late Friday afternoon, at which time each child's accumulated weekly points are tallied and reviewed during a scheduled meeting of all children. Children must initially spend their points for the maximum hours of home-pass time they have qualified for on the weeekend. Remaining points may be used for participation in the variety of planned weekend activities outlined on the board. These activities and their associated point values vary, as would be expected, from watching cartoons on Saturday morning (low-point cost) to going bowling or swimming followed by a picnic lunch (high-point cost). Special events are also available exclusively for the unit's top point earners each week. Each child thus elects how he or she will spend their earned points prior to each weekend. Aside from its primary purposes of providing delayed consequences for behavior during the week and promoting long-term goal attainment, this strategy teaches children important planning skills that may be used at home following discharge from the hospital.

Use of the Inpatient Management Point System. The entire schedule of daily and weekend activities, pass time earned, and participation in various events is based on precalculated, earn–loss point ratios that are intended to maximize therapeutic change. These ratios have been adjusted over the course of 3 years and represent a balance between the degree of adaptive behavior (which includes specific goal attainment) and positive control a child exerts over himself or herself on a daily and weekly basis, and his or her ability to engage in various events on and off the unit that require such control. Therefore, changes in the point system can impact potentially every child's life on a daily and weekly basis, and are not undertaken without critical concern for both its specific and overall effect on the inpatient management system.

One of the more unique features of the IMP is the wealth of information collected on each child that may be used for clinical decision-making as well as for research purposes. For example, an integral part of the IMP is the computerized assessment/tracking (CAT-P) program. All weekly ratings, daily living and personal goal points earned, points lost by category of inappropriate behavior, specialty scales and inventories, emergent symptoms, and individual testing data are entered and calculated weekly. This information, in turn, is used in weekly rounds in a manner such that 4 consecutive weeks are shown for each child across the broad categories of unit ratings (each shift individually and for all scale factors), teacher ratings, totals and percentages possible of earned daily living and goal points, separate and combined categories of points lost, passes earned, weekly visits by parents, and so on. This information can be used subsequently to assess multifaceted aspects of each child's behavior throughout the hospital stay and to adjust treatment interventions accordingly. For example, a particular treatment intervention and/or personal goals may be altered for a child showing an increase in points lost for physical aggression over 2 weeks. The CAT-P would provide detailed information regarding whether disturbed conduct and/or increased physical aggression were limited to a particular time of day (e.g., days vs. evenings) or setting (school vs. on-unit), which may be due to a time-limited factor or circumstance. Appropriate interventions can then be initiated and their therapeutic effects monitored. The breadth of information provided on each patient's daily and weekly functioning is also used during discharge planning. A child with ADHD, for example, who continues to exhibit a high frequency of aggressive behavior that necessitates placement in seclusion or restraints despite several weeks of normally potent combined treatment interventions may be considered for residential care as opposed to home placement following discharge. More detailed examples regarding the use of the IMP and CAT-P are highlighted in the case illustration that follows.

CASE HISTORY

Developmental, Educational, Familial, and Medical History

Steve is a 10-year-old Caucasian male with a history of severely hyperactive and impulsive behavior dating back to his toddler years. Although Steve's mother feels that he was unusually active and more difficult to control than either of his two brothers by the age of 3, it was not until kindergarten that intervention was necessary. During his kindergarten year, Steve's classroom teacher telephoned his mother repeatedly to report that Steve simply could not sit still long enough to complete any of the tasks given to the class. Instead, he would run around the room and try to climb on the window sills and cabinets. When his teacher attempted to redirect him, he responded first by laughing and running away, and when she persisted, by hitting and kicking her and then resuming his previous behavior. He was also unable to play cooperatively with any of the other children in the class because of his "bossiness," his inability to take turns and share materials, and his increasing frequency of aggressive behavior. Steve fought daily with at least one other child in the classroom. On several occasions, he had actually injured another child either accidentally through his quick and impulsive movements, or by design. Steve's mother initially considered her child's unmanageable and increasingly disruptive behavior "a phase" that he was going through in response to her recent divorce and the death of her father with whom Steve shared a close relationship. Steve's difficulties continued, however, and by the middle of the kindergarten year, the school indicated that he would require a psychiatric evaluation to determine whether alternative classroom placement and/or treatment was warranted.

Steve was evaluated by a psychiatrist and neurologist and diagnosed as having ADHD. His physical examination was unremarkable and the neurologic examination revealed no focal abnormalities; although he was felt to have poor fine motor coordination and to exhibit a "clumsy" way of moving. These abnormalities were not seen in conjunction with any other neurologic symptoms and were thus considered "soft signs."

Treatment was started with a stimulant class medication, methylphenidate (MPH), at a dose of 5 mg twice daily. An alternative learning environment was also recommended. Steve was placed subsequently in a special education classroom with a ratio of 12 students to 1 teacher and 1 teacher aide (12:1:1 classroom) where he remained for the next 4 years. Although he continued to be difficult to manage, Steve received no psychological follow-up. His medication was prescribed and adjusted periodically by his pediatrician. After several months, the MPH reportedly lost its effectiveness, dosage was increased numerous times, and eventually it was discontinued and replaced with a different stimulant, Cylert. Steve's mother was never able to discern whether or not the medication was beneficial to her son.

During the next 4 years, Steve was shuttled back and forth between his mother's and his father's home because of his increasingly difficult behavior. His contact with the nonresiding parent at any given time was limited and erratic, resulting from the lack of communication between parents following their divorce. While living with his mother, he would continually fight with his brothers and defy his mother's directives. He often became so enraged that he would threaten to kill her, then run into his room and destroy his furniture. When he was sent to live with his father, he worried excessively about his mother's welfare, fearing that she may die while he was away. His ability to concentrate diminished significantly while he was living in the father's home, and Steve reportedly began to pace nervously during much of the day and expressed feelings of hopelessness and despair. In school, he felt that he was disliked by everyone and seemed to have little success with reading or math. His grades were characteristically poor and he was continually in trouble because of his inattention and impulsive response style. When his teacher would try to help him, he would often become angry and storm out of the classroom. She would frequently find him in the bathroom weeping out of frustration.

Over the period of several months prior to admission, Steve became increasingly more irritable and anxious, as well as motorically agitated. He began to exhibit heightened fear of the dark, of being alone, and of being separated from his mother. He was forced to enroll in a different school on account of his mother's relocation of residence. Concomitant with this move, Steve began complaining of multiple aches and pains to avoid attending school. His relationship with his father continued to deteriorate and his interactions with his siblings were wrought with arguments and physical altercations. One week prior to admission, Steve began leaving notes around the house stating that he would be dead soon. In school, he reportedly began talking more excessively than usual with a corresponding diminution in concentration and academic functioning. When he took a knife from the school cafeteria and attempted to cut his wrists, his family was telephoned and he was brought to the hospital emergency room.

Admission for Inpatient Care

On admission, Steve presented as a small, thin boy who appeared younger than his stated age. He spoke rapidly, fidgeted continually, and denied that he had actually contemplated suicide. He admitted to sometimes "acting without thinking" and to being "moody," but denied feeling depressed presently. He reported that his biggest problem was that he "gets into trouble in school because he talks too much." His mood was dysphoric, characterized by anxiety and slight to moderate depression. There was no evidence of delusions or psychotic features.

The initial work-up included blood chemistries and physical examinations that were noncontributory. A neurologic examination confirmed the presence in Steve of poor coordination and clumsy movement, a dexamethasone suppression test (DST) that was negative, and an EEG that showed nonfocal slowing (considered a nonspecific abnormality). Family history was positive for bipolar illness in the maternal grandmother and a maternal aunt, alcoholism in the paternal grandfather, and hyperactivity/learning disabilities in both the father and paternal grandfather. Both of Steve's older brothers had positive histories of hyperactivity and marginal school performance, but were affected less seriously by comparison.

Psychometric testing revealed that Steve had a full-scale IQ of 102, with a verbal and performance IQ of 105 and 99, respectively. Significant variability was found among the performance subtests. Achievement testing revealed both math and reading levels to be between 1 and 2 years below grade expectation. Steve's performance on the Continuous Performance Test (CPT), a vigilance test, was characterized by a relatively high error rate that is usually associated with inattention (omission errors) and impulsiveness (commission errors). His impulsiveness with regard to visual problem-solving was also detected during administration of the Matching Familiar Figures Test (MFFT). He would gaze briefly at the target stimulus picture and rapidly select one of the six potential choice stimuli without regard for correctness or even a cursory attempt to utilize an organized search strategy. Consequently, his error rate and latency to initial response using age and gender norms were 96% (with 100% representing high error rates) and 39% (with 1% representing short latencies), respectively (i.e., a "fast-inaccurate" or impulsive response style). Steve's short-term memory and ability to learn new, unrelated associations between arbitrary letter pairs (bigrams) and numbers over a 15-minute time span were assessed using a computerized version of the Paired Associates Learning Test (K-PAL). The results revealed moderate to severe difficulties in this area (i.e., Steve could not recall an average of 1.5 for every 2.2 associations learned on a minute-to-minute basis). Similar results were obtained on the Stimulus Equivalence (SE) Paradigm, a measure sensitive to pharmacological interventions that provides information regarding the acquisition and long-term recall of both directly taught and untaught visual relationships (Vyse & Rapport, 1989).

A clinical psychiatric interview in conjunction with a structured interview (K-SADS) conducted separately with Steve and his mother reflected endorsement of several DSM-III-R diagnoses. These included Attention-

Deficit Hyperactivity Disorder (ADHD), Oppositional Defiant Disorder, and Dysthymic Disorder. According to his mother, Steve's symptoms of both depression and irritability waxed and waned over time, but she could not identify clear-cut cycles. Clinical interview and observations conducted during the initial 2 weeks of hospitalization also indicated the presence of several symptoms characteristic of overanxious disorder and mania, albeit insufficient to meet full diagnostic criteria for either disorder.

Behavioral and Pharmacological Treatment

Following the initial biopsychosocial evaluation and observation/assessment period, a comprehensive treatment program was developed for Steve. This included (1) pharmacological intervention, (2) specific and general behavioral and milieu therapies of an ongoing nature (see Inpatient Management Program, previous section), (3) individualized personal goals that were worked on daily and adjusted to accommodate and facilitate therapeutic progress throughout the course of hospitalization, and (4) specific management and emotional issues to be addressed in therapeutic sessions with the patient and both of his parents.

Given Steve's diagnosis of ADHD, history of severe and chronic impairment, and undocumented level of improvement when treated previously with stimulant medications, a brief trial of methylphenidate (MPH) was tried initially. His response to MPH treatment was characterized by clear reductions in gross motor activity and impulsiveness, increased attention, and corresponding improvement on several cognitive measures (e.g., CPT, MFFT, and PAL). Steve's emotional state with regard to the mixed picture of irritability, depressive phenomena, and overall emotional lability, however, remained unresponsive to treatment. Although Steve did not meet the criteria for Bipolar Disorder at the time, a trial of lithium ($LiCO_3$) was administered in the context of a double-blind, placebo-controlled, modified reversal (A-B-A-B) design owing to his continued display of mixed symptomatology and strong family history for bipolar illness. Following a week-long placebo trial, Steve was titrated to a blood level of 1.0 mmol/L (mg/dl), which required a dose of 1200 mg of lithium per day. Over the course of hospitalization, his daily lithium dosage remained constant with biweekly blood levels ranging from 0.8 to 1.0 mmol/L (mg/dl). Approximately 4 weeks after reaching therapeutic blood level, Steve was observed by staff to be calmer and less irritable, with a corresponding improvement in the frequency of his positive verbalizations regarding himself and his difficulties. He was less oppositional during passes with his family, and he seemed better able to deal with the chronic hostility between his parents. Although his peer relationships on and off the unit remained poor, he exhibited moderate improvement in his ability to listen to and utilize suggestions offered to him by peers and staff. Despite these improvements, Steve's attention and concentration in the unit's classroom remained deficient. Since he had exhibited a positive response in these areas during the brief trial of stimulant, differing dosages of MPH (10, 15, and 20 mg BID) were added to the lithium regimen for week-long trials. The effects were assessed using a modified reversal (A-B-A-B) design and compared to both placebo (one at the beginning, "P-1," and a second trial at the end, "P-2," to provide an estimate of behavioral/milieu effect over time) and lithium ($LiCO_3$) alone after 4, 8, and 10-weeks of continuous treatment.

To illustrate both the relative effectiveness of and manner in which clinical change was assessed during the various therapeutic conditions, several measures of Steve's behavior across the three microsettings (unit, school, and clinic-based assessment of cognitive functioning), as derived from the IMP's computerized assessment/tracking program (CAT-P), are depicted in Figures 1 through 5. The lower graphs in Figures 1 to 4 and both graphs in Figure 5 show Steve's behavior or performance (over and above the effects of the inpatient behavioral program that is administered continually throughout the course of a child's hospitalization) under each medication condition over time. The medication conditions occurred in the order shown, and each represents a week-long period of time. The initial lithium ($LiCO_3$) condition is also based on a week-long period of time (i.e., the 5th week), but represents behavior and performance *after* 4 consecutive weeks of lithium treatment (including initial titration to therapeutic level).

The primary purposes of these lower graphs are to (1) provide a general flavor for the similarities observed in the different microsettings despite weekly changes in medication status (e.g., compare unit and school TSCRS ratings of Steve's self-control in Figure 1); (2) demonstrate how closely weekly nursing staff ratings represent certain aspects of a child's behavior on the unit (e.g., see IGRS Conduct Factor and Daily Living Points lost for noncompliance during each week in Figure 2); (3) highlight particular constructs of behavior such as "attention" or "impulsiveness" that are measured by cognitive testing (e.g., the CPT and MFFT, respectively) and examine their relationship to nursing ratings (see IGRS Inattention Factor and CPT Errors in Figure 3) and the weekly frequency in which a standardized behavioral intervention for improving personal control on the unit is employed (see MFFT and Time-Outs in Figure 4); and (4) illustrate the time-course effects lithium may exert

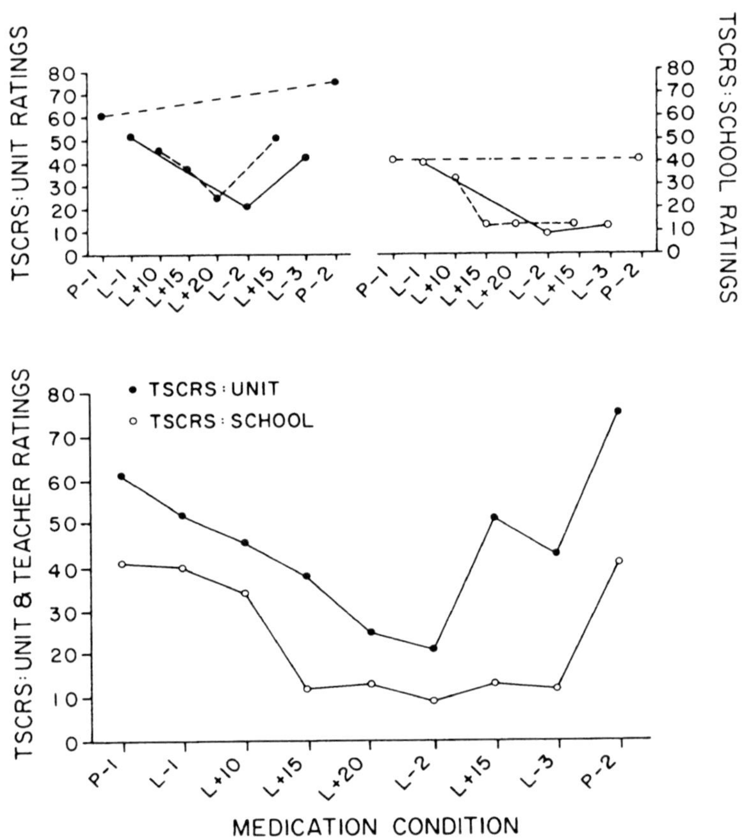

Figure 1. Dose-response curves of unit (nursing) and classroom Teacher Self-Control Rating Scale (TSCRS) scores across medication conditions. Scores are inverted such that lower scores or downward movement on the vertical axis indicates improved self-control. Dose-response curves of nursing (top left) and classroom (top right) TSCRS scores are depicted in isolated format above main graph to facilitate interpretation of medication × time effects for placebo (P − 1, P − 2), lithium alone (L − 1, L − 2, L − 3) at 5, 8, and 10 weeks, and combined lithium and methylphenidate (L + 10, L + 15, L + 20) treatment conditions. P = placebo; L = lithium ($LiCO_3$); +10, +15, and +20 = methylphenidate at 10-mg, 15-mg, and 20-mg BID dosages.

on certain aspects of a child's learning, and what occurs when MPH and lithium are combined in a treatment regimen (see Percentage Correct during the initial learning acquisition phase compared to the number of Learning Retention associations per minute during the recall phase in the top and lower portions of Figure 5, respectively).

The smaller subplots shown in the upper left- and right-hand cor-

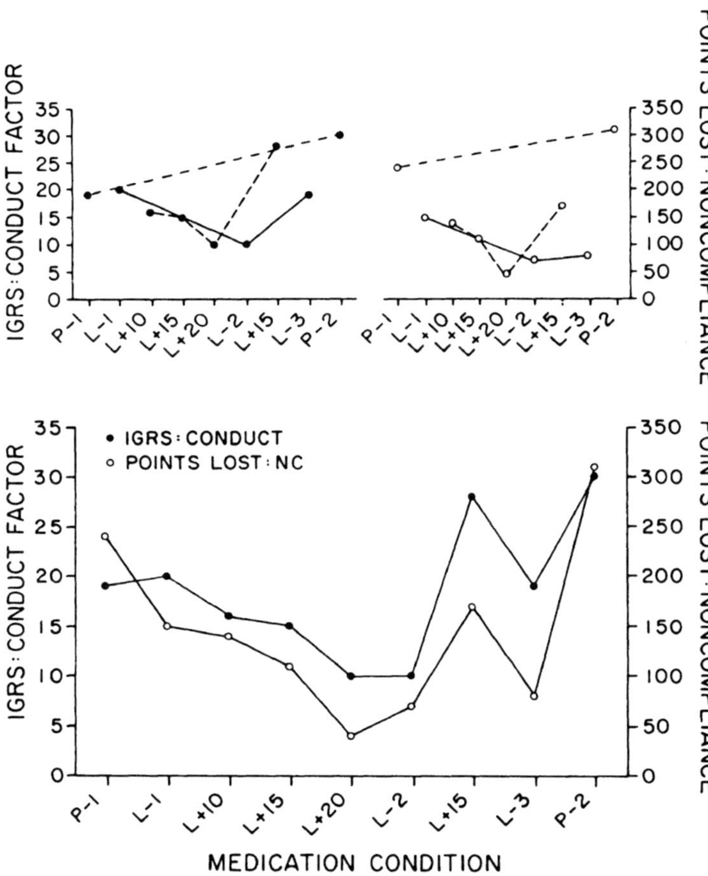

Figure 2. Dose-response curves of unit (nursing) Inpatient Global Rating Scale (IGRS) Conduct Factor scores and Daily Living Points (DLP) subtracted weekly for noncompliant behavior across all medication conditions. Improvement is indicated by downward movement on the vertical axis or by lower scores and fewer point losses. Dose-response curves of nursing IGRS scores (top left) and DLP losses (top right) are depicted in isolated format above the main graph to facilitate interpretation of medication × time effects for placebo (P − 1, P − 2), lithium alone (L − 1, L − 2, L − 3) at 5, 8, and 10 weeks, and combined lithium and methylphenidate (L + 10, L + 15, L + 20) treatment conditions. P = placebo; L = lithium ($LiCO_3$); +10, +15, and +20 = methylphenidate at 10-mg, 15-mg, and 20-mg BID dosages.

ners of the larger graphs were drawn to illustrate the effects of lithium with and without MPH compared to placebo (behavior/milieu therapy alone) over time. Although space limitations do not permit a detailed discussion, it is interesting to note the following effects in this particular individual: (1) lithium appears to exert an increasingly therapeutic effect

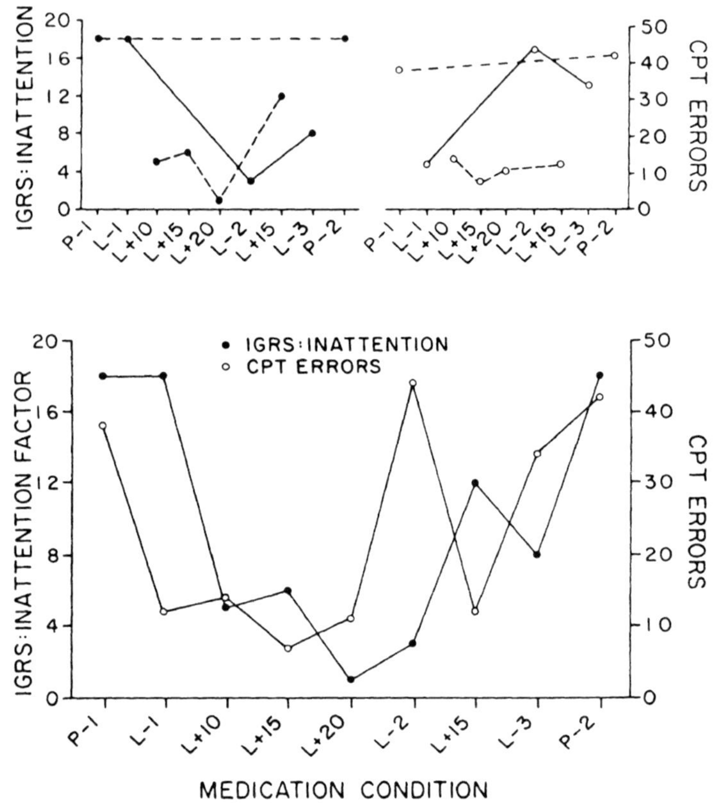

Figure 3. Dose-response curves of Continuous Performance Test (CPT) errors and nursing Inpatient Global Rating Scale (IGRS) Inattention Factor scores across all medication conditions. Improvement is indicated by downward movement on the vertical axis or by fewer errors (CPT) and lower IGRS scores. Dose-response curves of IGRS scores (top left) and CPT errors (top right) are depicted in isolated format above the main graph to facilitate interpretation of medication × time effects for placebo (P − 1, P − 2), lithium alone (L − 1, L − 2, L − 3) at 5, 8, and 10 weeks, and combined lithium and methylphenidate (L + 10, L + 15, L + 20) treatment conditions. P = placebo; L = lithium ($LiCO_3$); +10, +15, and +20 = methylphenidate at 10-mg, 15-mg, and 20-mg BID dosages.

compared to placebo as a function of time for both directly observed and rated behaviors regardless of setting (see the $LiCO_3$ line on each of the smaller graphs); (2) adding MPH to an ongoing lithium regimen during the initial 5 to 8 weeks results in either no appreciable effect (see unit TSCRS and IGRS conduct factor ratings in Figures 1 and 2), or in most cases, a synergistic[1] therapeutic effect under the higher 15- and 20-mg

[1]Although not depicted on the graphs, the effects of $LiCO_3$ + MPH on the child's behavior and performance for the variables shown were also greater than those observed under MPH alone during the initial 3-week stimulant trial.

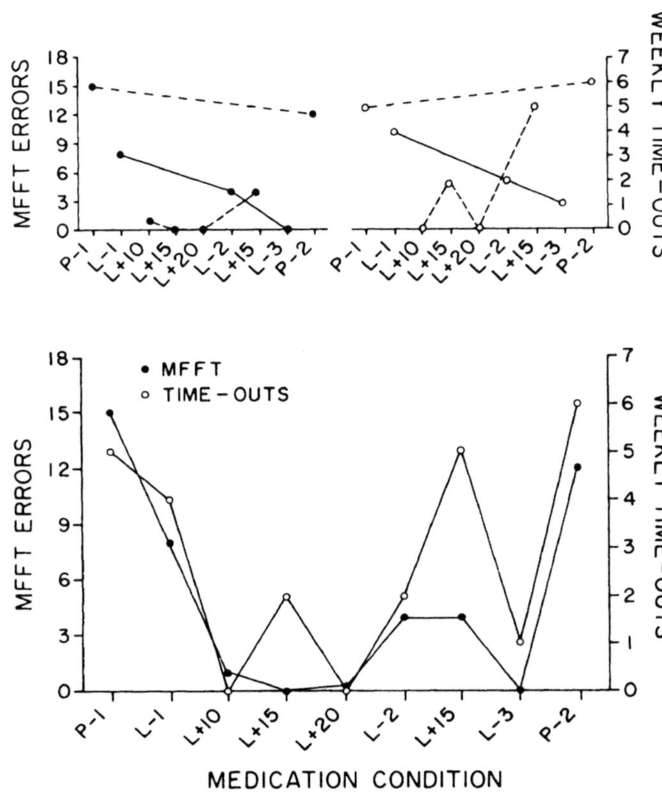

Figure 4. Dose-response curves of Matching Familiar Figures Test (MFFT) errors and time-out frequency (weekly) across all medication conditions. Improvement is indicated by downward movement on the vertical axis or by fewer errors and time-outs. Dose-response curves of MFFT errors (top left) and weekly time-outs (top right) are depicted in isolated format above the main graph to facilitate interpretation of medication × time effects for placebo (P − 1, P − 2), lithium alone (L − 1, L − 2, L − 3) at 5, 8, and 10 weeks, and combined lithium and methylphenidate (L + 10, L + 15, L + 20) treatment conditions. P = placebo; L = lithium ($LiCO_3$); +10, +15, +20 = methylphenidate at 10-mg, 15-mg, and 20-mg BID dosages.

MPH dosages (see TSCRS school ratings and Points Lost for Noncompliance in Figures 1 and 2; CPT/MFFT errors, weekly time-outs, and IGRS attention factor ratings in Figures 3 and 4); and (3) the addition of a 15-mg MPH dosage after 10 weeks of continuous lithium treatment no longer results in a synergistic effect and often reduces the clinical effectiveness of lithium alone.

Finally, the effects of lithium with and without MPH over time on Steve's ability to learn (acquisition phase) and remember (retention phase) visual relationships as assessed by the Stimulus Equivalence (SE) Paradigm (Vyse & Rapport, 1989) are depicted in Figure 5. During the

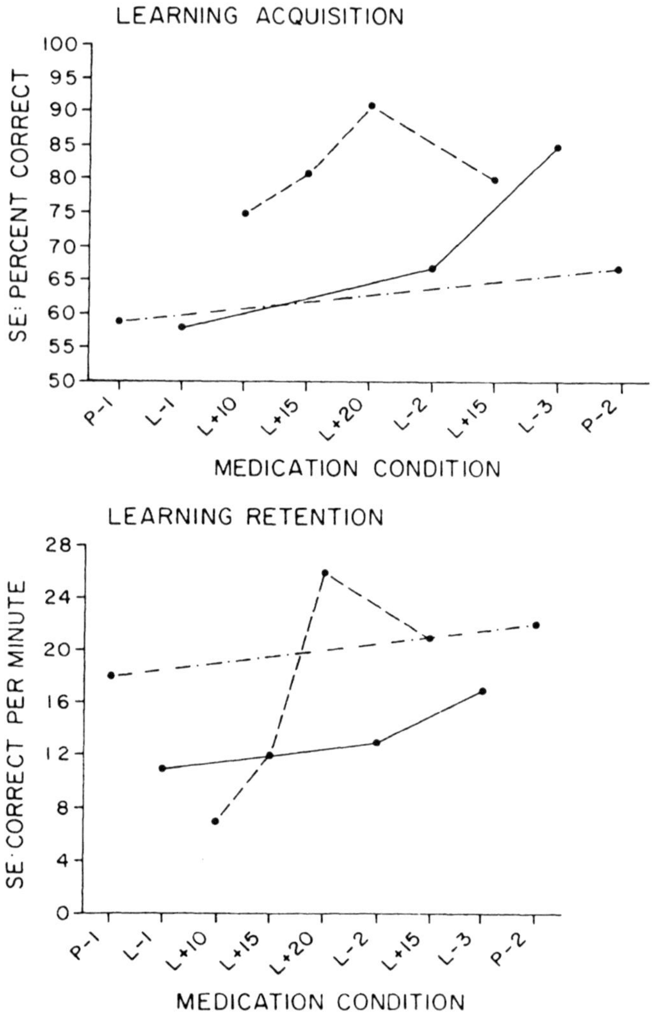

Figure 5. Dose-response curves of stimulus equivalence (SE) performance during the initial learning acquisition phase (top graph) and learning retention phase (bottom graph) are depicted to highlight medication × time effects for placebo (P − 1, P − 2), lithium alone (L − 1, L − 2, L − 3) at 5, 8, and 10 weeks, and combined lithium and methylphenidate (L + 10, L + 15, L + 20) treatment conditions. P = placebo; L = lithium ($LiCO_3$); +10, +15, +20 = methylphenidate at 10-mg, 15-mg, and 20-mg BID dosages.

initial 10 weeks of lithium treatment, Steve's ability to learn the visual relationships during the *acquisition phase* of the paradigm was relatively unaffected (see Percent Correct in top graph in Figure 5). His ability to remember these relationships 30 to 45 minutes later during the *retention phase,* however, was impaired moderately compared to the pre-post placebo line (see Correct Per Minute in bottom graph in Figure 5). After 12 weeks of continuous treatment with lithium, both acquisition and retention showed improvement, with performance during acquisition moving well above the pre-post placebo line. Inspection of raw score values indicates that Steve's reduced ability to retain newly learned information under lithium was due in part to slower response latencies (compared with placebo) which gradually shortened and approached placebo values with continued lithium treatment (despite dosage and blood level remaining constant over this time period). The "slowed effect" does not fully explain the results, however, in that the percentage of correctly remembered relationships during the retention phase remained low compared to placebo values even after the effects of response latency were removed (i.e., he simply did not remember as many of the relationships regardless of how long it took him to respond.

The addition of MPH to Steve's lithium regimen clearly facilitated his ability to learn new relationships and to retain this information under the higher 20-mg dosage condition. A synergistic effect appears to have occurred as both aspects of learning were improved over and above that observed under lithium alone and during the initial MPH alone trial (not shown).

Following his hospital course, Steve learned the unit's behavioral management system quickly and began to qualify for 10 to 12-hour weekend passes off the unit by his sixth week of hospitalization (i.e., an indirect measure of the sum of daily living points and personal goal points awarded less point reductions for inappropriate behavior during a given week). During the course of hospitalization, Steve's "personal goal points" were assigned primarily for (1) developing and improving prosocial/interpersonal behaviors with peers; (2) identifying events and situations in which he became frustrated or angry, reducing the likelihood of these events whenever possible, and "timing himself out" to maintain personal control under appropriate circumstances; and (3) working with various members of the treatment team to develop a realistic understanding regarding the conflict between his parents and its impact on himself as well as other members of the family, with a concomitant adoption of useful coping strategies. As with other children on the unit, personal goals were altered continually to reflect and promote therapeutic progress.

Discharge Planning

As discharge neared, Steve expressed concern that his family might not be able to carry out the behavioral program at home and that his previous gains and future efforts would be futile. His family was educated regarding the importance of providing daily structure, setting consistent limits that incorporated both positive and negative consequences, and, in general, child management skills. Although they were able to enact many of the management techniques while role-playing with staff, under direct supervision, and later during the 4 to 6-hour home passes, they appeared unable to use and/or apply the knowledge consistently as Steve began to qualify for more lengthy home passes. The discord and bitterness that existed between his divorced parents was unchanged at the end of his hospitalization.

Steve was discharged with an improved mood, significantly better impulse control, and a more stable/adaptive method of responding to the various stressors in his daily life. He had also shown moderate improvement in his peer and interpersonal relationships and was discharged on a combination of lithium and MPH. His family was provided with a detailed home care plan to serve as a guide for continuing the behavioral management plan that had been successful during his hospitalization. The recommendation was made for Steve to be placed in a small, therapeutic self-contained and highly structured day treatment/special education classroom. The family was given the suggestion that structured group sporting or other leisure activities would be beneficial in developing Steve's still deficient social skills. Finally, outpatient follow-up was recommended, including a child psychiatrist to monitor the medication and a behaviorally oriented therapist to help the family develop a more organized and consistent life-style (as well as to implement and monitor the behavioral interventions).

PROBLEM AREAS

There are a number of problem areas associated with this case, and, to some extent, a majority of cases seen in child psychiatry inpatient services. Among the most serious of these is the failure to generalize treatment effects to the child's natural environment and the capacity to maintain these effects over time. In the present case, for example, the child clearly benefited both from the daily behavioral management program (and its highly structured, consistent environment) and the individually regulated medication regimen of lithium and MPH. A vital element in discharge planning was thus to locate and/or establish environmental supports and resources that would provide the child with as many of the components as necessary for continued therapeutic progress. Steve was recommended and placed subsequently in a day treatment facility. This facility was able to address many of Steve's educational needs (e.g., individualized instruction within the confines of a small, structured 6:1:1 classroom that incorporated a system of consistent feedback), while concomitantly providing for ongoing medical consultation (psychiatric) and psychological intervention (both individual, group, and family training). The latter two services are critical for a majority of cases discharged from inpatient units as neither an "educational" model nor purely "psychotherapeutic" model can address adequately the multifaceted needs of these children. Many elements of the behavioral plan Steve worked on during the course of hospitalization were shared with the staff at the day treatment facility, who, in turn, incorporated them whenever possible into his new educational/behavioral goals to facilitate generalization and maintenance of treatment effects. Similarly, the consulting child psychiatrist at the facility continued to monitor Steve's medication status regularly to check for compliance and emergent symptoms (e.g., with lithium: polydipsia, polyuria, skin rashes, tremors) and regulate appropriate blood levels as required.

Establishing a social support network for both Steve and his family outside of the day treatment facility was not as successful due to a lack of easily accessible services available in the surrounding community as well as to continued familial chaos. Creating a "patchwork" network is wrought with difficulties, such as scheduling of multiple services, arranging transportation, communicating with different agencies, and the never ending need to reestablish the entire network on a not infrequent basis.

Similarly, the degree of conflict and animosity between Steve's parents and personal/interpersonal dysfunction among family members in the home waxed and waned over time but could never be considered as "improved." On follow-up, Steve appeared to be doing reasonably well in the day treatment program insofar as the stressors at home remained within reasonable limits. When the level of dysfunction within the familial environment worsened, Steve's behavior and ability to function at school worsened accordingly. It became readily apparent that, although a highly regulated and potent combination of behavioral and pharmacological intervention bolstered treatment gains under circumstances in which stressors remained within the mid-to-moderate range at home, the addition and/or exacerbation of existing stressors thwarted therapeutic efforts regularly. Recommendations to the parents to address these difficulties were rebuffed, often met with hostility, and frequently resulted in further noncompliance in Steve's treatment.

SUMMARY

Children with ADHD who are admitted to child psychiatry inpatient facilities nearly always present with co-occurring disorders, experience moderate to severe educational difficulties, and come from families characterized by disharmony, conflict, and stress. Although some cases appear intransigent to even the most comprehensive, multidisciplinary efforts during the course of hospitalization, a majority of children with ADHD who are admitted for inpatient care will likely show moderate to excellent progress. Usually, therapeutic intervention will involve a multifaceted but individually titrated treatment effort as these children are scourged by a complex disorder of brain, development, and behavior that brings them into direct and continual conflict with their environment. The effects of multimodal treatment observed during their course of hospitalization will frequently reveal the "optimal" level of functioning one can expect upon their discharge. However, in most cases, this will not subsequently carry over to the real life environment of these children.

Future work with these children need not further emphasize methods by which to increase "generalization" and "maintenance" of treatment effects of the traditional nature, as hospital-based interventions are routinely structured to facilitate transfer to external settings, and sufficient (albeit not "ideal") resources are available in the community that can be relied upon for continued therapy and monitoring. The enigma, however, more frequently involves *obtaining* these services for a particular child and increasing *compliance*. Efforts to create or establish interventions for parents or custodial care-givers of these children are sorely needed as traditional parent training and intervention models do not address their difficulties. Issues regarding the presence of psychopathology in individual members of the family, multiple acute and chronic environmental stressors of a moderate to severe nature, the absence of family/community support, and a life-style that perpetuates continued dysfunction all impinge upon treatment compliance and outcome.

REFERENCES

Achenbach, T. (1978). The Child Behavior Profile: I. Boys aged 6–11. *Journal of Consulting and Clinical Psychology, 46*, 478–488.

American Psychiatric Association. (1980). *Diagnostic and statistical manual of mental disorders* (3rd ed.). Washington, DC: Author.

American Psychiatric Association. (1987). *Diagnostic and statistical manual of mental disorders* (3rd ed., rev.). Washington, DC: Author.

Barkley, R. A. (1984). Hyperactivity. In E. J. Mash & L. G. Terdal (Eds.), *Behavioral assessment of childhood disorders* (pp. 127–184). New York: Guilford Press.

Carlson, G. A., & Rapport, M. D. (1989). Diagnostic classification issues in attention-deficit hyperactivity disorder. *Psychiatric Annals, 19,* 576–583.

Conners, C. K. (1985). IGRS (Inpatient Global Rating Scale). *Psychopharmacology Bulletin, 21,* 832–834.

Douglas, V. I. (1988). Cognitive deficits in children with attention deficit disorder with hyperactivity. In L. M. Bloomingdale & J. A. Sergeant (Eds.), *Attention deficit disorder: Criteria, cognition, intervention* (pp. 65–81). New York: Pergamon Press.

Edelbrock, C., & Achenbach, T. (1984). The teacher version of the Child Behavior Profile: I. Boys aged 6–11. *Journal of Consulting and Clinical Psychology, 52,* 207–217.

Geraty, R. (1989). Administrative issues in inpatient child and adolescent psychiatry. *Journal of the American Academy of Child and Adolescent Psychiatry, 28,* 21–25.

Gittelman, R., Mannuzza, S., Shenker, R., & Bonagura, N. (1985). Hyperactive boys almost grown up: I. Psychiatric status. *Archives of General Psychiatry, 42,* 937–947.

Harper, G. (1989). Focal inpatient treatment planning. *Journal of the American Academy of Child and Adolescent Psychiatry, 28,* 31–37.

Hinshaw, S. P. (1987). On the distinction between attentional deficits/hyperactivity and conduct problems/aggression in child psychopathology. *Psychological Bulletin, 101,* 443–463.

Humphrey, L. L. (1982). Children's and teacher's perspectives on children's self-control: The development of two rating scales. *Journal of Consulting and Clinical Psychology, 50,* 624–633.

Jemerin, J. M., & Philips, I. (1988). Changes in inpatient child psychiatry: Consequences and recommendations. *Journal of the American Academy of Child and Adolescent Psychiatry, 27,* 397–403.

Lahey, B. B., Piacentini, J. C., McBurnett, K., Stone, P., Hartdagen, S., & Hynd, G. (1988). Psychopathology in the parents of children with conduct disorder and hyperactivity. *Journal of the American Academy of Child and Adolescent Psychiatry, 27,* 163–170.

Loney, J. (1988). Hyperactivity and aggression in the diagnosis of attention deficit disorder. In B. B. Lahey & A. E. Kazdin (Eds.), *Advances in clinical child psychology* (Vol. II, pp. 99–135). New York: Plenum Press.

Loney, J., & Milich, R. (1982). Hyperactivity, inattention, and aggression in clinical practice. *Advances in Developmental and Behavioral Pediatrics, 3,* 113–147.

Mannuzza, S., Klein, R. G., Bonagura, N., Konig, P. H., & Shenker, R. (1988). Hyperactive boys almost grown up: II. Status of subjects without a mental disorder. *Archives of General Psychiatry, 45,* 13–18.

McConaughy, S., Achenbach, T., & Gent, C. (1988). Multiaxial empirically-based assessment: Parent, teacher, observational, cognitive, and personality correlates of Child Behavior Profiles for 6–11-year-old boys. *Journal of Abnormal Child Psychology, 16,* 485–509.

Milich, R., Widiger, T. A., & Landau, S. (1987). Differential diagnosis of attention deficit and conduct disorders using conditional probabilities. *Journal of Consulting and Clinical Psychology, 55,* 762–767.

Nurcombe, B. (1989). Goal-directed treatment planning and the principles of brief hospitalization. *Journal of the American Academy of Child and Adolescent Psychiatry, 28,* 26–30

Orvaschel, H., Puig-Antich, J., Chambers, L. W., Tabrizi, M. A., & Johnson, R. A. (1982). Retrospective assessment of prepubertal major depression with the Kiddie-SADS-E. *Journal of the American Academy of Child and Adolescent Psychiatry, 21,* 392–397.

Quay, H. C. (1986). Classification. In H. C. Quay & J. S. Werry (Eds.), *Psychopathological disorders of childhood* (3rd ed., pp. 1–34). New York: Wiley.

Quay, H. C. (1988). Attention deficit disorder and the behavioral inhibition system: The relevance of the neuropsychological theory of Jeffrey A. Gray. In L. M. Bloomingdale & J. A. Sergeant (Eds.), *Attention deficit disorder: Criteria, cognition, intervention* (pp. 117–125). New York: Pergamon Press.

Rapport, M. D. (1988). Hyperactivity and attention deficit disorders. In V. B. Van Hasselt, P. S. Strain, & M. Hersen (Eds.), *Handbook of developmental and physical disabilities* (pp. 295–315). New York: Pergamon Press.

Rapport, M. D., Kelly, K., Carlson, G. (1989). *The inpatient management program (IMP): A comprehensive system and computerized assessment/tracking program to facilitate patient care and research on child psychiatry inpatient units.* Unpublished manual and computerized assessment package (copyright pending).

Riddle, M. A. (1989). Research on a children's psychiatric inpatient service. *Journal of the American Academy of Child and Adolescent Psychiatry, 28,* 42–46.

Sergeant, J. (1988). From DSM-III attentional deficit disorder to functional defects. In L. M. Bloomingdale & J. A. Sergeant (Eds.), *Attention deficit disorder: Criteria, cognition, intervention* (pp. 183–218). New York: Pergamon Press.

Strayhorn, J. M. (1987). Medical assessment of children with behavioral problems. In M. Hersen & V. B. Van Hasselt (Eds.), *Behavior therapy with children and adolescents: A clinical approach* (pp. 50–74). New York: Wiley.

Taylor, E., Schachar, R., Thorley, G., & Wieselberg, M. (1986). Conduct disorder and hyperactivity: I. Separation of hyperactivity and antisocial conduct in British child psychiatric patients. *British Journal of Psychiatry, 149,* 760–777.

Trites, R. L., & Laprade, K. (1983). Evidence for an independent syndrome of hyperactivity. *Journal of Child Psychology and Psychiatry, 24,* 573–586.

Ullmann, R. K., Sleator, E. K., & Sprague, R. L. (1985). Introduction to the use of ACTeRS. *Psychopharmacology Bulletin, 21,* 915–920.

Vyse, S. A., & Rapport, M. D. (1989). The effects of methylphenidate on learning in children with ADDH: The stimulus equivalence paradigm. *Journal of Clinical and Consulting Psychology, 57,* 425–435.

Werry, J. S., Elkind, G. S., & Reeves, J. C. (1987). Attention deficit, conduct, oppositional, and anxiety disorders in children: III. Laboratory differences. *Journal of Abnormal Child Psychology, 15,* 409–428.

Werry, J. S., Reeves, J. C., & Elkind, G. S. (1987). Attention deficit, conduct, oppositional and anxiety disorders in children: I. A review of research on differentiating characteristics. *Journal of the American Academy of Child and Adolescent Psychiatry, 26,* 144–155.

Woolston, J. L. (1989). Transactional risk model for short and intermediate term psychiatric inpatient treatment of children. *Journal of the American Academy of Child and Adolescent Psychiatry, 28,* 38–41.

III

Treatment of Adolescents

10

Antisocial Behavior

JOHN E. LOCHMAN, KAREN J. WHITE, JOHN F. CURRY,
AND RICHARD R. RUMER

INTRODUCTION

This chapter will review literature that has examined the effectiveness of cognitive-behavioral and behavioral treatment procedures with antisocial children and adolescents in institutional settings. The construct of antisocial behavior refers to a broad range of actions "that reflect social rule violations and/or that are acts against others" (Kazdin, 1987a, p. 11). These actions include physical aggression (e.g., hitting, kicking, biting), verbal aggression (e.g., threatening others with use of force), and other contranormative or oppositional behaviors (e.g., lying, truancy, running away, theft, vandalism, fire setting). Certain of these behaviors represent criminal actions. However, although much of the literature on the characteristics and treatment of antisocial adolescents is derived from research on juvenile delinquency, the construct of antisocial behavior is certainly not restricted to delinquency. Some aggressive and oppositional behaviors are relatively common in mild forms during early childhood, but antisocial behaviors become clinically significant if certain

---

JOHN E. LOCHMAN, JOHN F. CURRY, AND RICHARD R. RUMER • Department of Psychiatry, Duke University Medical Center, Durham, North Carolina 27710. KAREN J. WHITE • Department of Psychology, University of Notre Dame, St. Joseph, Indiana 46556.

Inpatient Behavior Therapy for Children and Adolescents, edited by Vincent B. Van Hasselt and David J. Kolko. Plenum Press, New York, 1992.

behaviors still persist in later childhood, if they are highly intense, or if they occur with high frequency. Clinically significant antisocial behaviors occur in approximately 5% to 10% of children, and boys with antisocial behavior outnumber girls by about three to one (Kazdin, 1987b; Quay, 1986).

In addition to frequency and intensity, two other continua that have important implications for assessing antisocial behavior are the dimensions of overt to covert, and situational to cross-situational. Children and adolescents who engage in antisocial behavior may display aggression in direct, externalized, overt ways (assaults, threats), their behavior may be covert, often representing instrumental efforts to gain other valued goals (theft), or they may engage in both types of behavior. The latter youth are regarded as versatile, and they have the most chronic pattern of antisocial behavior (Loeber & Schmaling, 1985). Versatility across situations is also predictive of more severe levels of antisocial behavior. Those youth who display antisocial behavior in multiple settings are more at risk for continued disorder than are youth who are aggressive in only one setting, such as at school or at home (Loeber & Dishion, 1983).

CLINICAL DESCRIPTION

The antisocial behaviors referred to in this chapter commonly occur as symptoms of DSM-III-R (American Psychiatric Association, 1987) psychiatric disorders, such as Conduct Disorder or Oppositional-Defiant Disorder. However, aggressive behavior can occur with inpatients having a wide variety of diagnoses, ranging from pervasive developmental disorders to adjustment disorders. The behavioral interventions reviewed here are directed at behavioral patterns rather than at diagnostic entities, and thus can have application across a range of psychopathology. It should also be recognized that emerging research is indicating that aggression in children and adolescents is correlated with biochemical indices, such as plasma testosterone and dopamine-beta-hydroxylase (Mattsson, Schalling, Olweus, Low, & Svensson, 1980; Rogeness, Hernandez, Macedo, Mitchell, Amrung, & Harris, 1984). Although the direction of influence between these biological markers and aggressive behavior is still inconclusive in these correlational findings, researchers during the next decade will likely begin to examine ways in which biological interventions directed at hormonal or neurotransmitter levels might augment the effectiveness of behavioral interventions.

This chapter reviews the assessment of conduct disorders and behavioral, cognitive-behavioral, and social skills treatment studies with antisocial children and adolescents who were placed in inpatient and other institutional settings. The latter sections of the chapter outline impediments and obstacles that interfere with the use of behavior therapy in inpatient settings for children and adolescents, and then summarize the results of behavior therapy research in these settings.

PSYCHIATRIC AND BEHAVIORAL ASSESSMENT

In their comprehensive chapter on the assessment of conduct disorders, McMahon and Forehand (1988) pointed out the need for continued improvement of assessment procedures. In acknowledging the complexity of assessing conduct disorders (CD), McMahon and Forehand suggested 3 foci for evaluation: (1) child behavior *per se,* within an interactional context, (2) other child characteristics, and (3) familial and extrafamilial factors.

Presented in this section is an overview of the most commonly used, well-established instruments, including (1) behavioral checklists/rating scales, (2) interview techniques, and (3) direct observation. The appropriateness of standardized intellectual and academic assessment, and evaluation of other cognitive factors (e.g., problem-solving skill, attributional style) is discussed with respect to developing a comprehensive understanding of conduct-disordered children.

Behavioral Checklists and Rating Scales

The advantages of using checklists have been well documented (Barkley, 1984; McMahon, 1984). They are particularly helpful given the wide range and impact of problem behaviors among CD children. Among the most solidly researched checklists is the Child Behavior Checklist (CBCL) (Achenbach & Edelbrook, 1983). Age (2 to 16 years) and sex norms are available for parent and teacher forms. A variety of uses of the CBCL are possible because of the equivalent forms for multiple informants and the provision of both broad-band (e.g., externalizing-internalizing) and narrow-band (e.g., aggression) syndromes. As McMahon (1984) pointed out, the CBCL is one of the few rating scales that evaluates for prosocial behavior, too.

The Revised Behavior Problem Checklist (RBPC) (Quay & Peterson, 1983) has been successfully employed as both a screening and treatment-outcome measure. Norms are available for teacher's ratings of children in kindergarten through grade 12 and mothers' ratings of children whose ages range from 5 through 16. McMahon and Forehand noted as drawbacks of the RBPC the limited number of dimensions of child behavior disorders and the lack of assessment of appropriate or prosocial behaviors.

The Eyberg Child Behavior Inventory (ECBI) (Eyberg, 1980) generally assesses overt conduct disorder behavior, with very few "covert" behavior items included. It nicely combines a two-dimensional yes or no rating of "problem present" and a 7-point rating of "intensity." Age norms are available for 2 to 12 year olds and adolescents (13 to 16 years), but norms for sex are not available.

Other checklists frequently used in assessment of CD children include those developed by Conners (1969, 1970, 1973) with parent and teacher forms. Two scales derived from the revised version (Goyette, Conners, & Ulrich, 1978) of the Conners, each consisting of 10 items are particularly useful: the Abbreviated Symptom Questionnaire (ASQ) (Conners, 1973) and the Iowa Conners Teacher Rating Scale (IOWA CTRS) (Loney & Milich, 1982). Each of these instruments is helpful in identifying problems in hyperactivity and conduct disorder.

A number of checklists have been developed to assess familial and extrafamilial factors, such as parental perceptions of child behavior (e.g., Parent Attitudes Test—Cowen, Huser, Beach, & Rappaport, 1970), parents' personal and marital adjustment (e.g., Beck Depression Inventory—Beck, Rush, Shaw, & Emery, 1980; and Locke's Marital Adjustment Test—Locke & Wallace, 1959), and parental stress (e.g., Parenting Stress Index—Abidin, 1983). McMahon and Forehand (1988) provided a discussion of empirical findings linking conduct-disordered behavior and aspects of parent modeling and home events. In addition, the relationship between parent extrafamilial support and CD child behavior has been elucidated by Wahler's work on the "insular" mother by using a brief checklist (Community Interaction Checklist—Wahler, Leske, & Rogers, 1979).

Behavioral Interviews

Behaviorally oriented interviews are a critical component to the assessment of conduct disorders, especially in understanding the interactional patterns and social perceptions among family members. Typically, interviews can be conducted with a focus on functional analysis of the problem behaviors. However, several researchers have developed structured interviews involving checklist formats (e.g., Forehand &

McMahon, 1981; Patterson & Bank, 1986; Wahler & Cormier, 1970), some of which allow for distinction of overt/covert behavior problems (e.g., Interview for Antisocial Behavior—Kazdin & Esveldt-Dawson, 1986). Other interviews are structured with respect to diagnostic criteria and are administered to parents, child, or both (e.g., Diagnostic Interview for Children and Adolescents—Herjanic & Reich, 1982; Diagnostic Interview Schedule for Children—Costello, Edelbrock, Dulcan, & Kalas, 1984; and Child Assessment Schedule—Hodges, Kline, Fitch, McKnew, & Cytryn, 1981). The degree of agreement between parents and children about externalizing and internalizing symptoms is an important clinical consideration and heuristically valuable research area. As noted in the introduction, making distinctions among patterns of covert, overt, and "mixed" conduct disorders yields a wealth of information regarding family structure and functioning, likely targets for intervention, and important assessments of risk status and treatment outcome. In addition, assessing for the presence of attentional problems and depression is also critical (see McMahon & Forehand, 1988, for discussion).

Behavioral Observation

As McMahon and Forehand (1988) explained, behavioral observations probably yield the most valid information regarding family interaction patterns (as opposed to interviews, questionnaires). When used in combination with other sources, better decisions can be made with respect to the target of intervention (e.g., child behavior, parent perception or adjustment). McMahon and Forehand reviewed a variety of observational systems for use in the clinic, home, and school, with detailed information on psychometric properties and relationship with other measures.

Standardized Testing and Assessment of Other Cognitive Factors

It is important to recognize that CD children often have serious academic problems that may influence their attitudes not only about learning, but about themselves, authority figures, and peers. Learning problems, especially reading disabilities (Sturge, 1982), are not uncommon. Therefore, a psychoeducational evaluation is usually critical in identifying a very important risk factor—poor academic progress. Other cognitive and/or affective factors that have been shown to yield useful information (e.g., treatment goals, response to intervention) have included those assessing attributional biases (e.g., Dodge & Frame, 1982;

Lochman, 1987), and social problem-solving skill and self-esteem (e.g., Lochman & Lampron, 1986). As yet, further psychometric development is required, but the measures used by the above researchers supply valuable empirical findings and rich clinical information.

TREATMENT APPROACHES

Contingency Management and Token Economy Programs

The use of behavioral treatment approaches for aggressive children and adolescents in inpatient or residential settings emerged in the mid 1960s and seemed to be motivated in part by the apparent frustration with "traditional" or analytically oriented approaches with institutionalized adolescents (e.g., Burchard & Tyler, 1965). In addition, contingency management techniques were proposed as a means by which to combat the powerful influences of peer reinforcement of inappropriate behavior (e.g., Meichenbaum, Bowers, & Ross, 1968; Sanson-Fisher, Seymour, & Baer, 1976) that is nearly inescapable with groups of adolescents housed together, especially those exhibiting antisocial behavior problems.

The studies to be reviewed in this section include investigation of contingency management in group homes for delinquents (e.g., Achievement Place), adolescent wards in state mental hospitals, and child and adolescent units in psychiatric hospitals. Interestingly, the majority of empirical investigations have been conducted in group home settings, specifically the Achievement Place/Teaching-Family model which originated at the University of Kansas (Phillips, 1968). Remarkably few studies regarding behavior management of aggressive children or adolescents in psychiatric settings have been conducted, despite the recognized need for effective treatment of this potentially dangerous behavior pattern.

In 1965, Burchard and Tyler provided a convincing demonstration of the positive results of contingency management with an institutionalized 13-year-old boy. The subject had received a wide range of diagnostic labels during 4 years of continuous hospitalization. For 2 years prior to this study, he had been involved in "regressive therapy." His high rates of aggressive and antisocial behavior were responded to with an overuse of seclusion. In the year preceding this project, the subject had spent a total of 200 entire days in isolation. Through the systematic use of time-out and differential reinforcement of appropriate behaviors, significant decreases in inappropriate behavior were obtained and the time the subject spent on the ward increased substantially. This study serves as a preliminary example of the importance of teaching and directing staff to use basic contingency management techniques.

In another early study, Meichenbaum *et al.* (1968) modified the disruptive classroom behavior of 10 adolescent females in a training school by reinforcing a strictly defined set of behaviors considered to be appropriate in the instructional setting. This group of girls ($\bar{X} = 15 - 4$) had been institutionalized for an average of 240 days. Significant reductions in disruptive behavior were obtained as a function of providing fixed internal schedules of feedback and reward (once per hour) regarding the percentage of time engaged in appropriate behavior. "Feedback slips" were exchangeable for cash. Further reductions in disruptive behavior were obtained with the use of a variable schedule of feedback and by giving feedback in the form of the amount of money earned (as opposed to the percentage of appropriate behavior observed). The last phase of the study combined reinforcement and response-cost contingencies yielding a reduction in inappropriate behavior that approached that of a group of 12 noninstitutionalized adolescent girls who were used as a comparison group.

"Within-institution" behavior change (Graziano & Mooney, 1984) has been reported in a number of residential and detention homes for delinquent adolescents. Emshoff, Redd, and Davidson (1976) compared the effects of "generalized" versus "constant" training for positive verbalizations in four subjects from a residential home for delinquent and disturbed adolescents. Two subjects received constant training (seven 30-minute sessions during a 2-week period) in which their positive comments were rewarded with points redeemable for small amounts of cash, and with verbal praise. In the generalized training condition, two other subjects received the same type of reward contingency, but the activity, location, trainer, and time of day varied. Both pairs of subjects showed increases in positive comments during training sessions, but the generalized training group showed a tendency to increase positive comments in settings in which the trainers were not present. This study is one of the few early investigations of contingency management for delinquents in which generalization was addressed.

In a study (Sanson-Fisher *et al.*, 1976) in which adolescent delinquents' verbal behavior was evaluated, the actual "instruments" of the intervention were staff members who were trained to respond differentially to verbal statements made by the subjects. The subjects were 12 delinquent adolescent females (ages 14 to 18 years), all of whom had been previously institutionalized. One group of staff members ($n = 5$)

were instructed to deliver and record positive attention (e.g., praise or approving statements) to the girls' prosocial conversation and ignore antisocial verbalizations. Another group of staff (n = 6) were asked to deliver negative attention (e.g., disapproving statements) to the girls' antisocial remarks. In general, positive comments made by the subjects increased only during treatment sessions. Probably the most important finding was that the girls made fewer positive comments to staff in the condition in which both positive and negative staff attention was employed. This finding suggests that the subjects withdrew from staff when their antisocial conversation elicited staff disapproval. The authors noted that staff attempts to alter peer group reinforcement patterns can have undesirable effects and suggested that enlisting peers as the behavior change agents (e.g., Fixsen, Phillips, & Wolf, 1973) may produce more desirable results. As Graziano and Mooney (1984) noted, however, marked differences between groups on pretraining (baseline) levels of verbalization type (especially antisocial) limit the comparisons that can be made between the two interventions.

Several studies have evaluated the effects of token economy programs on a variety of target behaviors. In a multiple, return to baseline design, Barkley, Hastings, Tousel, and Tousel (1976) measured changes in performance of daily chores, littering in the house, and school performance (indexed by teacher evaluation). The eight subjects were older (ages 15 to 18), "difficult" delinquent males whose offenses included drug and alcohol abuse, breaking and entering, petty theft, and grand larceny. Completion of chores increased and littering decreased as a function of reinstating the reward and fines, respectively. Removal and reinstatement of feedback and rewards for school performance were evaluated with only two of the eight subjects because of concerns about the possible negative responses of adolescents who had been in the program for shorter periods of time. Interestingly, no changes in academic performance were observed with removal of the rewards for teacher evaluation. The authors hypothesized that the daily teacher evaluation (even without rewards) may have been sufficiently reinforcing for these students to maintain their performance.

Achievement Place Programs. One of the most influential forces in the development of treatment for juvenile delinquents and children with externalizing disorders was the development of the Teaching-Family or Achievement Place program. These programs are carried out in family-style, community-based group homes for delinquents. In these programs, an average of six youths live with a married couple, "teaching parents," who receive about 1 year of professional pre- and in-service training. Consistent with a social learning perspective, the goal is to encourage achievement and to teach "situation-relevant" behavior patterns, norms, and decision-making skills (Braukmann, Kirigin, & Wolf, 1980). There are four main elements of the program: (1) instruction in fundamental skills and discriminations in areas of interpersonal relations, academic tasks, and self-care; (2) development of rewarding relationships between teaching parents and adolescents; (3) motivation through a flexible, individualized token economy; and (4) mediation of peer consequences through constructive, self-government procedures.

The Achievement Place series of investigations highlights the importance of controlling access to "naturally occurring" positive events in the environment through the use of a token economy. Early investigations (e.g., Phillips, 1968) demonstrated very good responses to the token economy with respect to a variety of "within-home" target behaviors (e.g., aggressive verbalizations, bathroom cleaning, punctuality, homework completion). In other studies (i.e., Phillips, Phillips, Fixsen, & Wolf, 1971), the importance of flexibility by thinning the schedule of reinforcement in a token economy system was illustrated.

In addition to some attention to "within-institution" maintenance, a couple of studies evaluated the effects of social influences (as opposed to tangible reinforcers) in the adolescents' environment. Phillips (1968) determined that the person responsible for the delivery of reinforcers and fines was an important factor. In comparing two conditions in which the "manager" of a bathroom cleaning duty varied between house parent and peer, subjects performed at a more efficient level when the manager was a peer.

Another Achievement Place study (Fixsen *et al.*, 1973) evaluated the "semi-self-government" system in which residents learned about the process of democratic decision-making. In this aspect of the program, youths were encouraged to establish rules, monitor their peer's behavior, and determine consequences for rule violations. In two experiments, different factors or procedures were manipulated to evaluate the boys' participation in self-government exercises (family meetings, or "trials" as the boys called them). In Experiment One, comparisons were made between conditions in which peers or the teaching parents had complete responsibility for determining consequences for rule-breaking. Subjects ($n = 7$) indicated that greater participation in discussions occurred when peers were responsible for delivering consequences. Also, violations reported by the boys (vs. teaching parents) were more likely to result in trials (i.e., tended to be more serious violations). In Experiment Two, it was found that more trials were called when teaching parents (vs. adolescents) were responsible for that task. When subjects were awarded points for calling trials, the average number of trials per day increased, but more trivial violations were reported.

In these experiments (Fixsen *et al.*, 1973; Phillips, 1968), important influences on delinquents' within-institution behavior are addressed. Obviously, peer approval (e.g., Phillips, 1968) has a powerful impact on youths' behavior and can be channeled in positive directions. Allowing adolescents to evaluate their peers' behavior (within a supportive, structured environment) tends to promote higher degrees of involvement in decision-making exercises (Fixsen *et al.*, 1973). Unfortunately, there appear to be no reports of these types of manipulations in such settings as psychiatric units for adolescents.

In a review of behavior modification/token economy interventions with aggressive/delinquent populations, Davidson and Wolfred (1977) made note of important issues in evaluating the studies mentioned above. First, long-term maintenance of improvements is rarely assessed and second, within-institution change programs fail to demonstrate that these changes are effective in reducing delinquency. However, two more recent evaluations of the Teaching-Family/Achievement Place model made more reasonable attempts to address these concerns.

An evaluation of the overall effectiveness of the Teaching-Family approach was conducted comparing the "prototype" of Achievement Place, a number of replication programs, and other group home programs (Braukman *et al.*, 1985). Measures included the percentage of subjects with criminal and noncriminal offenses before, during, and 1 year after treatment. Criminal and noncriminal offense rates (number of offenses committed) per subject were also assessed, as well as records of commitments to institutions at the three time periods. Consumer satisfaction rating scales were completed by the subjects, their parents and teachers, group home personnel and the boards of directors, and juvenile court and social welfare personnel. The sample included adolescents from the original Achievement Place (AP), 12 "replication" group homes, and 9 conventional non-Achievement Place programs in Kansas. All subjects were court-adjudicated delinquents (ages 12 to 16). One hundred forty adolescents (102 male, 38 female) from Achievement Place homes were compared with adolescents from the conventional group homes. AP subjects were significantly less likely to commit offenses during treatment than non-AP subjects, but these differences were not maintained at the 1-year follow-up. Interestingly, the offense rate for non-AP subjects was also significantly higher than their own pretreatment scores. Similar patterns were observed for males and females.

Regarding the consumer satisfaction ratings, AP programs consistently obtained higher scores. These ratings were also used to validate treatment-outcome measures. The Achievement Place philosophy is that more involvement with and instruction from group home parents reduce the likelihood of delinquent behavior. From the subjects' point of view then, higher satisfaction with their relationship with teaching parents would be related to lower offense rates. Significant negative correlations between offense rate and consumer satisfaction (with teaching parents) supported this hypothesis.

The authors addressed the lack of maintenance at posttreatment by pointing to the need to intervene with the posttreatment placement environments. No discussion of the apparent failure to "internalize" AP values was provided. However, this study was exemplary for its use of clinically relevant outcome measures and the attempt to measure consumer attitudes as an index of "process" variables relating to outcome.

Braukman and colleagues (1985) later addressed some other very important measures of delinquents' response to the AP program, use and abuse of alcohol and drugs, and prosocial behaviors (both via self-report measures). Three groups of adolescents were compared: those in Teaching-Family (AP model) group homes (n = 82), adolescents in conventional non-AP homes (n = 103), and friends of both the AP (n = 28) and non-AP subjects (n = 32). Measures obtained before, during, and after treatment (at 1-month intervals up to 1 year posttreatment) were collected. A summary of the findings revealed lower rates of drug use and higher rates of prosocial behavior were obtained during treatment for the AP versus the non-AP subjects. No significant differences were obtained in the MANOVA for posttreatment group differences. Comparison between AP subjects and their matched "friend" pairs (who were not in institutions) revealed a similar pattern of significant differences during treatment, but not posttreatment, on measures of drug use and prosocial behavior. Non-AP adolescents were not different from their friends on any measure either during or after treatment.

Comparisons regarding process variables revealed that subjects in both types of group homes reported that the staff cared about their behavior at equal levels. However, the AP subjects saw their group home parents as more involved, as more likely to detect inappropriate behavior (drug use), and as having stronger reactions to the discovery of drug use than their non-AP delinquent peers in conventional group homes. Regression analyses revealed that a significant proportion of the variance of "during treatment" outcome variables was explained by some of the process variables; specifically, staff reinforcing value, staff's likely reaction to drug use, and, to a lesser extent, staff teaching.

The authors commented that the failure to obtain posttreatment differences in comparisons between treatment groups or between AP subjects and their friends indicates a strong need for drug and alcohol treatment components in delinquent treatment programs. Development of new behavior change strategies that would have long-term effects on drug use are also needed. The study was notable for its attempt to construct reasonable comparison groups, although the authors addressed some significant pretreatment group differences that may have biased the outcome in favor of the AP program. However, other factors (e.g., subject selection) are identified that may produce opposite effects. The authors also advocated the use of other corroborative measures of drug use, such as school and work problems, physical illness, and urine tests. Overall, the study is a very respectable attempt to address clinically meaningful, difficult to measure, outcome variables.

Application of Achievement Place Model in an Inpatient Setting. Elder and his colleagues (Elder, Plants, Welch, & Feindler, 1983) took on the ambitious task of implementing an Achievement Place program in an adolescent unit of a state mental institution. The project was initiated at the request of hospital administrators in response to unacceptably high rates of residents' fighting, self-abuse, and accidents, as well as a lack of treatment programming. The unit staff (12 psychiatric aides, a social worker, a psychiatric nurse, and 3 special education teachers) were trained as "teaching parents" and learned operant behavior management techniques (including implementation of a point and level system, and social skills training). This program evaluation covered a year and a-half period during which time 43 adolescents (ages 12 to 17) were hospitalized in this 10-bed unit.

Program evaluation measures included the cost of running the program, the number of "incidents" (injuries to staff and patients), ratings of staff competence, improvements in classroom environment and teacher satisfaction, rates of aggressive behavior, and changes in discharge rates, elopement, and recidivism. In general, positive changes were obtained in all areas when comparing a 9.5-month pretraining period to a 7.5-month period during which the Achievement Place model had been implemented. Of particular importance were significant reductions in injuries and repair-related man hours, and increases in both staff competence and adolescent discharge rates. Although this hospital-based program cost about five times that of a typical Achievement Place group home, the authors noted that the alternative would have meant closing down the adolescent unit and reallocating funds to other hospital programs. It was noted that the hospital unit had a 2 to 1 staff–patient ratio as compared to a 0.43 to 1 ration in a group home.

Hospital program costs included the salaries of all staff members as well as physicians.

Time-out and Seclusion in Child/Adolescent Inpatient Units. Time-out and/or seclusion procedures are included in most inpatient programs. Reports on the efficacy of these techniques are rare, even though they are considered to be integral parts of the treatment program. This section reviews the effects of differential time-out duration and factors (e.g., diagnostic category) associated with the frequency and duration of seclusion.

The effect of differential time-out duration (15, 30, 45, 60, and 90 minutes) on assaultive behavior was evaluated in a group of 13 psychiatrically hospitalized 9 to 17 year olds (Benjamin, Mazzarine, & Kupfersmid, 1983). The investigators found that the longer the amount of time given for the time-out (TO), the longer the period needed for patients to become settled, suggesting that longer TOs promote assaultiveness. The authors hypothesized that with longer TOs, children and adolescents may be more likely to continue physical violence, rather than cooperate and take the TO of their own accord.

In another study (Thomas & Maus, 1983), the imposition of an arbitrary time requirement was examined. A release criterion of 5 minutes of quiet time was implemented in a residential treatment facility for "behavior problem" children and adolescents (of mildly retarded or below average intellectual functioning). The average duration of TOs for 431 patients was 19.6 minutes. Over 68% of TOs were terminated within 15 minutes and 95% were terminated within 1 hour. Again, these findings suggest that if contingencies are clearly stated, time-out does not have to result in unusually long periods of isolation for the patients. These studies also suggest that patients' perceptions of the procedures (i.e., time-limited and/or somewhat under their control) may be important factors to consider in designing TO to be an effective treatment procedure.

Reports on seclusion (as distinguished from time-out) are characterized by rather vague explanations about procedure and treatment objectives. Reasons for its use are often primarily stated in terms of protection of patients and staff. Some investigators (Oates & Cooper, 1983) proposed that the seclusion period may be appropriate for "instruction" on more appropriate behavior. Frequency and duration of seclusions (e.g., Erickson & Realmuto, 1983) can be affected by such factors as underuse of antipsychotic medication and inappropriate staff response to adolescents' limit testing.

Atkins and Riccuiti (1989) reported on setting and patient characteristics affecting the use of seclusion in a state inpatient facility for children and adolescents, over half of whom received a diagnosis of a disruptive behavior disorder (attention-deficit hyperactivity disorder, conduct disorder, oppositional-defiant disorder). Subjects' (n = 408) average age was 15 years; 62% were male and 33% were black. Average length of stay during a calendar year was 144 days. With this sample, the average duration of seclusion was 5 hours, with males having significantly more seclusions than females. Blacks had almost twice the seclusion rate relative to whites. High-rate secluders tended to be younger, had more prior admissions, and were more likely to have a disruptive behavior disorder diagnosis and were less likely to have a concurrent diagnosis of anxiety or depression. Interestingly, use of a variety of interventions prior to seclusion (e.g., PRN medication, restraints, other punishers, rewards, and individual attention) were more frequently reported for low-rate secluders. If this report is representative of seclusion use with aggressive children in psychiatric facilities, there appears to be a number of important issues ripe for investigation. The interaction of diagnostic category, responsiveness to alternatives/preventive procedures and racial/cultural staff–patient differences all need to be investigated more carefully.

Cognitive-Behavioral Therapy and Social Skills Training

The set of procedures identified as cognitive-behavioral therapy (CBT) are designed to have an impact on children's and adolescents' cognitive processing of the frustrating and provocative situations they encounter. CBT outcome studies with aggressive youth have primarily been directed at children in outpatient clinics or school settings (e.g., Lochman, 1990), although some research has begun to be directed at clients with more severe conduct disorder who are being treated in inpatient or residential settings. In this section of the chapter, we will focus only upon the latter studies.

A particular strength of the CBT approach is that these therapies can be directed toward the deficits and distortions that have been identified in the social-cognitive processes of aggressive children. Although this research has been conducted with children in noninstitutional settings with only a few exceptions (e.g., Slaby & Guerra, 1988), the resulting information-processing models have clear implications for treatment of social-cognitive dysfunctions of institutionalized children and adolescents. Within these models, children's aggressive behavior is assumed to result from their idiosyncratic perceptions of social situations, which, in turn, influence the arousal they experience and the decisions they make about how to react to the situations. These moment-by-moment aspects of social-cognitive processing are assumed to be influenced by the children's prior state (e.g., arousal from earlier in the day), traits (e.g., low self-esteem; expectations for successfully attaining reinforcements using given behavior), and learning history (e.g., prior reinforcements and punishments received for certain behaviors) (Lochman, Nelson, & Sims, 1981). Dodge (1986) has suggested a 5-step model of social-cognitive processes in which children can have difficulties in (1) attending to and encoding elements of the social situation, (2) interpreting the meaning of others' intentions, (3) generating a set of competent solutions to a problem, (4) considering consequences for various solutions and deciding upon a best solution, and (5) behaviorally enacting chosen solutions. These steps are expected to operate in a sequential fashion, so that distortions or deficits at one step (e.g., making attributions) affect subsequent steps (e.g., deciding which solution to use).

Empirical support exists for these models, since aggressive children have been found to be overly selective in attending to hostile cues in social situations, to over-infer that others have hostile intentions in ambiguous situations, to be relatively unaware of their own level of aggressiveness in early stages of conflict, thus attributing less responsibility for conflict to themselves, and to generate problem solutions that are more action-oriented and aggressive, with fewer verbal assertion strategies, in comparison to nonaggressive children (Dodge, 1986; Lochman, 1987; Lochman & Lampron, 1986). Aggressive children's social problem-solving deficiencies have been found to be influenced by other factors as well, including (1) their characteristic style of retrieving salient strategies from their memory, (2) their tendency to generate more maladaptive problem solutions following arousal related to rejection, owing to their apparent inability to modulate the effects of the arousal as quickly as nonaggressive children, and (3) their social goals which are more oriented to achieving dominance and revenge and less oriented to achieving affiliation than those of nonaggressive adolescents (Lochman, Meyer, Rabiner, & White, 1991). All these interacting social-cognitive processes can become the focus of intervention, and most CBT interventions emphasize at least several processes in the models. Thus, CBT can include components directed at social perspective-taking, social problem-solving training, self-instruction training, accurate awareness of physiological arousal and affective state, relaxation training to promote control over physiological arousal, and moral reasoning training. Social skills training (SST) is also often included as a component of CBT programs, to facilitate children's competent enactment of the problem solutions they choose. CBT and SST use similar therapy procedures, such as modeling and role-played behavioral rehearsal, during sessions. CBT focuses more on cognitive processes, and SST emphasizes overt behavior, but there is considerable overlap in the implementation of these procedures. In this section, we will review recent CBT and SST studies with children and adolescents in inpatient settings, and with adolescents in other residential or institutionalized settings.

Cognitive Behavior Therapy with Child Psychiatric Inpatients. Kazdin, Esveldt-Dawson, French, and Unis (1987b) randomly assigned 56 children on a psychiatric inpatient unit to one of three conditions: (1) problem-solving skills training (PSST), (2) relationships therapy (RT), and (3) treatment-contact control (TCC). The children ranged in age from 7 to 13, and included 11 girls and 45 boys; all were referred for treatment of overt (e.g., fighting, unmanageability at home or at school) or covert (e.g., stealing, running away, truancy) antisocial behavior. Sixty-nine percent of the children had diagnoses of conduct disorders, with the other children having diagnoses of depression, attention-deficit disorder, adjustment disorder, or other disorders. All children were rated above the 98th percentile on either the Aggression or Delinquency scale of the Child Behavior Checklist, using parent ratings. Due to attrition of the sample, 47 children were available for posttesting and 42 for the 1-year follow-up. PSST and RT were administered individually in 20 45-minute sessions. PSST included social problem-solving and self-instruction training, and RT provided empathy, unconditional positive regard, and warmth in nondirective format. TCC provided for the treatment of the usual ward routine and of nonspecific therapist contact. At both the posttreatment assessment and at the 1-year follow-up, the children receiving PSST had significantly more reductions in ratings of externalizing problem behavior by parents and teachers than did children in the other two conditions. Despite this indication of treatment gains over time for PSST, the children in this condition had not been able to move into a normal range by follow-up, and the magnitude of treatment gains was less than desired.

Similar results were reported in a second study by Kazdin, Esveldt-Dawson, French, and Unis (1987a) in which the problem-solving skills training was combined with parent behavioral management training (PSST and PMT) for half of the 40 child inpatients, while the other half were randomly assigned to treatment-contact control (TCC). Children were again aged 7 to 12, and were referred for antisocial behavior. The combined PSST and PMT condition produced significantly greater reductions in parents' and teachers' ratings of externalizing behavior at posttreatment and at the 1-year follow-up, in comparison to TCC. However, the magnitude of the treatment effects was quite similar to the PSST condition in the Kazdin *et al.* (1987b) study, indicating that the parent management training may have added little to the effects of the problem-solving training alone, for this inpatient sample.

Cognitive Behavior Therapy with Adolescent Psychiatric Inpatients. More research on the effectiveness of cognitive-behavioral and social skill therapies have been conducted with inpatient adolescents than with inpatient children. However, the overall quality of research with adolescents varies from simple demonstration reports to controlled studies. Corder, Whiteside, and Haizlip (1986) provided an example of a descriptive demonstration report. Thirteen adolescents in a state psychiatric hospital (ages 13–18; 6 male, 7 female) participated in nine weekly sessions. Their intellectual abilities ranged from low to high average, and their diagnoses ranged from character disorder to borderline psychosis, with most of the adolescents having a history of sporadic, destructive, acting-out behavior. The training program included both group and individual sessions and focused on cognitive training involving the use of subvocal self-instructions, on recognition of cues for arousal, and on relaxation training through muscular relaxation exercises and galvanic skin response biofeedback. In addition, the adolescents received an unspecified number of sessions of social problem-solving training which used didactic training, role-play, and discussion groups. Although this demonstration project illustrated a multifaceted cognitive-behavioral program which included biofeedback and relaxation exercises, the usefulness of this program remains unclear, since it only summarized anecdotal positive statements of staff.

Of the three studies that have used experimental designs in which treatment conditions were compared to untreated conditions, two studies have produced equivocal results. Saylor, Benson, and Einhaus (1985) randomly assigned 14 male patients in a state psychiatric hospital to either an Anger Management (AM) or an Attention Control (AC) condition. The patients ranged in age from 9 years-8 months to 14 years-8 months, and 29% had nonwhite racial status. Although diagnoses were not reported, all boys had identified initial problems of excessive anger, difficulty with anger management, or physical and verbal aggression. The AM condition was conducted in 18 individual, half-hour sessions over 9 weeks, with clinical psychology graduate students as therapists. The sessions provided instruction on the determinants of anger, relaxation training, imaginal coping with provocations while relaxed, and modeling and faded rehearsal of self-statements. With the latter skills, the therapist first modeled the use of coping self-statements when provoked and in ensuing sessions children repeated audibly and then silently these self-statements. In the last sessions, the children role-played their use of these coping skills. The AC children met with therapists for the same number of individual sessions as in the AM condition, but the children discussed emotions other than anger in the AC condition. At posttesting, the AM boys had significant reductions in their self-reported anger on the Children's Inventory of Anger, in comparison to the AC boys. However, there were no significant treatment effects found in staff or teacher behavioral ratings, or in direct observations of behavior on the unit or in gym classes.

Tisdelle and St. Lawrence (1988) provided interpersonal problem-solving skill training to eight male inpatients (ages 13 to 19) at a state psychiatric hospital, and compared their acquisition of problem-solving skills to a social validation sample of 20 normal high school students. The inpatient adolescents all had diagnoses of CD and had IQ scores ranging from 70 to 109. They met in 13 twice-weekly group sessions. Examining responses to hypothetical social problems, the treated adolescents demonstrated improvement in the problem-solving skills of problem identification, goal definition, generation of alternatives, comparison of consequences, and selection of the best alternative. These improvements were evident both in the repeated administration of the measure to the patients over the course of the multiple-baseline design, and in comparison to the social validation group. Although the two subject groups were significantly different in self-reported problem-solving skills at pretesting, the inpatients had improved to be within a normal range by posttesting. However, there were no accompanying changes in staff ratings of adolescents' problem behavior on the Missouri Children's Behavior Checklist, and there was little generalization to actual problem-solving behavior in role-played problems with staff.

Although these two studies indicated that adolescents could improve in social problem-solving skills and in self-reported anger arousal following treatment, these gains in cognitive controls did not generalize to out-of-session behavior. In contrast, Feindler, Ecton, Kingsley, and Dubey (1986) have found behavioral as well as social-cognitive changes. Feindler *et al.* (1986) randomly assigned 10 adolescents within one unit of a psychiatric treatment facility to anger control training (ACT), and 11 adolescents in another unit to wait list control (WLC). All patients were male, were 13 to 18 years old, and had been identified by staff as having problems with aggressive, explosive behavior. Sixteen of the adolescents had diagnoses of Conduct Disorder. Although both subject groups had similar levels of low-average intelligence, the ACT boys were slightly younger (15.4 years vs. 16.9 years), and had fewer black youth (1 vs. 6) than did the WLC boys. These pretest differences were not tested to see if they were significant. The ACT was provided in 12 sessions over 8 weeks, and focused on identifying situational "triggers" to anger, relaxation training, use of "hassle sheets" to self-monitor their daily anger arousal, self-instruction training, training of assertion responses, and anticipation of consequences of actions. In comparison to WLC, the ACT adolescents (1) had become less cognitively impulsive, as indicated by fewer errors and longer latencies on the Matching Familiar Figures Test, (2) had higher staff ratings of adolescents' self-control, (3) increased their rates of appropriate requests and decreased their rates of inappropriate/hostile comments and negative physical contact during videotaped role-played conflicts with male confederates, and (4) decreased their rates of dorm violations. Although it cannot be conclusively determined why the Feindler *et al.* (1986) study produced more significant behavioral generalization than did the Tisdelle and St. Lawrence (1988) and Saylor *et al.* (1985) studies, the Feindler *et al.* program included a wider array of problem-solving, self-instruction training, relaxation training, and self-monitoring components, and the study included a somewhat larger sample, making testing of statistical significance easier. The monitoring of behavior by self and others outside of the treatment sessions may be a particularly important means of promoting generalization (e.g., Lochman, Burch, Curry, & Lampron, 1984).

Social Skills Training in Child and Adolescent Inpatient Psychiatric Settings. One approach to the treatment of aggressive children and adolescents—social skills training—has been rooted in the assumption that aggressive behavior may be a function of a social skills deficit. When individuals with skill deficits experience frustration, one response may be aggression. A number of studies investigated the effects of social skills training on aggressive behavior patterns.

A group of four children (2 boys, 2 girls, ages 8 to 12) on an inpatient psychiatric unit were provided with an "assertive" skill training program (Bornstein, Bellack, & Hersen, 1980) in three specific skills: eye contact, tone of voice, and requests for new behavior. No diagnoses were provided for the subjects, but they were all described as having aggressive interpersonal styles. IQs ranged from 83 to 91. A multiple-baseline (across behaviors) design was employed in which the children were trained in a group for three consecutive sessions on one behavior at a time. Measures included pre- and posttesting on the Behavioral Assertiveness Test for Children (BAT—C) (Bornstein, Bellack, & Hersen, 1977) with thrice-weekly assessment probes during baseline, treatment, and a follow-up. Pre- and posttreatment observations were conducted of the subjects' interactions with other children in a group therapy context. Training involved enactment of the BAT—C scenes with repeated therapist feedback, role-play, modeling, instruction, and rehearsal. Positive changes were obtained for each subject on each target behavior following training for that behavior. One out of four subjects showed evidence of generalization across settings (i.e., the group therapy context). Unfortunately, no measures of aggressive behavior or general functioning on the ward were collected. Interestingly, the authors commented on the importance of cognitions (e.g., a subject's belief that threats were important to maintain status) in developing future treatment programs.

A similar approach was implemented with a group of four adolescents ($M = 98.5$, range = 78–108) on an adolescent unit in a large state psychiatric hospital (Elder, Edelstein, & Novick, 1979). All subjects evidenced problems in verbal and physical aggression. One improvement over the previous study was that target behaviors were determined on the basis of staff-rated problems on the Jesness Behavior Checklist. The target behaviors included interruptions, responses to negative communication (teases, threats), and requests for behavior change. A multiple-baseline (across behaviors) design was employed. Measures included in-group session ratings of target behaviors, direct observations in extra-group settings, and changes in the number of fines for each of the target behaviors. Treatment consisted of 14 group social skills training sessions, conducted four times a week for 45 minutes. Therapists (2 female staff members) provided instruction, modeling, and feedback regarding appropriate execution of each skill. Meaningful improvements in the target behaviors were obtained with in-group ratings and extra-group observations. In addition, reductions in seclusion rates and in fines incurred for inappropriate behavior were obtained. At a 3-month follow-up, three subjects had been discharged and all were still in the community at a 9-month interval. The fourth subject had regressed to pretreatment levels of functioning.

Kolko, Dorsett, and Milan (1981) implemented a similar SST program with three aggressive adolescents (ages 14, 15, and 16) on an inpatient unit. Several aspects of the treatment addressed issues that the authors had identified as weaknesses in previous SST research reports. Care was taken to implement *in vivo* simulations on the unit with confederate staff members and peers before and after training. Multiple (vs. single) response role-plays were used to approximate a more "natural" flow of interaction. The social validity of training effects was assessed via ratings by a staff and a group of "naive" evaluators (hospital staff members unfamiliar to the subjects). A multiple-baseline (across subjects and skills) design was employed. Training focused on five aspects of behavior (eye contact, response latency, facial expression, voice loudness, and verbal response). Behavioral observations revealed marked improvement in all subjects for each trained behavior in both training and *in vivo* simulations. Significant improvement was noted in staff ratings of subjects' responses to training and novel situations. Randomized ratings by the naive evaluators also indicated reliable improvements in the before and after videotapes of the subjects. Effects were maintained at 1 to 3 posttreatment sessions. Unfortunately, no follow-up data or ratings of aggressive behavior were collected.

Jamison and his colleagues (Jamison, Lambert, & McCloud, 1986) modeled their training program after that of Kolko *et al.* (1981). However, they employed a group design ($n = 12$) with adolescents (age range 15 to 17) diagnosed with Conduct Disorder ($n = 9$) or Adjustment Disorder ($n = 3$) who were hospitalized at a state psychiatric institute. The five-session (1 hr per week) program incorporated the same training procedures as Kolko *et al.* (1981), but behaviors were not trained sequentially (à la multiple-baseline design). In addition, homework assignments were used (e.g., observe/record two instances of nonverbal communication). No *in vivo* simulations were conducted. The control group received only the "regular hospital treatment." Analysis of variance of ratings of nonverbal and verbal behavior (pre- and posttreatment) indicated significant changes in eye contact (but not facial expression) and verbal assertiveness for the treatment group only.

Cognitive Behavior Therapy and Social Skills Training in Other Institutional Settings. Research on the effects of cognitive-behavioral therapy and social skills training has also been conducted with children and adolescents in residential school, group home, and training school settings, and these results can have some implications for inpatient treatment. The four studies reviewed here are representative of these studies. They have documented positive changes that were due to the treatments, but the results are again mixed. Bell, Mundy, and Quay (1983) randomly assigned boys in a private residential school for severely retarded and seriously disturbed youth to either an experimental treatment condition (E) or a control condition (C). The intellectual abilities of the boys ranged from the low-average to the high-average range ($\bar{X} = 89$), the boys all had histories of impulsive and antisocial behavior, and they ranged in age from 10 to 16. The E program was provided to 24 boys and consisted of 14 twice-weekly sessions in which the boys received self-instruction training on five steps that they could use on cognitive tasks ("Find out what I'm supposed to do," "Look at all the possibilities," etc.) to reduce their impulsive responding. This program was similar to the Kendall and Braswell (1985) cognitive-behavioral treatment and used the same four-stage faded rehearsal format, in which treatment proceeds from therapists' overt modeling to children's overt and then covert rehearsal of the self-instructions. The C program was provided to 21 boys, and reinforced the children for correct responses on the same cognitive tasks, but without self-instruction training. The E group demonstrated greater reduction in impulsive responding after the intervention period than did the C group on the Porteus May Q score, but not on the Matching Familiar Figures Test latency score. Thus, the results suggested that the treated boys had a decrease in impulsivity on one of the two measures, although the generalization of this effect to behavior on the unit was not tested.

In a preliminary effort to teach another social-cognitive skill—social problem-solving—to delinquent adolescents living in a therapeutic group home, Hains (1984) implemented a brief intervention with four adolescent males (ages 14 to 17). The group home used a Teaching-Family Achievement Place model, and this study represented an initial effort to integrate a cognitive-behavioral component into this well-established behavioral model. The intervention itself was a minimal one, since it consisted of one educational session about antecedents of problems, means of resolving problems, and consequences, followed by the adolescents' rehearsal of these skills on hypothetical dilemmas for two to four more sessions. Using a multiple-baseline design, the adolescents were found to increase their quantitative rates of antecedents, solutions, and consequences on hypothetical problems, but only a minimal amount of transfer was evident to adolescents' discussions of their personal social problems. The weak generalization of treatment effects may have been partially due to the brevity and narrowness of the treatment program.

A larger number of studies have examined the utility of social skills training with delinquents in residential, noninpatient settings, and these results have been reviewed by Goldstein, Glick, Reiner, Zimmerman, and Coultry (1987). Among the best of these studies, Ollendick and Hersen (1979) randomly assigned 27 male adolescent delinquents (ages 13 to 16) to one of three conditions: social skills (SS), discussion (D), or control (C). The three conditions were matched on age, IQ scores, and number of arrests. This sample was selected from a larger population of 73 delinquents in a training school, and represented the individuals with the most external locus of control scores. The training school unit also had a token economy and behavioral contracting system. The SS program met in weekly group sessions for 10 weeks. The adolescents discussed current interpersonal problems in the sessions.

They received instructions on alternative ways of responding, rehearsed the situations, observed the modeling of group leaders and peers, received feedback on their behavior, received social reinforcement, and were instructed to practice their new responses between sessions. It should be noted that this kind of social skills training program is highly similar to social problem-solving training programs, although the social skills training programs place more emphasis on direct instruction about solutions rather than encourage brainstorming from group participants about an array of possible solutions. The D program also met for 10 weekly group sessions. The primary group leaders had an eclectic orientation, encouraged discussion of interpersonal problems, but did not use the behavioral training techniques. The C condition did not augment the basic behavior modification programs with additional group treatment. Changes before and after the program were examined. In comparison to both the D and C conditions, the SS adolescents demonstrated improvements on self-report measures (reduced state anxiety, more internal locus of control), in role-played scenes (shorter response latency, more eye contact, more positive behavior, less aggressive content, more adaptive requests for new behavior from others), and in the number of points they earned in the unit's token economy. Although the social skills training did not produce reductions in the number of disruptive behavior incidents on the unit, the program did have relatively broad effects on the adolescents in the other domains that were assessed.

Glick and Goldstein (1987; Goldstein *et al.*, 1987) have assembled and evaluated an Aggression Replacement Training (ART) program for delinquents. This wide-ranging program has both social skills training and cognitive-behavioral components, including Structured Learning Training (Goldstein's previously evaluated social skills training program which had social problem-solving elements), Anger Control Training (the Feindler *et al.*, 1986, Anger Control program), and Moral Education (using Kohlberg-style moral dilemmas, based on Arbuthnot and Faust, 1981). The focuses of these components, especially the first two, overlap to a moderate degree. During the ART program, each of these three units are presented in a weekly group session. Over the 10-week program period, 30 sessions are held. Glick and Goldstein (1987) evaluated ART by presenting it to adolescent male delinquents (ages 13 to 21) at two residential correction facilities. The youth had histories of criminal behavior, but all were not necessarily aggressive. In the study at the first residential facility, 60 delinquents were randomly assigned by units to ART (n = 24), to Brief Instruction Control (BIC) (n = 24), and to No-treatment Control (NC) (n = 12). The BIC youth did not have group sessions, but prior to posttesting they received test instructions which described the nature and value of the skills involved. In comparison to the two control conditions at posttest, the ART youth displayed significant improvements in the structured learning skills (e.g., how to express a complaint, handle stressful conversation, respond to anger, respond to group pressure), had lower staff ratings of impulsiveness on the Kendall-Wilcox Self-Control Scale, and had a reduction in the number and intensity of staff ratings of acting-out behavior. In the second correctional facility, 51 youth were assigned to ART and C conditions. The ART-treated delinquents again demonstrated improvements in structural learning skills, had reductions in staff ratings of impulsiveness, and had higher staff ratings of prosocial behavior. However, in the second facility, staff ratings of antisocial behavior did not improve for ART youth. In addition to the mixed findings on this primary outcome variable for acting-out behavior, the study had several other weaknesses, including potential bias in ratings by staff who were apparently not blind to treatment conditions, and lack of assessment of interrater reliability. The findings were encouraging but mixed, in a manner similar to most studies reviewed in this section.

Challenges to Implementation of and Research on Behavior Therapy in Inpatient Settings

Impediments to the use of behavior therapy in inpatient settings must be distinguished from impediments to systematic research on the effectiveness of behavior therapy in such settings. Impediments to research are more extensive than impediments to the use of behavior therapy techniques, but only behavioral interventions that have been evaluated will appear in the scientific literature. Our review of literature reveals a relative lack of well-designed outcome studies on behavioral intervention with inpatient children and adolescents. In contrast, many, if not most, inpatient programs utilize a structured environment, milieu, or set of environmental contingencies to manage the behavior of hospitalized youths. In this section, we will review some challenges to the implementation of behavior therapy programs in inpatient settings and then examine the impediments to systematic research on such interventions.

Challenges to the implementation of behavior therapy in an inpatient setting can derive from theoretical or programmatic factors. At a theoretical level, inpatient programs vary in the degree to which they emphasize nurturance versus behavioral control. Within the programs' staff, there are likely to be significant variations in supportiveness for the adolescent's struggle toward autonomy and in the perceived importance of behavior control. This issue, which is central to a parental role in normal familial settings (Minuchin, 1974), is heightened in inpatient settings, because a major function of the milieu is containment (Gunderson, 1978). This is particularly the case with regard to potentially assaultive or suicidal youths. On the other hand, programs which stress behavioral control to an extreme degree will be perceived by youngsters as demanding only conformity without internalization and generalization of new learning. At the theoretical level, therefore, behavior therapy programs need to reflect the shared assumptions of program staff in the degree to which they demand behavioral control or permit a wide latitude of expressiveness.

Several programmatic factors also influence the feasibility of developing behavioral interventions in inpatient settings. One factor is the presence of multiple, simultaneous, therapeutic modalities. In keeping with the attempt to offer comprehensive biopsychosocial assessment and intervention, inpatient programs often include individual, group, family, milieu, recreation, and art therapy, and medication when appropriate. A behavioral treatment can function either as the overall matrix in which these modalities occur (e.g., a comprehensive token economy) or as one additional component of treatment (e.g., stress management training). Primarily behavioral programs tend to use behavior therapy as a comprehensive matrix, whereas more eclectic programs add it to the mix of modalities.

A second programmatic issue affecting implementation of behavior therapy is the structure of the inpatient unit. Some units have a centralized, fairly uniform program, so that almost all children or adolescents admitted to the program participate in a relatively standardized assessment and treatment protocol, lasting an expectable duration of time. On the other hand, decentralized units are those in which the assessment and treatment protocol and, to some extent, the length of stay are determined by the primary clinician, the attending doctor, or by external constraints on length of stay. Although individualized behavioral treatment plans may be implemented in the latter type of structure, group or milieu behavioral treatment is much more difficult to implement.

If the program staff members are able to surmount the challenges to implementing the behavioral treatment outlined above, the next set of challenges to be faced are those to systematic research on such interventions. In general, controlled comparisons between different treatments are difficult to implement within an inpatient program. As a function of multiple, simultaneous, therapeutic modalities, it is difficult to link specific therapeutic gains with a specific therapeutic modality. In addition, the closed nature of inpatient settings makes it impossible to assure that subjects in the "alternate" treatment condition have not received part of the "experimental" treatment through exposure to subjects in that condition. Yalom (1983) has discussed this problem with reference to inpatient group psychotherapy, but his discussion of constraints on research design is equally pertinent to the study of any component of an inpatient program. As Yalom noted, one solution to this set of constraints is the use of a sequential treatment comparison model (Beutler, Frank, Schieber, Calvert, & Gaines, 1984). In this model, participants in the inpatient program during a set period of time receive the usual treatment protocol or the usual treatment plus treatment A. Later, the participants receive the usual treatment plus treatment B. Lack of overlap between the subject groups in their presence in the programs is a control for "contamination" across groups.

The clinical demand for comprehensive care can also conflict with the research demand for clarity of effects. Many children and adolescents in inpatient settings present with more than one major problem or diagnosis (Carlson & Cantwell, 19809; Geller, Chestnut, Miller, Price, & Yates, 1985). An adolescent with conduct problems, family conflict, and major depression, for example, may be treated on clinical grounds with a trial of antidepressant medication and with cognitive or interpersonal psychotherapy, functional family therapy, and a behavioral milieu program. Successful outcome would then not clearly be attributable to any one component. Between subjects comparisons within comprehensive care programs, however, can be used to determine what kinds of youths are most likely to benefit from the program as a whole (Gossett, 1977).

Finally, there are a set of general administrative, financial, and personnel issues that must be addressed for successful research to occur on behavioral inpatient treatment. Gossett (1977) has outlined guidelines for outcome research in clinical settings which pertain to behavioral research as well as to other treatment outcome studies. They include the need for administrative support for outcome research, the need to obtain funding to support research personnel, the need for consistent research project leadership, the importance of obtaining informed consent, and the need to return feedback to cooperating clinicians. Failure to meet these guidelines would be likely to preclude long-term or routinized outcome research on behavioral interventions, whereas adherence to them will greatly facilitate the research process.

CASE HISTORY

The following case study illustrates several central issues in implementing behavior modification programs to manage antisocial and self-destructive behavior in an inpatient setting. General issues, rather than specific components of the behavioral program, will be emphasized.

F. R. was a 13-year-old white male of superior intellectual ability who had a past history of hyperactivity. He was admitted to an inpatient unit because of the recent onset of severe depression with suicidal ideation and suicide threats. His history also included "concealing" conduct disordered behavior, such as stealing and spending money belonging to family members and neighbors. His diagnosis included both a conduct disorder and a major affective disorder.

Because of his refusal to comply with normal ward expectations and because of his destruction of property and self-mutilating behavior in the ward, F. R. was placed in an individualized behavior modification program. The program, which was developed by a staff member and then given to the patient, required that F. R. attend school on time, complete all homework, engage in "relevant" and not "superficial" individual treatment sessions, refrain from cursing, lying, kicking, smoking, fighting, destroying property, cutting or scratching himself, and "manipulating others." Any failure to abide by these requirements resulted in a response cost, such as restriction from social activities, loss of "category" or level of freedom for one day, or a lengthy time-out (1 hour or more). These consequences were provided through a seven-level category system, in which adolescents received more and less freedom to engage in on-ward and off-ward activities, depending on staff judgments of their behavior after each shift.

F. R.'s reaction to this program was extremely negative. His noncompliance increased. He perceived the program as an effort by staff to control him and stated that he refused to compromise with staff because to do so would result in loss of self-respect. The intensity of the power struggle between F. R. and the treatment staff was recognized, and consultation was requested.

After interviewing F. R. and the staff members, the consulting psychologist, with guarded optimism, made three suggestions to the treatment staff. The recommendations were accompanied by direct recognition of the dynamics in which the staff were trapped: F. R. demanded complete autonomy yet threatened and engaged in self-destructive behavior. Therefore, staff members were understandably anxious about allotting him more freedom and were simultaneously angered by his destructive behavior and unwillingness to compromise.

The three recommendations were: (1) to allow F. R. to write his own

> program, which would then have to be approved by the treatment team; (2) to limit target behavior to no more than five clearly observable behaviors, and to avoid inferential judgments about such behavior as "manipulative" and "superficial" interactions; and (3) to focus the program in terms of positive reinforcers rather than response cost. The treatment staff agreed to try this recommendation, and F. R. subsequently wrote his program with enthusiasm. It focused on compliance with ward routines and on avoidance of destructive or self-destructive behavior. The program was supported by F. R.'s psychiatrist and by his primary nurse who co-signed the program.
>
> F. R. then proceeded to abide by the program very consistently. As a result, the therapeutic alliance with F. R. was greatly improved, the power struggle greatly reduced, and the attitude of the staff toward F. R. became much more positive.

In this case the issue of establishing a therapeutic alliance was probably the most critical issue. In addition, this case illustrates the importance in implementing behavior therapy procedures by avoiding such pitfalls as focusing on too many behaviors at once and not evaluating beforehand the adolescent's perception and interpretation of various positive reinforcements, response-cost procedures, and time-out. The case also emphasizes the need for continuous monitoring of staff understanding of behavior modification principles, especially on inpatient units such as this one that do not use behavior therapy as the primary treatment modality. Finally, addressing adolescent developmental issues related to autonomy, by involving the adolescent in the design of the behavioral program, appeared to improve markedly not only the response to the behavior therapy, but also to other modalities of therapy offered by the program. The complex, potentially very dangerous problems presented by F. R., could then be addressed by use of a full range of services, including appropriate medication for his affective disorder and family therapy to address major power struggles within the family.

CONCLUSIONS

Summary of Findings

Unfortunately, our conclusions about the utility of behavioral and cognitive-behavioral therapy procedures with inpatient antisocial youth have to be advanced cautiously. It is remarkable that there are few controlled studies of behavior therapy in inpatient settings, and the studies that have been conducted have produced quite an array of mixed results, in contrast to the generally more positive results of behavior therapy with outpatient and community samples (Lochman, 1990; McMahon & Wells, 1992). Studies that have used behavioral management principles and social skills training to alter antisocial behavior have generally been successful, but much of this research has not been conducted in inpatient settings. These social skill training studies that were done in inpatient settings are limited with regard to sample size (predominant use of single-subject designs), uneven use of socially valid measures of behavior changes (in social skill and aggression), and assessment of generalization. Among those that did address generalization (e.g., Elder *et al.*, 1979), minimal attention was given to the possible factors that were responsible for this generalization. Is generalization strictly attributed to learning of specific behaviors and changes in environmental contingencies? Or are there changes in the subject's social perceptions, attributions, and problem-solving skills?

Research conducted with cognitive-behavioral techniques in inpatient units has produced decidedly mixed outcomes. The strongest cognitive-behavioral treatment results emerged from several of the studies with the most stringent designs using comparison groups and follow-up assessment. Social problem-solving training with inpatient children (Kazdin *et al.*, 1987a,b) and a multifaceted anger control program for inpatient adolescents (Feindler *et al.*, 1986) were found to effectively reduce staff ratings of youths' aggression and disruption. Less effective cognitive-behavioral programs were generally presented for shorter lengths of time or included fewer elements of cognitive-behavioral treatment.

Although the results of behavior therapy with inpatient antisocial youth are promising, further research is clearly necessary. More rigorous and intensive studies need to be conducted. These studies should include: (1) large enough sample sizes to provide sufficient statistical power to test fairly for treatment effects, (2) randomly assigned minimal treatment and untreated comparison conditions to demonstrate conclusively the utility of treatment, (3) follow-up assessments, and (4) the use of independent, unbiased behavioral observers so that staff ratings are not the sole measures of behavioral change. All these design suggestions are more difficult to implement in inpatient than in outpatient settings, but it is imperative that the utility of behavioral therapy techniques be clearly demonstrated with the severely disturbed children and adolescents in inpatient settings, rather than merely be assumed. Several of the most prominent, specific gaps in the treatment research are noted below.

Foci for Future Research

Behavioral Parent Training. With the exception of the Kazdin *et al.* (1987a) study, no research has examined the effects of collateral behavioral parent training for antisocial inpatient children and adolescents. This gap in the behavioral therapy literature is particularly striking since behavioral parent training and behavioral family therapy have produced the currently most consistent treatment effects among the behavioral methods for conduct-disordered, aggressive youth (Kazdin *et al.*, 1987b; Lochman, 1990; McMahon & Wells, 1989). Conducting behavioral parent training while a child is in an inpatient unit is assuredly a difficult procedure, since the parents are unable to begin practicing immediately the behavioral techniques with the target child in their home setting. However, parents could begin trying out more consistent, positive behavioral management procedures with their other children, they could observe staff use of behavioral management procedures, and the parents' and child's behavior during the inpatient family sessions could be modified by therapists to improve their conflict management and social problem solving behaviors.

Time-out and Seclusion. Even though time-out and/or seclusion procedures are included in most inpatient programs for children and adolescents (along with token economics), the efficacy of these procedures with inpatient antisocial youth has not been clearly documented. One of the most critical needs arising from this review is for immediate outcome research of time-out effects. Does time-out effectively reduce antisocial behavior on inpatient units? What are the most optimal means of structuring time-out (e.g., length of time-out period, behavioral contingencies)? A comprehensive scientific analysis of the efficacy of time-out is essential, so that the use and effects of time-out can be differentiated from the frequently used seclusion procedures on inpatient units (Varley, 1984). Time-out is an extinction procedure in which reinforcers are removed from an individual for a short period of time immediately after the occurrence of a target act by the individual. Seclusion is a ward action that is often meant to be a punishment to a patient, to remove the patient from excess stimulation by others on the unit, or to protect the other patients and staff from a patient's acutely assaultive behavior. Although a clear need exists for seclusion procedures on inpatient units, seclusion should not be regarded as a behavior therapy technique. Only when the parameters of effective time-out, in combination with comprehensive behavior management procedures (e.g., reward, contracting), have been researched can we begin to cogently examine the similarities and differences between time-out and seclusion on inpatient settings.

Prescriptive Treatment Planning. Since the general state of research on inpatient behavioral therapy with antisocial youth is still in early stages of development, it is not surprising that researchers have not yet tackled the questions of which behavioral therapy techniques work best for which types of inpatients. Such studies will require an increasingly sophisticated ability to identify meaningful subtypes and dimensions of youth with antisocial behavior. For example, preliminary research with a psychoeducational, residential re-ed treatment facility for assaultive youth found that children and adolescents with higher initial staff ratings of internalizing behaviors (e.g., anxiety, depression) made the most improvements in their externalizing, aggressive behaviors during the course of treatment (Lochman, Bennett, & Simmers, 1988). In more finely differentiated dimensional studies with noninpatient samples, aggressive boys with initially low levels of social problem-solving skills have been found to make more behavioral gains following cognitive-behavioral treatment than boys with better problem-solving skills. Families of aggressive boys with depressed, insular parents who have high levels of marital discord are less likely to benefit from behavioral parent training than are other parents (Lochman, 1990; McMahon & Wells, 1989).

Sexual offenders are one example of an unresearched subtype of antisocial youth who present special concerns about both the utility and the appropriateness of behavioral treatments. Cognitive-behavioral therapy and social skills training would appear to be useful in helping offenders to reframe distorted cognitions about their behavior and its impact on their victims, to recognize the cycle of violence that is associated with sexual offending and to seek alternative coping strategies (Agee, 1979).

Although these techniques could be adapted to the treatment of sexual disorders with relatively little controversy, the use of sexually explicit behavior modification techniques with minor clients may be more problematic. For example, adolescent offenders may need to be instructed to practice verbal satiation of deviant fantasies rather than use adult-oriented techniques (Salter, 1988; Witt & Sager, 1988), such as masturbatory satiation with fantasies (Becker & Kavoussi, 1988). As behavioral therapy research develops with antisocial child and adolescent inpatients, we anticipate these studies will address the differential effectiveness and appropriateness of behavior therapy techniques with a variety of specific types of antisocial inpatients.

ACKNOWLEDGMENTS

The preparation of this chapter was supported in part by a grant from the National Institute of Mental Health (MH-39989) to the first author. We gratefully acknowledge the assistance of Dorothy Rummel in the final typing of this manuscript.

REFERENCES

Abidin, R. R. (1983). *Parenting Stress Index—Manual*. Charlottesville, VA: Pediatric Psychology Press.

Achenbach, T. M., & Edelbrock, C. S. (1983). *Manual for the Child Behavior Checklist and Revised Child Behavior Profile*. Burlington: University of Vermont, Department of Psychiatry.

Agee, V. L. (1979). *Treatment of the violent incorrigible adolescent*. Lexington, MA: Lexington Books.

American Psychiatric Association. (1987). *Diagnostic and statistical manual of mental disorders* (3rd ed., rev.). Washington, DC: Author.

Arbuthnot, Y., & Faust, A. (1981). *Teaching moral reasoning: Theory and practice*. New York: Harper and Row.

Atkins, M. S., & Riccuiti, A. (1989). *Characteristics of locked door seclusion in a children's psychiatric hospital*. Unpublished manuscript, Medical College of Pennsylvania at Eastern Pennsylvania Psychiatric Institute.

Barkley, R. A. (1984). *A review of child behavior rating scales and checklists for research in child psychopathology*. Rockville, MD: Center for Studies of Child and Adolescent Psychopathology, Clinical Research Branch, National Institute of Mental Health.

Barkley, R. A., Hastings, J. E., Tousel, R., & Tousel, S. E. (1976). Evaluation of a token system for juvenile delinquents in a residential setting. *Journal of Behavioral and Experimental Psychiatry, 7*(3), 227–230.

Beck, A. T. (1978). *Depression inventory*. Philadelphia: Center for Cognitive Therapy.

Becker, J. V., & Kavoussi, R. J. (1989). Diagnosis and treatment of juvenile sexual offenders. In R. Rosner & H. I. Schwartz (Eds.), *Critical issues in American psychiatry and the law:* Juvenile psychiatry and the law (Vol. 4. pp. 133–143). New York: Plenum Press.

Bell, C. R., Mundy, P., & Quay, H. C. (1983). Modifying impulsive responding in conduct-disordered institutionalized boys. *Psychological Reports, 52*, 307–310.

Benjamin, R., Mazzarine, H., & Kupfersmid, J. (1983). The effect of timeout (TO) duration on assaultiveness in psychiatrically hospitalized children. *Aggressive Behavior, 9*, 21–27.

Beutler, L., Frank, M., Schieber, S. C., Calvert, S., & Gaines, J. (1984). Comparative effects of group psychotherapies in a short-term inpatient setting: An experience with deterioration effects. *Psychiatry, 47*, 66–76.

Bornstein, M., Bellack, A., & Hersen, M. (1980). Social skills training for highly aggressive children. *Behavioral Modification, 4*, 173–186.

Bornstein, M. R., Bellack, A. S., & Hersen, M. (1977). Social skills training for unassertive children: A multiple baseline analysis. *Journal of Applied Behavior Analysis, 10*, 183–195.

Braukmann, C. J., Kirigin, K. A., & Wolf, M. M. (1980). Group home treatment research: Social learning and social control perspectives. In T. Hirschi & M. Gottfredson (Eds.), *Understanding crime: Current theory & research* (pp. 117–130). Beverly Hills: Sage Publications.

Braukman, C. J., Bedlington, M. M., Belden, B. D., Braukman, P. D., Husted, J. J., Ramp, K. K., & Wolf, M. M. (1985). Effects of community based group home treatment programs on male juvenile offenders' use and abuse of drugs and alcohol. *American Journal of Drug and Alcohol Abuse, 11*(3&4), 249–278.

Burchard, J. D., & Tyler, V. O. (1965). Modification of delinquent behavior through operant conditioning. *Behavior Research and Therapy, 2*, 245–250.

Carlson, G., & Cantwell, D. P. (1980). Unmasking masked depression in children and adolescents. *American Journal of Psychiatry, 137*, 445–449.

Conners, C. K. (1969). A teacher rating scale for use in drug studies with children. *American Journal of Psychiatry, 126*, 884–888.

Conners, C. K. (1970). Symptom patterns in hyperkinetic, neurotic and normal children. *Child Development, 41*, 667–682.

Conners, C. K. (1973). Rating scales for use in drug studies with children. *Psychopharmacology Bulletin, 9*, 24–84.

Corder, B. F., Whiteside, R., & Haizlip, T. (1986). Biofeedback, cognitive training and relaxation techniques as multimodal adjunct therapy for hospitalized adolescents: A pilot study. *Adolescence, 21*, 339–346.

Costello, A. J., Edelbrock, C. A., Dulcan, M. K., & Kalas, R. (1984). *Testing of the NIMH Diagnostic Interview Schedule for Children (DISC) in a clinical population* (Contract No. DB-81-00217. Final report to the Center for Epidemiological Studies, National Institute for Mental Health). Pittsburgh: University of Pittsburgh.

Cowen, E. L., Huser, J., Beach, D. R., & Rappaport, J. (1970). Parental perceptions of young children and their relation to indexes of adjustment. *Journal of Consulting and Clinical Psychology, 34*, 97–103.

Davidson, W. S., & Wolfred, T. R. (1977). Evaluation of a community-based behavior modification program for prevention of delinquency. *Community Mental Health Journal, 13*, 296–306.

Dodge, K. A. (1986). A social information-processing model of social competence in children. In M. Perlmutter (Ed.), *Minnesota symposium on child psychology* (Vol. 18, pp. 77–125). Hillsdale, NJ: Lawrence Erlbaum.

Dodge, K. A., & Frame, C. L. (1982). Social cognitive biases and deficits in aggressive boys. *Child Development, 53*, 620–635.

Elder, J. P., Edelstein, B. A., & Novick, M. M. (1979). Adolescent psychiatric patients: Modifying aggressive behavior with social skills training. *Behavior Modification, 3*(2), 161–178.

Elder, J. P., Plants, D., Welch, H. J., & Feindler, E. L. (1983). Achievement place in a psychiatric setting: Program evaluation. *Journal of Psychiatric Treatment and Evaluation, 5*, 337–344.

Emshoff, J. G., Redd, W., & Davidson, W. S. (1976). Generalization training and the transfer of prosocial behavior in delinquent adolescents. *Journal of Behavior Therapy and Experimental Psychiatry, 7*, 141–144.

Erickson, W. D., & Realmuto, G. (1983). Frequency of seclusion in an adolescent psychiatric unit. *Journal of Clinical Psychiatry, 44*(7), 238–241.

Eyberg, S. M. (1980). Eyberg Child Behavior Inventory. *Journal of Clinical Child Psychology, 9*. 19.

Feindler, E. L., Ecton, R. B., Kingsley, D., & Dubey, D. R. (1986). Group anger-control training for institutionalized psychiatric male adolescents. *Behavior Therapy, 17*, 109–123.

Fixsen, D. L., Phillips, E. L., & Wolf, M. M. (1973). Achievement place: Experiments in self-government with predelinquents. *Journal of Applied Behavior Analysis, 6*, 31–47.

Forehand, R., & McMahon, R. J. (1981). *Helping the noncompliant child: A clinician's guide to parent training*. New York: Guilford Press.
Geller, B., Chestnut, E. C., Miller, M. D., Price, D. T., & Yates, E. (1985). Preliminary data on DSM-III associated features of major depressive disorder in children and adolescents. *American Journal of Psychiatry, 142*, 643–644.
Glick, B., & Goldstein, A. P. (1987). Aggression replacement training. *Journal of Counseling and Development, 65*, 356–362.
Goldstein, A. P., Glick, B., Reiner, S., Zimmerman, D., & Coultry, T. (1987). *Aggression replacement training*. Champaign, IL: Research Press.
Gossett, J. T. (1977). Guidelines for research in a clinical setting. *National Association of Private Psychiatric Hospitals, 10*, 19–27.
Goyette, C. H., Conners, C. K., & Ulrich, R. F. (1978). Normative data on revised Conners Parent and Teacher Rating Scales. *Journal of Abnormal Child Psychology, 6*, 221–236.
Graziano, A. M., & Mooney, K. C. (1984). *Children and behavior therapy*, New York: Aldine.
Gunderson, J. G. (1978). Defining the therapeutic processes in psychiatric milieus. *Psychiatry, 41*, 327–335.
Hains, A. A. (1984). A preliminary attempt to teach the use of social problem-solving skills to delinquents. *Child Study Journal, 14*, 271–285.
Herjanic, B., & Reich, W. (1982). Development of a structured psychiatric interview for children: Agreement between child and parent on individual symptoms. *Journal of Abnormal Child Psychology, 10*, 307–324.
Hodges, K., Kline, J., Fitch, P., McKnew, D., & Cytryn, L. (1981). The Child Assessment Schedule: A diagnostic interview for research and clinical use. *Catalog of Selected Documents in Psychology, 11*(3), 56.
Jamison, J. N., Lambert, W., & McCloud, D. J. (1986). Social skills training with hospitalized adolescents: An evaluative experiment. *Adolescence, 21*(81), 55–65.
Kazdin, A. E. (1987a). *Conduct disorders in childhood and adolescence*. Newbury Park, CA: Sage Publications.
Kazdin, A. E. (1987b). Treatment of antisocial behavior in children: Current status and future directions. *Psychological Bulletin, 102*, 187–203.
Kazdin, A. E., & Esveldt-Dawson, K. (1986). The interview for antisocial behavior: Psychometric characteristics and concurrent validity with child psychiatric inpatients. *Journal of Psychopathology and Behavioral Assessment, 8*(4), 289–303.
Kazdin, A. E., Esveldt-Dawson, K., French, N. H., & Unis, A. S. (1987a). Effects of parent management training and problem-solving skills training combined in the treatment of antisocial child behavior. *Journal of the American Academy of Child and Adolescent Psychiatry, 26*, 416–424.
Kazdin, A. E., Esveldt-Dawson, K., French, N. H., & Unis, A. S. (1987b). Problem-solving skills training and relationship therapy in the treatment of antisocial child behavior. *Journal of Consulting and Clinical Psychology, 55*, 76–85.
Kendall, P. C., & Braswell, L. (1985). *Cognitive-behavioral therapy for impulsive children*. New York: Guilford Press.
Kolko, D. J., Dorsett, P. G., & Milan, M. A. (1981). A total-assessment approach to the evaluation of social skills training: The effectiveness of an anger control program for adolescent psychiatric patients. *Behavioral Assessment, 3*, 383–402.
Lochman, J. E. (1987). Self and peer perceptions and attributional biases of aggressive and nonaggressive boys in dyadic interaction. *Journal of Consulting and Clinical Psychology, 55*, 404–410.
Lochman, J. E. (1990). Modification of childhood aggression. In M. Hersen, R. Eisler, & P.

Miller (Eds.), *Progress in behavior modification* (Vol. 25, pp. 47–85). Newbury Park, CA: Sage Publications.

Lochman, J. E., & Lampron, L. B. (1986). Situational social problem-solving skills and self-esteem of aggressive and nonaggressive boys. *Journal of Abnormal Child Psychology, 14*, 605–617.

Lochman, J. E., Nelson, W. M. III, & Sims, J. P. (1981). A cognitive behavioral program for use with aggressive children. *Journal of Clinical Child Psychology, 10*, 146–148.

Lochman, J. E., Burch, P. R., Curry, J. F., & Lampron, L. B. (1984). Treatment and generalization effects of cognitive behavioral and goal setting interventions with aggressive boys. *Journal of Consulting and Clinical Psychology, 52*, 915–916.

Lochman, J. E., Bennett, C. L., & Simmers, D. A. (1988). Residential re-ed treatment of highly aggressive youth: Preliminary indications of effectiveness and the precursors of improvement. *Education and Treatment of Children, 11*, 52–62.

Lochman, J. E., Meyer, B. L., Rabiner, D. L., & White, K. J. (1991). Parameters influencing social problem-solving of aggressive children. In R. J. Prinz (Ed.), *Advances in behavioral assessment of children and families* (pp. 31–63). Greenwich, CT: JAI Press.

Locke, H. J., & Wallace, K. M. (1959). Short marital-adjustment and prediction tests: Their reliability and validity. *Marriage and Family Living, 21*, 251–255.

Loeber, R., & Dishion, T. J. (1983). Early predictors of male delinquency: A review. *Psychological Bulletin, 94*, 68–99.

Loeber, R., & Schmaling, K. B. (1985). Empirical evidence for overt and covert patterns of antisocial conduct problems: A meta-analysis. *Journal of Abnormal Child Psychology, 13*, 337–352.

Loney, J., & Milich, R. S. (1982). Hyperactivity, inattention, and aggression in clinical practice. In M. Wolraich & D. K. Routh (Eds.), *Advances in developmental and behavioral pediatrics* (Vol. 2, pp. 113–147). Greenwich, CT: JAI Press.

Mattsson, A., Schalling, D., Olweus, D., Low, H., & Svensson, J. (1980). Plasma testosterone, aggressive behavior, and personality dimensions in young male delinquents. *Journal of the American Academy of Child Psychiatry, 19*, 476–490.

McMahon, R. J. (1984). Behavioral checklists and rating scales. In T. H. Ollendick & M. Hersen (Eds.), *Child behavioral assessment: Principles and procedures* (pp. 80–105). New York: Pergamon Press.

McMahon, R. J., & Forehand, R. (1988). Conduct disorders. In E. J. Mash & L. G. Terdal (Eds.), *Behavioral assessment of childhood disorders* (2nd ed., pp. 105–153). New York: Guilford Press.

McMahon, R. J., & Wells, K. C. (1989). Conduct disorders. In E. J. Mash & R. A. Barkley (Eds.), *Behavioral treatment of childhood disorders* (pp. 73–132). New York: Guilford Press.

Meichenbaum, D. H., Bowers, K. S., & Ross, R. R. (1968). Modification of classroom behavior of institutionalized female adolescent offenders. *Behavior Research and Therapy, 6*, 343–353.

Minuchin, S. (1974). *Families and family therapy.* Cambridge: Harvard University Press.

Oates, J. A., & Cooper, G. D. (1983). Characteristics of secluded children in a residential treatment center. *Residential Group Care and Treatment, 1*(3), 43–54.

Ollendick, T. H., & Hersen, M. (1979). Social skills training for juvenile delinquents. *Behavior Research and Therapy, 17*, 547–554.

Patterson, G. R., & Bank, L. (1986). Bootstrapping your way in the nomological thicket. *Behavioral Assessment, 8*, 49–73.

Phillips, E. L. (1968). Achievement place: Token reinforcement procedure in a home-style rehabilitation setting for predelinquent boys. *Journal of Applied Behavior Analysis, 1*, 213–223.

Phillips, E. L., Phillips, E. A., Fixsen, D. C., & Wolf, M. M. (1971). Achievement place: Modification of the behaviors of predelinquent boys within a token economy. *Journal of Applied Behavior Analysis, 4,* 45–59.

Quay, H. C. (1986). Conduct disorders. In H. C. Quay & J. S. Werry (Eds.), *Psychopathological disorders of childhood* (3rd ed., pp. 35–72). New York: Wiley.

Quay, H. C., & Peterson, D. R. (1983). *Interim manual for the Revised Behavior Problem Checklist.* Unpublished manuscript, University of Miami.

Rogeness, G. A., Hernandez, J. M., Macedo, C. A., Mitchell, E. L., Amrung, S. A., & Harris, W. R. (1984). Clinical characteristics of emotionally disturbed boys with very low activities of dopamine-beta-hydroxylase. *Journal of the American Academy of Child Psychiatry, 23,* 203–208.

Salter, A. C. (1988). *Treating child sex offenders and victims: A practical guide.* Beverly Hills, CA: Sage Publications.

Sanson-Fisher, R. W., Seymour, F. W., & Baer, D. M. (1976). Training institutional staff to alter delinquents' conversation. *Journal of Behavioral Therapy and Experimental Psychiatry, 7,* 243–247.

Saylor, C. F., Benson, B., & Einhaus, L. (1985). Evaluation of an anger management program for aggressive boys in inpatient treatment. *Journal of Child and Adolescent Psychotherapy, 2,* 5–15.

Slaby, K. G., & Guerra, N. G. (1988). Cognitive mediators of aggression in adolescent offenders: 1. Assessment. *Developmental Psychology, 244,* 580–588.

Sturge, C. (1982). Reading retardation and antisocial behavior. *Journal of Child Psychology and Psychiatry and Allied Disciplines, 23,* 21–31.

Thomas, D. R., & Maus, M. E. (1983). Duration characteristics of locked-room time-out with behavior contingent release: A seven-year analysis. *Behavioral Engineering, 8*(3), 116–121.

Tisdelle, D. A., & St. Lawrence, J. S. (1988). Adolescent interpersonal problem-solving skill training: Social validation and generalization. *Behavior Therapy, 19,* 171–182.

Varley, W. H. (1984). Behavior modification approaches to the aggressive adolescent. In C. R. Keith (Eds.), *The aggressive adolescent: Clinical perspectives.* New York: Free Press.

Wahler, R. G., & Cormier, W. H. (1970). The ecological interview: A first step in out-patient child behavior therapy. *Journal of Behavior Therapy and Experimental Psychiatry, 1,* 279–289.

Wahler, R. G., Leske, G., & Rogers, E. S. (1979). The insular family: A deviance support system for oppositional children. In L. A. Hamerlynck (Ed.), *Behavioral systems for the developmentally disabled: Vol. 1. School and family environments* (pp. 102–127). New York: Brunner/Mazel.

Witt, P., & Sager, W. (1988). Procedures for treating deviant sexual arousal patterns. In P. A. Keller & S. R. Heyman (Eds.), *Innovations in clinical practice: A source book* (Vol. 7, pp. 89–98). Sarasota, FL: Professional Resource Exchange.

Yalom, I. D. (1983). *Inpatient group psychotherapy.* New York: Basic Books.

11

Inpatient Behavioral and Cognitive Therapy for Substance Abuse in Adolescents

YIFRAH KAMINER AND OSCAR G. BUKSTEIN

INTRODUCTION

Substance abuse, or chemical dependency, continues to be a major public health problem, with substance use or abuse among adolescents occupying increasing national attention and concern. In the United States, overall drug use in young people is the highest among the industrialized nations, despite recent statistics indicating a continued trend of gradual decline (Johnston, Bachman, & O'Malley, 1988). In this highly quoted annual (1987) survey of high school seniors, over half (57%) of the seniors reported having tried an illicit drug and 92% reported some experience with alcohol. The seniors indicated a daily use of 4.8%, 3.3%, and 0.3% of alcohol, marijuana, and cocaine, respectively (Johnston *et al.*, 1988). Adolescents who use alcohol or other drugs have an increased vulnerability to accidents, injuries, and a variety of dangerous behav-

YIFRAH KAMINER • Center for Alcohol and Addictions Studies, Brown University, and Adolescent Substance Abuse Intervention Center, Emma Pendleton Bradley Hospital, East Providence, Rhode Island 02915. OSCAR G. BUKSTEIN • Department of Psychiatry, Western Psychiatric Institute and Clinic, 3811 O'Hara Street, Pittsburgh, Pennsylvania 15213.

Inpatient Behavior Therapy for Children and Adolescents, edited by Vincent B. Van Hasselt and David J. Kolko. Plenum Press, New York, 1992.

iors. Alcohol-related motor vehicle accidents are the leading cause of death among American youth between the ages of 15 and 24, and increased alcohol levels are found in victims of suicide and homicide (American Academy of Pediatrics, 1987). Clearly, with increasing recognition of this serious problem, society in the United States now directs more resources toward the treatment of chemically dependent adolescents. In this chapter, we hope to describe the entity of adolescent chemical dependency and to discuss assessment methods and appropriate behavioral treatment modalities as applied to hospitalized adolescents with alcohol and/or drug use problems.

Clinical Description of the Disorder

Diagnosis

Defining exactly what behaviors and symptoms constitute substance abuse (SA) is a problematic proposition. Most efforts at establishing a diagnostic classification for pathological substance use have been concerned with adults, and the reader should be cautioned that, despite almost universal application of these same criteria to adolescents, many differences exist between adolescents and adults in a variety of substance use characteristics, including use patterns and consequences (Blane, 1979; Wechsler, 1979). Although adult criteria may provide a reasonable point of departure for making a diagnosis of SA in adolescents, further research is necessary to establish a valid classification system for pathological substance use in this group.

The unitary disease model, historically promoted by Jellinek (1960), remains the most important influence on the popular conception, definition, and ultimate treatment approach for both alcohol and drug abuse. In this model, the alcoholic or drug abuser is different from those without the disease, and these differences are manifested in the diseased individual by a craving and/or loss of control. However, the validity and usefulness of these symptoms, as well as any unitary model, are suspect, despite their widespread acceptance by the public and many in the treatment community (Pattison, 1985). Criteria established by the National Council on Alcoholism (NCA) represent another prominent example of an attempt to establish diagnostic criteria for a substance use disorder (National Council on Alcoholism, 1972). However, an overemphasis of the physical consequences of alcohol use and on the later stages of the "illness" (Chafetz, 1972) call into question the value of using the NCA criteria to diagnose adolescents.

Recent efforts in the classification of substance abuse are reflected in the diagnoses of substance abuse and dependence in the *Diagnostic and Statistical Manual of Mental Disorders,* 3rd edition (DSM-III) (American Psychiatric Association, 1980) and of psychoactive substance abuse and dependence in the DSM-III-R (American Psychiatric Association, 1987). In the DSM-III, substance abuse is defined in terms of pathological use and impairment in social or occupational functioning that is due to substance use. Substance dependence is defined by the presence of tolerance or withdrawal and either of the primary criteria for substance abuse. Among the criticisms directed at the DSM-III substance use disorders are the lack of specificity in what constitutes tolerance (Rounsaville, 1987) and the rare occurrence of physiological withdrawal in adolescents (Vingilis & Smart, 1981). A reliance on impairment in function is also problematic as a primary criterion. Inclusion of criteria for impairment in social functioning often assumes that negative consequences are the result of substance use and are not due to preexisting factors, such as coexisting psychopathology or environmental disorganization. By virtue of restrictions in age and legal status, alcohol and drug use by adolescents is almost always illicit, and certain negative consequences follow from this proscription rather than necessarily from the properties of the substance being used. For example, interpersonal consequences are often due to the intolerance of the family or the individual's social system and thus can vary widely between adolescents.

The DSM-III-R psychoactive substance use disorders represent a change from the DSM-III in broadening the concept of dependence to include clinically significant behaviors, cognitions, and symptoms indicating a substantial degree of involvement with a psychoactive substance (Rounsaville, Spitzer, & Williams, 1986). The Alcohol Dependence syndrome, proposed by Edwards and Gross (1976), and its companion diagnosis with Drug Dependence syndrome (Skinner & Goldberg, 1986) form the model for the DSM-III-R. The Alcohol Dependence syndrome is based on seven essential elements including tolerance, withdrawal, and compulsion to use, each of which exists to varying degrees in an individual, and provides a range of severity and a dimensional system based on empirical clustering of the essential elements. Not all of the elements are necessary for an individual to qualify for the syndrome. Indeed, alcohol-related problems, including social, occupational, physical, or psychological consequences of use, form a second but related axis.

The classification systems noted previously do not make a distinction between the diagnosis of substance use disorders in adulthood and in adolescence. Several researchers have attempted to operationalize problem drinking (Donovan & Jessor, 1978; Rachal *et al.*, 1980). Criteria from the definitions use drunkenness and/or negative consequences related to alcohol use, despite evidence indicating a fairly weak association between intoxication and alcohol-related problems, which suggests that these two variables represent two distinct dimensions of adolescent problem drinking (Rachal *et al.*, 1980; White, 1987).

Because of the problematic nature of existing definitions and the absence of valid diagnostic criteria for adolescent substance abuse, and the existence of various co-morbid psychiatric disorders (Bukstein, Brent, & Kaminer, 1989), clinicians should exercise much care in making a determination of the existence and the severity of a substance use disorder and related problems. Specifically, overreliance on quantity, frequency, or problems related to substance use may result in overdiagnosis and referral to inappropriate treatment settings.

BEHAVIORAL AND COGNITIVE FACTORS

Before reviewing the inpatient behavioral treatment of SA in adolescents, it is imperative to illustrate particular behavioral and cognitive concepts and to highlight their possible role in the etiology and pathogenesis of this dependence. The Drug Dependence syndrome, based on the Alcohol Dependence syndrome proposed by Edwards and Gross (1976), implicates both biological processes and learning. The rapid reinstatement of tolerance and withdrawal symptoms with resumption of the drug and alcohol habit in afflicted individuals suggested a biological process, whereas the use of alcohol and drugs to relieve withdrawal symptoms and craving in response to internal or external cues seemed more consistent with a learning process (Meyer, 1986). The elements of the syndrome that represent a clinical-behavioral construct with hypothetical biological dimensions were utilized as guidelines for the criteria for psychoactive substance abuse disorders in the DSM-III-R (Kosten, Rounsaville, Babor, Spitzer, & Williams, 1987).

Traditional views of tolerance assume that the physiological changes underlying tolerance result simply from past exposure to the drug *per se*. However, Pavlovian conditioning models of tolerance (Siegel, 1973) and relapse incidence (Wikler, 1965) based on animal as well as human data indicate that environmental cues present at the time of drug administration contribute to tolerance. Drugs are external agents that can produce disturbances in homeostatic systems. Animals appear to react to the effects of many drugs with compensatory mechanisms that reduce their effects.

In addition to reacting to disruptions of homeostatic systems, animals also respond to anticipation of important environmental events, as was exemplified by Pavlov in his studies of salivary conditioning in dogs (Pavlov, 1927). The analogy to drug administration in human subjects is clear, and the potential for the establishment of anticipatory responses is inherent in drug administration procedures. Specifically, any external cue, such as a bottle, a needle, the drug-related environment, or people, which invariably accompanies drug administration, can serve as a conditioning stimulus in that it may reliably precede the effects of the drug and thus can act as an unconditioned stimulus.

Subsequent to the development of experimental cognitive psychology in the 1970s, cognitive and learning factors were introduced to the field of SA (Wilson, 1987). The following theories involve learning in the development of SA models that have received more attention in the last two decades.

Modeling

Although it is important in the initiation and maintenance of substance abuse (Wilson, 1987), modeling is also extensively used in the prevention, treatment, and Relapse Prevention of SA. In the initiation of use, family members, peers, and celebrities often serve as models of behavior which the adolescent imitates. Although such other factors as tension reduction and expectancies may eventually make the chemical use problematic, the model is often responsible for initiation of use. For prevention and treatment, models of positive, prosocial behaviors are emphasized.

Tension Reduction

Tension reduction is another theory that has been proposed to account for such addiction disorders as bulimia nervosa, cigarette smoking, and drug/alcohol abuse and dependency. Tension is extensively perceived as a stress by patients as well as therapists, and consequently chemicals are ingested in order to alleviate its impact (Wilson, 1982).

Cognitive Social Learning Theory

Cognitive social learning theory holds that both anxiety and avoidance behavior are related coeffects of a person's level and strength of perceived self-efficacy (Bandura, 1977). The stress-dampening effect of drugs and alcohol is expected to boost self-efficacy and also to directly alter the encoding of negative social feedback even though the feedback is accurately identified as inherently negative (Yankofsky, Wilson, Adler, Hay, & Vrana, 1986).

People learn to predict the effects of drug and alcohol soothing on personal distress and acquire a learned outcome expectation regarding its consequences. A contingency relationship is learned, but it is cognitively mediated and not automatically conditioned. Many variables, such as the social setting and the amount consumed, may significantly moderate drug and alcohol effects on self-efficacy (Wilson, 1982).

Self-Awareness Model

Alcohol disinhibits social behavior by reducing an individual's level of self-awareness (Hull, 1981). Thus, alcohol and other drugs are said to reduce tension by their primary effect on cognitive processes by disrupting the encoding of self-relevant information that then affects affective reactions and provides a source of psychological relief.

Marlatt's Expectancy Model

Alcohol and drugs are known to induce a distortion of higher cognitive processes. Alcohol is known to impair memory, and this may help to account for why alcoholics hold positive expectations of drinking even when their actual experiences are negative. Marlatt (1982) postulated that people learn to expect short-term positive consequences in order to be freed from the inhibitory effect of past negative experiences. It is also interesting to note that adolescent problem drinkers and alcohol abusers, in contrast to their peers who are not problem drinkers, expect that alcohol will improve their cognitive and motor functioning.

Self-Handicapping Theory

The self-handicapping theory holds that individuals who are unsure about their competence in certain situations will consume alcohol in advance of the situation in order to perform poorly so that their social failure can then be attributed to their intoxicated state and not to their actual competence (Jones & Berglas, 1978; Tucker, Vuchinich, & Sobell, 1981). This theory may explain why abstinent relapse is often in response to success experiences rather than failure experiences.

Lastly, certain drugs, especially cocaine, are so reinforcing and the immediate affective state is so positively experienced by the user that self-administration becomes a targeted behavior (Fischman, 1988). This subjective feeling is far beyond the social, sexual, and other common claims made about performance enhancement attributed to drugs and alcohol. The drug-seeking behavior is maintained on account of the positively reinforcing effects of the drug.

BEHAVIORAL AND PSYCHIATRIC ASSESSMENT

As suggested by the preceding discussion, the optimal clinical evaluation of adolescents should involve multiple domains and methods of assessment. Several screening measures that were originally developed for adults are available. The Michigan Alcoholism Screening Test (MAST) (Selzer, 1971), its companion, the Drug and Alcohol Screening Test (DAST) (Skinner, 1982), and the MacAndrew Alcoholism Scale (MAC) (MacAndrew, 1979) represent three of the more commonly used instruments. Several studies suggest that the MAC, taken from the MMPI, may be helpful in discriminating groups of adolescents with and without substance abuse (Klinge, Lachar, Grisell, & Berman, 1978; Wolfson & Erbaugh, 1984). The Adolescent Alcohol Involvement Scale (AAIS) (Mayer & Filstead, 1979) is a short, 14-item screening instrument developed to detect adolescent alcohol misuse. This instrument possesses acceptable reliability and validity (Moberg, 1983); however, the lack of stability of both the drinking patterns and the problems of adolescents should caution the clinician from using the test for exclusive cross-sectional interpretations. The Addiction Severity Index (ASI) (McLellan, O'Brien, & Woody, 1980) measures several dimensions of the social consequences of addictive behaviors.

Both clinicians and researchers are currently attempting to develop and refine a number of comprehensive instruments or batteries to assess substance use behaviors and related problems (Henly & Winters, 1988; Oetting, Beauvais, Edwards, & Waters, 1984). For example, the Drug and Alcohol Assessment System (Oetting *et al.*, 1984) is a 39-page, self-report measure of multiple areas of drug and alcohol use and related problems that produces a profile or style of the drug user for the clinician. The use of structured or semistructured interviews and the demonstrated reliability and validity of such instruments for adult alcoholics (Schuckit, Irwin, Howard, & Smith, 1988) may portend the use of similar instruments, such as the K-SADS (Puig-Antich, Orvaschel, Tabrizi,, & Chambers, 1980), for adolescents. As suggested by Schuckit *et al.* (1988), these interviews may be valuable for determining the chronology of the substance use disorder as well as coexisting psychiatric syndromes.

Although these diagnostic instruments play a role in the assessment of drug and alcohol problems, clinicians should measure multiple areas of the individual's functioning as well as aspects of the drug and alcohol use behavior in several relevant domains. In the behavioral treatment of substance-abusing adolescents, optimal clinical assessment involves a functional analysis of the individual adolescent's substance use directed toward the antecedent factors, target behavior factors, and consequences or reinforcers of substance use. A detailed analysis of these factors is necessary because it provides information essential to the development of appropriate treatment goals and the selection of treatment modalities in a specific setting.

Antecedents

Environmental antecedents are among the more robust predictors of adolescent drinking and drug-taking behavior, with parental attitudes and behavior being the most significant among these factors (Kandel, 1982). In addition to parental role-modeling, the quality and consistency of family communication and parent behavior management are strong predictors of substance use (Kandel, Kessler, & Margulies, 1978). Thus, assessment for adolescents in an inpatient program should include a detailed description of family functioning, including prevailing behavior management, communication within the family, parental and sibling substance use history, the presence of current family crises, as well as other parental or parent–child conflicts. Family variables are important not only in the prediction of adolescent chemical use but also in the prediction of the response to treatment and in the follow-up maintenance of treatment gains. For example, alcoholic parents may not be invested in the treatment of their children or may attend family-oriented treatment modalities in an intoxicated state. Obviously, family variables also offer a specific target for treatment, including improving family communication, strengthening behavioral management, changing parental attitudes through psychoeducation, or referring parents for chemical dependency or psychiatric treatment. Peer factors also are strong predictors.

Among peer-related factors shown to have predictive value are peer drug-use behaviors and attitudes (Kandel *et al.*, 1978) and perceived use of substances by peers (R. Jessor & S. L. Jessor, 1978). Peer relationships are also a relevant area for assessment. Although using the adolescent's peers as actual informants is problematic, the adolescent and his or her family can provide useful information about the attitudes of specific friends and whether they are involved in substance abuse. The clinician should ask who the adolescent's close friends are and what they do together, including the use of substances. Because of the influence of peers upon substance use, most treatment programs work toward changing the adolescent's prevailing peer network, asking that the adolescent not associate with chemical-using peers. The adolescent's participation in self-support groups and association with abstinent peers should further reinforce a decision of abstinence.

Individual factors, including beliefs, attitudes, substance use-related expectancies, and preexisting psychopathology, are implicated as antecedents of adolescent substance use and abuse. Examples of attitudes include acceptable uses of various substances. Expectancies are the adolescent's anticipation of the effects of substance use, including intoxication, improved social performance, and attractiveness. Preexisting and current beliefs about alcohol are associated with current drinking patterns (Christiansen, Goldman, & Inn, 1982). Favorable attitudes about drug use preceding initiation appear to facilitate the beginning of drug use (Kandel *et al.*, 1978). Substance use-related expectancies, the effects attributed to a substance that the individual adolescent anticipates when using that substance, are related to future substance use (Brown, 1985) as well as to current use patterns (Christiansen, Goldman, & Brown, 1985). The Alcohol Expectancy Questionnaire (AEQ) (Brown, Christiansen, & Goldman, 1987) is a 90-item self-report instrument designed to measure the degree to which adolescents expect alcohol to produce a variety of general and specific effects. Its use, along with other inquiry into attitudes, beliefs, and expectancies regarding substance use, might increase an understanding of the antecedent factors in the individual. Attitudes and expectancies about chemical use are salient targets for treatment. Documenting any change in these variables can provide the clinician with an index of treatment progress.

Preexisting as well as coexisting psychopathology in the adolescent is all too often neglected as an antecedent factor. Antisocial behavior often predicts adolescent substance use (Johnston, O'Malley, & Eveland, 1978; Kandel *et al.*, 1978) with delinquency occurring prior to substance use. Other studies suggest that depression (Deykin, Levy, & Wells, 1987) and attention-deficit disorder (Gittleman, Mannuzza, Shenker, & Bonagura, 1985) may precede substance use or abuse. Therefore, evaluation of past psychiatric history and of current psychiatric status is essential for all substance abuse treatment programs. The clinician may also wish to consider self-report and parent report measures, such as the Child Behavior Checklist (CBCL) (Achenbach & Edelbrock,

1983). Questions about family psychiatric history may also prove useful in elucidating the individual adolescent's current psychiatric status in addition to any vulnerability to psychiatric disorder.

Target Behaviors

Substance use is, of course, the target behavior whose patterns must be detailed in terms of identification of drugs used, quantity and frequency of each drug used, routes of administration, last use, perceived effects, motivation, location and context of use, as well as the presence or absence of tolerance, dependence, or withdrawal states. In addition to quantity and frequency data, variability in use patterns must also be assessed because adolescents often follow an irregular use pattern with a tendency to weekend binge use. Time line methods may be useful in facilitating patient recall.

Information provided by collateral informants and the use of toxicology screens for illicit substances may address reliability issues brought on by the adolescent's denial of any problem or the general recall problems that are often seen with substance abusers.

Consequences of Substance Abuse

Generally, substance use behavior may be categorized in terms of positive consequences, which may reinforce the substance use behavior, or negative consequences, which may have presented the adolescent for clinical assessment. The clinician must be certain to document possible reinforcers for continued substance use. Positive reinforcers include enjoyment of pharmacological action of the substance, perceived pleasurable actions of the substance, avoidance of possible difficulties in initial abstinence, including withdrawal symptoms, maintenance of peer social relationships, and assumption of the sick role. Identification of such positive reinforcers is critical because treatment must find replacement behaviors to achieve these reinforcers without chemical use or other deviant behaviors. Developing replacement, prosocial behaviors should be an important component of treatment. Assessment may include evaluation of social skills.

Negative consequences are the usual reason for the adolescent's entry into treatment and will form, in addition to measures of subsequent substance use, the basis for assessment of treatment success upon posttreatment follow-up. Assessment of problems in various areas—family, school, legal, medical, interpersonal interactions, and psychological functioning—is necessary to ascertain the need for treatment and to establish a baseline to measure treatment effects. Suicidal and homicidal risk should always be assessed in substance-abusing patients. One must exercise caution in not confusing negative consequences with antecedents of substance use or possibly with coexisting but unrelated problems.

Most existing instruments that are used in the assessment of substance abuse in adults measure the psychosocial and/or physical consequences of substance use. MAST (Selzer, 1971) and DAST (Skinner, 1982) assess a variety of consequences related to substance use, whereas the ASI (McLellan *et al.*, 1980) and the AAIS (Mayer & Filstead, 1979) measure problem severity. The instruments pertinent to the assessment of adolescent substance abuse were reviewed recently (Tarter, 1990). Among these instruments is a teen version of the ASI, known as the T-ASI (Kaminer, Bukstein, & Tarter, 1991), which assesses the following domains: (1) substance abuse, (2) family function, (3) legal status, (4) peer social relationships, (5) psychiatric status, and (6) school or employment status.

Of related interest to the assessment of the consequences of substance use are prior treatment attempts as either self-directed efforts or in formal treatment settings. The clinician should also obtain a detailed list of the various treatment modalities employed in addition to periods of abstinence.

Assessment of antecedent, behavioral, and consequent or reinforcing factors are rarely isolated from each other and often continue into the treatment period. Initial treatment efforts to minimize or eliminate denial serve to elicit further information about antecedents, substance use behavior, and consequences. The assessing clinician should also make every effort to detail and quantify assessment data so that follow-up and assessment of treatment outcome can be more easily determined. Quantitative assessment data offer a clear statement of improvement or lack thereof. The clinician can demonstrate small increments of positive change to the adolescent and positively reinforce efforts at behavior change and maintenance of abstinence.

BEHAVIORAL TREATMENTS

Recent challenges to the effectiveness of various treatment modalities of SA suggest that the benefits of many of these treatments are modest at best (Cummings, 1979; Edwards *et al.*, 1977). In view of even more recent later findings that neither the intensity nor the type of treatment facility is a good predictor of success with unselected groups of patients (Holden, 1987), it is therefore not surprising that the Institute of Medicine report of 1980 concluded that "the best predictor of patient outcome is the patient." These legitimate questions regarding the treatment of the syndrome reflect how little is known about the natural history of chemical dependency, and make it extremely difficult to judge whether an outcome measure of either a program and/or of a patient is indeed a measure of treatment effectiveness. The role of nontreatment factors, such as maturation, spontaneous remission, and regression, which can account for much of the observed improvements, needs to be determined (Armor, Polich, & Stambul, 1978; Simpson, Savage, & Sells, 1978).

The conservative approach toward the treatment of chemical dependency still dominates the field. This treatment package, built around the recovery principles of such self-help organizations as Alcoholics Anonymous (AA) and Narcotics Anonymous (NA), consists of providing a standard treatment regimen of services to all patients who are diagnosed as chemically dependent. However, exclusive or preferential reliance on either AA and/or the prevailing therapeutic approach (known also as the "shotgun" approach) is not justified by present knowledge (Craig, 1987; Miller & Hester, 1980).

A current conceptualization for the treatment of chemical dependency, known as the "treatment-matching" approach, heralds a new and a more advanced attitude. The basic idea of this program is to provide the type of treatment required for a particular type of patient (Craig, 1987). This therapeutic concept is supported by studies which suggest that certain types of patients do better with certain kinds of treatment. For example, chemical dependency patients with midrange psychiatric severity show differential outcomes following alternative treatments, especially bolstered by specific patient–program matches (McLellan, Luborsky, O'Brien, Woody, & Druley, 1983; Rounsaville, Kosten, Weissman, & Kleber, 1986). Adolescents with moderate to severe chemical use, social functioning, or psychiatric status would be matched to an inpatient program whereas those with less severe pathology may be maintained as outpatients. Certain types of patients may benefit from self-support group attendance while others may not. Psychotherapy may also be useful with certain populations. Within the adolescent age group, no significant data are available to guide the clinician in treatment matching, although matching may more successfully allocate limited treatment resources in the future. If outcome is more likely to be influenced by the type of intervention with a particular patient population (Miller & Hester, 1986), the real issue is one of finding out "what modes of intervention bring out what kinds of changes in what kind of patients under what kind of circumstances" (Craig, 1987).

Inpatient Programs

Inpatient programs for substance abuse adolescents are usually hospital-based, closed (i.e., locked) units that provide a relatively brief but highly structured experience, lasting several weeks to 2 months as an average. Further treatment, such as outpatient aftercare or residential treatment, is often required after discharge.

There are no specific empirically based criteria for admission of adolescents to a SA inpatient unit. Usually the types of patients requiring admission include dually diagnosed patients with moderate to severe psychiatric disorder, patients with past treatment failure, IV drug and cocaine freebase abusers, and patients with psychical dependence requiring medical supervision.

The treatment package for substance abuse adolescents usually includes various combinations of family therapy, self-support group activities, individual psychotherapy, and different group therapies and activities. A list of common group therapies and activities that often integrate cognitive-behavioral therapy principles and techniques (Kaminer & Frances, 1991) follows.

The Therapeutic Environment and Process

It is important to define the goals of inpatient behavioral treatment to substance abuse adolescents as well as to inform them about the process of change that subsequently occurs. The process is composed of three stages: (1) initial commitment to change; (2) cessation of drug use, and (3) maintenance of abstinence. The role of the inpatient unit is to facilitate and consolidate the patient's initial commitment to change.

The behavioral and cognitive therapeutic process should be perceived as part of a comprehensive treatment regime within the inpatient adolescent substance abuse unit. Certain behavioral or cognitive modalities, such as social skills training, when added to a comprehensive treatment program, can contribute to improvements in the targeted behaviors (Chaney, O'Leary, & Marlzit, 1978; Oei & Jackson, 1982). There are two dimensions to the behavioral and cognitive therapeutic process within the unit. The first one is inherent within the structure of such a program since the highly demanding and structured program keeps the youngsters busy around the clock. At admission, a contract is usually signed by the patient, assuring his or her commitment to comply with the program. Rules and regulations are then introduced and the level system (a bidirectional graded evaluation system) is constantly used in order to monitor the patient's progress or regression. The patient is aware of these unit rules and that noncompliance with policies and regulations will warrant immediate staff response. For example, a patient knows that body and room searches as well as random urine analysis for drugs are mandatory and that positive findings of such a search will initiate in most programs administrative discharge. Reinforcement and punishment in a token economy are commonly used to modulate compliance with the level system.

The second dimension of behavioral or cognitive treatment is more of a part of the conventional therapeutic process. Encounters with explicit therapeutic goals are inherent in this dimension. Common interventions with behavioral or cognitive components for adolescents are: contingency contracting, social skills learning, extinction of conditioned responses, and contract groups and other interventions that are aimed toward achieving and maintaining abstinence and/or reducing drug-related problems. Aversion therapy techniques, while used commonly with SA adults, appears to be rarely used with adolescents. Family therapy, especially when incorporating parent management techniques, is a commonly used SA modality that may utilize behavioral principles (Reuger & Liberman, 1984).

Behavioral and Cognitive Elements in Chemical Dependency Treatment Modalities

AA Meetings and Principles. Support groups, such as AA and Alateen for adolescents, have inherent behavioral elements. AA members undergo cognitive restructuring. Scheduled weekly meetings, mutual aid phone calls, and loading of language are heavily tooled with cognitive-behavioral interventions. An AA meeting could be summarized as an event where symptoms and discomfort are initiated (by using cues). Identifying anger and identifying a person's common experience are preplanned goals. AA members learn how to identify cues that endanger abstinence. Avoidance is copiously used and even a Pavlovian paradigm is implemented. An AA aim is to break the sequence, and this process demands that the patient develop a procedure that will intervene between the conditioned stimulus (i.e., the places and situations where craving may occur) and the conditioned response (i.e., the drinking). However, the behavioral elements in self-support groups are largely secondary phenomena to the supportive goals of these groups.

Contingency Contracting. In most therapies, a contract is negotiated and signed by the patient and the therapist. In this contract, the patient specifies goals in terms of planned incremental behavior changes; that is, short-range approximations of the eventual goal(s). Goals cover relevant domains of the adolescent's life (e.g., family, school, antisocial behaviors) and especially drug/alcohol use with treatment compliance as a specified goal. Specific criteria are set for time and frequency limitations which constitute the behavior stated on the contract and the behaviors must be observable and, preferably, measurable. Specified positive reinforcement in the way of privileges are granted upon fulfillment of criteria and penalties or negative consequences are given upon failure to meet criteria. Upon attainment or maintenance of the goals, contracts are usually renegotiated to require further approximation toward a final desired behavioral goal. For example, an adolescent might initially contract for (1) negative random drug screens, (2) 90% school attendance, (3) 10 P.M. curfew on weekends, (4) responsibility for four specific chores at home, and (5) daily self-support group attendance. Upon satisfactory attainment of these goals within a 6-week period, the goals would be reset to 100% school attendance, 11 P.M. curfew, 6 specific home chores, and 3 self-support groups a week. This is a frequently used method in chemical dependency treatment. Such an approach is very helpful, especially to highly motivated patients who need to be constantly challenged.

Extinction of Conditioned Responses. Childress, McLellan, and O'Brien (1986) described this extinction technique whereby the patient, who is placed in an inpatient treatment program and thus is protected from using drugs, is then presented with the stimuli that often provoke cravings or impulses to use drugs. With repetition and without receiving the drug itself, the responses to these stimuli are diminished. The types of stimuli used in the extinction program should be tailored to each individual patient in order to reduce chances of relapse. Examples of stimuli might include heavy-metal music, conflict situations, and specific social situations with same and different-gender peers. Treatment may also develop replacement behaviors, such as social skills training and interest in prosocial activities as nondeviant responses to these stimuli. Relapse prevention (Marlatt & Gordon, 1985) contains elements for the extinction of such responses.

Recreation Time Planning and Contract Groups. These therapeutic activities provide the adolescent with alternative skills and interests to prevent boredom, anxiety, depression, and other stressful cues that may lead to drug-seeking behavior, or to association with peers who might eventually persuade or influence the patient to resume his or her drug habits. An emphasis on goal achievement is strongly recommended during these meetings, and constant positive peer pressure reinforces the patients to complete time-planned assignments. This program is similar to and often involves contingency contracting.

Social Skills Training (SST). The literature supports a negative relationship between social competence and chemical dependency (Levine & Zigler, 1973). Adolescent problem drinkers have difficulty in forming and maintaining social relationships, probably because of inadequately learned social responses (O'Leary, O'Leary, & Donovan, 1975). Social skills training is based upon the theoretical and experimental research done by Bandura (1977). Four major components are often employed in the process: (1) role-modeling, (2) reinforcement, (3) establishment of normative expectations, and (4) coping with social pressure. Such a group could be run by the patients themselves after a short training phase by staff and could be widely used for primary prevention as well. In fact, much of the sparse data regarding outcome in SST for adolescents comes from prevention or early intervention studies (Botvin, Baker, Renick, Filazzola, & Botvin, 1984). Social skills training interventions for the prevention of smoking and alcohol abuse are reported for younger adolescents (Flay, 1975; Perry, Kullen, Slinkard, & McAlister, 1980).

Among the most frequently targeted skills are assertiveness, anger control, and initiating conversation. Assertiveness training, consisting of both general assertiveness training and drug/or alcohol specific training, has shown promise (Horan & Williams, 1982; Watson & Maisto, 1983).

Problem-Solving Skill Training. Such social skills as interpersonal problem-solving and social network development intervention may enhance treatment maintenance and generalization and produce positive change in the social performance of substance abuse patients (Hawkins, Catalano, & Well, 1986). Satisfactory solution of problems may reduce the need to use drugs and alcohol in stressful situations.

Marlatt and George (1984) stated that the relapse prevention model is designed to teach individuals how to anticipate and cope with the problem of relapse. From the initiation of sobriety to its maintenance, each intervention or a combination of the interventions noted above can contribute toward the goal of relapse prevention. Marlatt and Gordon (1985) emphasized these prevention elements: (1) identifying situations that pose a high risk of relapse and preparing the patient to deal with them effectively, (2) dealing constructively with relapses, and (3) learning to view a relapse as a learning experience rather than a pronounced personal failure.

In their cognitive-behavioral model of relapse prevention, Marlatt and Gordon (1985) indicated how important the role of expectations is in determining relapse. Their approach is consistent with findings that support self-efficacy and beliefs as indices or predictors of relapse (Killen, Maccoby, & Taylor, 1984; Rist & Watzl, 1983). The availability of several treatment options is an issue that needs to be addressed. Sobell, Sobell, and Nirenberg (1982) argued that when relapse occurs, the costs of the various treatment strategies should be evaluated in relation to the client's life-style, values, and resources.

Assessing clients' resources was suggested by Sanchez-Craig (1984) as a method of helping clients to identify naturally occurring, successful coping responses. Monitoring progress during therapy is crucial in order to evaluate behavior change. If progress is not evident or is unreasonably slow, the therapist and client should be prepared to assess the situation (Sobell, Sobell, & Nirenberg, 1988).

Behavioral and Cognitive Therapy and Psychopharmacology. Currently, cocaine is the target of many pharmacological experiments. Pharmacotherapy was found to facilitate initiation of abstinence in cocaine abusers and chemical dependent individuals. However, at this stage, pharmacotherapy alone does not seem to eliminate cocaine abuse but may allow patients to generate more benefit from other therapeutic approaches (Gawin & Ellenwood, 1988). Bromocriptine, tricyclic antidepressants, carbamazepine, amantadine, lithium, Ritalin, and other dopamimetic agents have shown some efficacy in the treatment of cocaine craving (Gawin, Kleber, & Byck, 1989). In most reports, the number of subjects was too small to reach valid conclusions, and there was a lack of double-blind, methodologically sound studies; however, desipramine appeared to be the most promising agent tested for the treatment of cocaine craving in a double-blind, placebo-controlled, design study (Gawin *et al.*, 1989). Perhaps the optimal use of pharmacotherapy is for the treatment of coexisting psychiatric disorders and symptoms with indications for specific pharmacological intervention. The combination of various treatment modalities (e.g., behavioral, cognitive, and pharmacological) may be essential to achieve satisfactory outcomes in this resistant population.

CASE HISTORY

Background

Susie was a 14-year-old female who was referred to an inpatient psychiatric facility for adolescent substance abusers because of her increasing use of alcohol and other drugs, her disruptive behavior, and her suicidal ideation.

Susie's problems began at age 12 with her deteriorating school grades, truancy, a change in friends, and an increase in fighting with both peers and family. Also, she began to use diet pills up to three times a day in order to lose weight. Although she was referred for outpatient treatment at that time, Susie was soon hospitalized because of her suicidal ideation and a suicidal gesture. Upon her discharge, Susie was diagnosed as having an Adjustment Disorder with mixed disturbance of conduct and emotion. However, she did not attend her outpatient follow-up, and her behavior continued to deteriorate. Susie also made threats of suicide and had taken some nonlethal gestures. She began to drink alcohol, eventually progressing to such large quantities as to reach intoxication four to five times a week. She reported experiencing alcohol "black-outs" several times. Occasionally, she also used marijuana. Susie's significant family history data include her mother who was actively alcoholic by self-report and her biological father who had a prison record.

Assessment

Perhaps the most salient reason for inpatient hospitalization of the adolescent substance abuser is his or her removal from an often chaotic environment where many elements reinforce the substance use. Achieving even a brief period of abstinence is necessary to evaluate psychiatric symptoms and behavior in order not to be confused by the intoxicated states and acute and chronic withdrawal. Assessment is also a time for engaging the adolescent and his or her family into treatment, often by confronting a substantial amount of denial. For Susie, this meant separation from her alcoholic mother and substance-abusing friends, a complete evaluation of her presenting depressive symptoms and suicidality, and confronting her denial with the assessed consequences of her substance use. Upon initial inpatient assessment, Susie displayed poor insight, low self-esteem, and hopelessness regarding her future given the family's history of alcoholism and antisocial behavior. She was reluctant to cooperate, showing a significant denial of her problems. Staff noted no pervasive depressive anxiety or psychotic symptoms, although Susie did report transient but severe periods of dysphoric mood and hopelessness. Despite a moderately attractive appearance, Susie felt she was fat and unattractive. Additional target problems for Susie's inpatient treatment plan were interpersonal conflict with her family and her fear of the unknown. Final diagnostic formulation included the DSM-III diagnoses of Conduct Disorder and Alcohol Abuse. Staff noted that the patient appeared to be a "follower" who was significantly influenced by both the good and bad behaviors of her peers. By her own report, Susie had a limited ability to interact comfortably with peers when she was not drinking.

Treatment

Susie worked separately with a member of the staff to develop an overall treatment plan and also an individual contract that specified her problems in several domains (e.g., family, school, and peers), her short- and long-term goals to alleviate these problems, and the methods she would use to achieve these goals. Susie identified family issues and fear of the unknown as prominent long-term issues. Fear of the unknown is common in children of alcoholics because they have had to live with sudden, unexpected changes in their parent's behavior. Short-term goals are usually referenced to such behaviors as following unit roles and regulations and making small steps to achieving more effective communication with family members. For example, Susie would specify in her contract expectations that she would follow a specific unit rule without needing redirection and would call her mother daily and then appropriately end the conversation if her mother was intoxicated. Compliance with the contract would be reviewed not only by the staff but also by a peer group who would provide feedback as to the achievement of her stated goals. Individual work with the staff also focused on her negative cognitions of herself. Eventually, Susie was able to verbalize a difference between her mother and herself and her family. Following an initial period of resistance, Susie displayed slow but steady progress in achieving short-term goals on her contract. A sense of mastery over these goals resulted in observations of improved self-image.

Most of the therapeutic interventions are conducted in a group format. The group format allows adolescents to understand their common experiences and to provide peer feedback regarding an individual's cognitions or behaviors. These groups have significant cognitive-behavioral themes.

In the contract group, Susie presented her contract and received peer feedback and reinforcement for her behaviors toward fulfilling the contract. In a semistructured social skills group, Susie was able to learn and practice techniques toward (1) controlling her anger, (2) being assertive in a variety of situations, and (3) developing conversational and nonverbal communication skills. Through the use of modeling, role-playing, problem-solving procedures, and appropriate reinforcement, Susie was noted to be more assertive and proficient in her interactions with peers and family. She was able to confront her mother's drinking and to resist following or accepting peer's inappropriate behavior.

An inpatient program directs much attention toward meeting the treatment needs of the entire family unit. In addition to psychoeducation about the nature of substance abuse in the adolescent, Susie's family attended sessions in which they were taught how to control her oppositional behaviors using child management techniques, behavioral contracting, and positive-reinforcement skills. Susie's mother was directed to a treatment program for her own substance abuse problems. Susie attended a number of additional modalities, including self-help groups (e.g., Alcoholics Anonymous and Narcotics Anonymous), process-oriented groups, and psychoeducational groups. These modalities assisted staff in breaking through Susie's denial, and she was eventually able to acknowledge her drinking habit as well as other problems.

Follow-up

Discharge planning and follow-up for Susie included continued contracting, attendance at self-help groups, and participation in a semistructured group which was designed to prevent relapse by discussing and identifying antecedents to relapse into substance use behaviors. Unfortunately, Susie's mother continued to drink. The ensuing poor supervision allowed Susie to resume contact with substance-abusing peers and eventually to resume use herself. Her mother's continued failure to control her own drinking reinforced Susie's own sense of tenuous control and her hopelessness about the future. School officials noted Susie's increasing truancy and finally found her in an intoxicated state at school. Fortunately, school officials quickly identified her relapse, and she was readmitted to the inpatient program where she was originally treated. Following resolution of dispositional issues, that is, a recommendation for her placement outside the home, Susie continued to work toward maintenance of her abstinence from substance use.

Susie's case illustrates many of the typical features of an adolescent's presenting with substance abuse. These include oppositional behavior, poor school performance, and psychiatric or emotional disturbance, such as depression or suicidality. A comprehensive assessment includes a thorough evaluation of the multiple domains of the adolescent's life. Treatment is likewise directed toward improving function in multiple domains. Susie's case also illustrates the frequent occurrence of relapse and the often overwhelming effects of environmental factors, such as parental substance use and lack of supervision. Comprehensive treatment requires not only continuous vigilance for relapse but also the willingness to make radical changes in the adolescent's environment, if necessary.

PROBLEM AREAS

There are a number of areas in the treatment of chemically dependent adolescents that remain controversial or problematic, especially for the clinician.

Definition and Measurement of the Disorder

As previously noted, there are no current diagnostic criteria for adolescent substance abuse or chemical dependency with established validity. Clinicians and researchers must question the application of identical criteria for both adult and adolescent substance abuse.

The clinician must also be able to define specific, relevant behaviors as the focus of intervention. A broad range of appropriate outcome criteria should be designated: reduction in chemical use, completion of a treatment program, reduction in associated antisocial behaviors, or improved performance in one or more of a variety of domains in the adolescent's life. Although a focused behavioral/or cognitive intervention may have relatively restricted or narrow outcome criteria, families and society usually ask for more pervasive change across several areas of problem behavior directly or indirectly associated with adolescent chemical dependency. Again, such pervasive change may require a combination of modalities or a higher "dose" of a particular intervention. In addition, how the clinician measures change in target behaviors is also an area of concern with self-reports, parent reports, school reports, and direct observation all having significant limitations in terms of reliability and generalization over various situations in the adolescent's life.

Treatment Using Behavioral or Cognitive Modalities or Techniques

The clinician must be cautioned about the use with adolescents of behavioral or cognitive techniques that are described in the adult literature. Differences in the nature of the disorder between adolescents and adults, differences in their cognitive development, and differences in their life-style may make transposing behavioral or cognitive techniques designed for adults difficult to apply to adolescents. Developmentally appropriate modifications need to be made. Such modifications include simpler language and simpler, age-appropriate behavioral tasks, such as the use of parent provocations in anger control training. Contingency contracting concerning household chores, school performance, and abstinence from substance use also serve as examples of age and developmentally appropriate behavioral techniques.

Although various aspects of treatment planning and goal setting with cigarette users or alcohol abusers might be viewed as easily and logically extendable to drug abusers, caution must be exercised in doing so, because empirical support for such an extension is not presently available. Obviously, treatment efforts with the more prevalent problems of cigarette and alcohol abuse provide a departure point for treatment trials with abusers of other drugs. Behavioral and cognitive techniques should be modified according to the background of the patient and the difficulties presented by the specific drug or drugs involved. For example, the social and economic background of the crack user and the strong reinforcement properties of crack make a prospective behavioral intervention different from an intervention attempted with an upper middle-class adolescent who abuses marijuana.

Clinicians may also have problems in the primary application of behavioral and cognitive techniques described in prevention research for the treatment of adolescents who are already abusing drugs or alcohol.

Inpatient interventions and the resulting changes may not generalize to the outpatient or home settings. The clinician may have to consider continuation of behavioral and cognitive interventions in the outpatient setting and in booster sessions to help maintain treatment results, especially when the adolescent is exposed to the unconditional stimuli to SA in his natural environment.

We still do not know what is the relative weight of behavioral and cognitive treatment within the total therapeutic passage, milieu, and inpatient treatment of adolescents with substance abuse. Future research is warranted in order to provide answers to these questions. Although the behavioral and cognitive theories and techniques mentioned here are becoming widely used and accepted, investigators need to study these techniques further, especially with the clinical population of adolescents who are substance abusers. Collecting extensive data on admission, treatment, discharge, and follow-up, and investigating various therapeutic interventions will result in valuable data. It is also crucial for clinicians to define appropriate and specific problems and goals so that they are amenable to measurement and evaluation.

SUMMARY

Although there is increasing evidence for the effectiveness of behavioral and cognitive therapy in the treatment of substance abuse, there is little research in the adolescent age group. The sparse data that exist convey general optimism for behavioral and cognitive treatments, especially when combined with other modalities in a comprehensive program. Clinicians and researchers will have a better understanding of the problem and of the successful treatments when more clinical and research experience is accumulated.

REFERENCES

Achenbach, T. M., & Edelbrock, C. S. (1983). *Manual for the Child Behavior Checklist and Revised Child Behavior Profile*. Burlington: University of Vermont, Department of Psychiatry.

American Academy of Pediatrics, Committee on Adolescence. (1987). Alcohol use and abuse; A pediatric concern. *Pediatrics, 79,* 450–453.

American Psychiatric Association. (1980). *Diagnostic and statistical manual of mental disorders* (3rd ed.). Washington, DC: Author.

American Psychiatric Association. (1987). *Diagnostic and statistical manual of mental disorders* (3rd ed., rev.). Washington, DC: Author.

Armor, D. J., Polich, J. M., & Stambul, H. B. (1978). *Alcoholism and treatment*. Santa Monica, CA: Rand Corporation.

Bandura, A. (1977). *Social learning theory.* Englewood Cliffs, NJ: Prentice Hall.

Blane, H. (1979). Middle-aged alcoholics and young drinkers. In H. T. Blane & M. E. Chafetz (Eds.), *Youth, alcohol, and social policy* (pp. 102–124). New York: Plenum Press.

Botvin, G., Baker, E., Renick, N., Filazzola, N., & Botvin, A. (1984). A cognitive behavioral approach to substance abuse prevention. *Journal of Addictive Behaviors, 9,* 137–147.

Brown, S. A. (1985). Reinforcement expectancies and alcoholism outcome after a one year follow-up. *Journal of Studies on Alcohol, 46,* 305–308.

Brown, S. A., Christiansen, B. A., & Goldman, M. S. (1987). The alcohol expectancy questionnaire: An instrument for the assessment of adolescent and adult alcohol expectancies. *Journal of Studies on Alcohol, 48,* 483–491.

Bukstein, O. G., Brent, D. A., & Kaminer, Y. (1989). Comorbidity of substance abuse and other psychiatric disorders in adolescents. *American Journal of Psychiatry, 146,* 1131–1141.

Chafetz, M. E. (1972). Alcoholism criteria: An important step. *American Journal of Psychiatry, 129,* 214–215.

Chaney, E. F., O'Leary, M. R., & Marlzit, G. A. (1978). Skill training with alcoholics. *Journal of Consulting and Clinical Psychology, 46,* 1092–1104.

Childress, A. R., McLellan, A. T., & O'Brien, C. P. (1986). The role of conditioning factors in the development of drug dependence. *Psychiatric Clinics of North America, 9,* 413–426.

Christiansen, B. A., Goldman, M. S., & Inn, A. (1982). Development of alcohol-related expectancies in adolescents: Separating pharmacological from social learning influences. *Journal of Consulting and Clinical Psychology, 50,* 336–344.

Christiansen, B. A., Goldman, M. S., & Brown, S. A. (1985). The differential development of adolescent alcohol expectancies may predict adult alcoholism. *Journal of Addictive Behaviors, 10,* 299–306.

Craig, R. J. (1987). *Clinical management of substance abuse programs*. Springfield, IL: Charles C Thomas.
Cummings, N. A. (1979). Turning bread into stones: Our modern anti-miracle. *American Psychologist, 34*, 1–8.
Deykin, E. Y., Levy, J. C., & Wells, V. (1987). Adolescent depression, alcohol and drug abuse. *American Journal of Public Health, 77*, 178–182.
Donovan, J. E., & Jessor, R. (1978). Adolescent problem drinking—psychosocial correlates in a national sample study. *Journal of Studies on Alcohol, 39*, 1506–1524.
Edwards, G., & Gross, M. M. (1976). Alcohol dependence: Provisional description of a clinical syndrome. *British Journal of Medicine, 1*, 1058–1061.
Edwards, G., Orford, J., Egert, S., Guthrie, S., Hawker, A., Hensman, C., Mitcheson, M., Oppenheimer, O., & Taylor, C. (1977). Alcoholism: A controlled trial of "treatment" and "advice." *Journal of Studies on Alcohol, 38*, 1004–1031.
Fischman, M. W. (1988). Behavioral pharmacology of cocaine. *Journal of Clinical Psychiatry, 49* (Suppl. 2), 7–10.
Flay, B. (1975). What do we know about the social influences approach to smoking prevention? Review and recommendations. In C. Bell & R. Bettles (Eds.), *Prevention research; Deterring drug abuse among children and adolescents* (pp. 67–112). Washington, DC: NIDA Research Monogram.
Gawin, F. H., & Ellenwood, E. H. (1988). Cocaine and other stimulants: Actions, abuse, and treatment. *New England Journal of Medicine, 18*, 1173–1182.
Gawin, F. H., Kleber, H. D., & Byck, R. (1989). Desipramine facilitation of initial cocaine abstinence. *Archives of General Psychiatry, 46*, 117–121.
Gittleman, R., Mannuzza, S., Shenker, R., & Bonagura, N. (1985). Hyperactive boys almost grown up: I. Psychiatric status. *Archives of General Psychiatry, 42*, 937–947.
Hawkins, J. O., Catalano, R. F., & Well, E. A. (1986). Measuring effects of a skill training intervention for drug abusers. *Journal of Consulting and Clinical Psychology, 54*, 661–664.
Henly, G. A., & Winters, K. C. (1988). Development of problem severity scales for the assessment of adolescent alcohol and drug abuse. *International Journal of the Addictions, 23*, 65–85.
Holden, C. (1987). Is alcoholism treatment effective? *Science, 236*, 20–22.
Horan, J. J., & Williams, J. M. (1982). Longitudinal study of attention training as a drug abuse prevention strategy. *American Educational Research Journal, 19*(3), 341–351.
Hull, J. (1981). A self-awareness model of the causes and effects of alcohol consumption. *Journal of Abnormal Psychology, 90*, 586–600.
Jones, E. E., & Berglas S. (1978). Control of attributions about the self through self-handicapping strategies: The appeal of alcohol and the role of underachievement. *Personality and Social Psychology Bulletin, 4*, 200–206.
Jellinek, E. M. (1960). *The disease concept of alcoholism*. New Haven: College and University Press.
Jessor, R., & Jessor, S. L. (1978). Theory testing on longitudinal research. In D. B. Kandel (Ed.), *Longitudinal research on drug use: Empirical findings and methodological issues* (pp. 41–71). Washington, DC: Hemisphere-Wiley.
Johnston, L., O'Malley, P., & Eveland, L. (1978). Drugs and delinquency: A search for causal connections. In D. B. Kandel (Ed.), *Longitudinal research on drug use: Empirical findings and methodological issues* (pp. 137–156). Washington, DC: Hemisphere-Wiley.
Johnston, L. D., Bachman, J. G., & O'Malley, P. M. (1988). *Press release*. Ann Arbor: University of Michigan News and Information Service.
Kaminer, Y., & Frances, R. J. (1991). Adolescent substance abuse and comorbid psychiatric disorders: Inpatient treatment. *Hospital and Community Psychiatry, 42*, 951–953.

Kaminer, Y., Bukstein, O. G., & Tarter, R. E. (1991). The Teen Addiction Severity Index (T-ASI): Rationale and reliability. *International Journal of the Addictions, 26,* 219–226.
Kandel, D. B. (1982). Epidemiological and psychosocial perspectives on adolescent drug use. *Journal of the American Academy of Child Psychiatry, 21,* 328–347.
Kandel, D. B., Kessler, R. C., & Margulies, R. Z. (1978). Antecedents of adolescent initiation into stages of drug use: A developmental analysis. In D. B. Kandel (Ed.), *Longitudinal research on drug use: Empirical findings and methodological issues.* Washington, DC: Hemisphere-Wiley.
Killen, J. D., Maccoby, N., & Taylor, C. B. (1984). Nicotine gum and self-regulation training in smoking relapse prevention, *Behavior Therapy, 15,* 234–248.
Klinge, V., Lachar, D., Grisell, J., & Berman, W. (1978). Effects of scoring norms on adolescent psychiatric drug users' and nonusers' MMPI profiles. *Adolescence, 13,* 1–10.
Kosten, T. R., Rounsaville, B. J., Babor, T. F., Spitzer, R. L., & Williams, J. B. W. (1987). Substance-use disorders in DSM-III-R. *British Journal of Psychiatry, 151,* 834–843.
Levine, J., & Zigler, E. (1973). The essential-reactive distinction in alcoholism: A developmental approach. *Journal of Abnormal Psychology, 81,* 242–249.
MacAndrew, C. (1979). On the possibility of the psychometric detection of persons who are prone to the abuse of alcohol and other substances. *Addictive Behaviors, 4,* 11–20.
Marlatt, G., & George, W. H. (1984). Relapse prevention: Introduction and overview of the model. *British Journal of Addiction, 79,* 261–275.
Marlatt, G. A. (1982). Relapse prevention: A self-control program for the treatment of addictive behaviors. In R. B. Stuart (Ed.), *Adherence, compliance and generalization in behavioral medicine* (pp. 329–378). New York: Brunner/Mazel.
Marlatt, G. A., & Gordon, J. R. (1985). *Relapse prevention: Maintenance strategies in the treatment of addictive behaviors.* New York: Guilford Press.
Mayer, J. E., & Filstead, W. J. (1979). Empirical procedures for defining adolescent alcohol abuse. *Journal of Studies on Alcohol, 40,* 291–300.
McLellan, A. T., O'Brien, C. P., & Woody, G. (1980). An improved diagnostic evaluation instrument for substance abuse patients: The addiction severity index. *Journal of Nervous and Mental Disease, 168,* 26–33.
McLellan, A. T., Luborsky, L., O'Brien, C. P., Woody, G. E., & Druley, K. A. (1983). Is treatment for substance abuse effective? *Journal of the American Medical Association, 247,* 1423–1428.
Meyer, R. E. (1986). Old wine, new bottle: The alcohol dependency syndrome. *Psychiatric Clinics of North America, 9,* 435–453.
Miller, W. R., & Hester, R. K. (1980). Treating the problem drinker: Modern approaches. In W. R. Miller (Ed.), *The addictive behaviors: Treatment of alcoholism, drug abuse, smoking and obesity* (pp. 11–141). New York: Pergamon Press.
Miller, W. R., & Hester, R. K. (1986). Inpatient alcoholism treatment: Who benefits? *American Psychologist, 41,* 794–805.
Moberg, D. P. (1983). Identifying adolescents with alcohol problems: A field test of the Adolescent Alcohol Involvement Scale. *Journal of Studies on Alcohol, 44,* 701–721.
National Council on Alcoholism. (1972). Criteria for the diagnosis of alcoholism. *American Journal of Psychiatry, 129,* 127–135.
Oei, T. P. S., & Jackson, P. R. (1982). Social skills and cognitive behavioral approaches to the treatment of problem drinking. *Journal of Studies on Alcohol, 43,* 532–546.
Oetting, E. R., Beauvais, F., Edwards, R., & Waters, M. (1984). *The Drug and Alcohol Assessment System.* Fort Collins, CO: Rocky Mountain Behavioral Science Institute.
O'Leary, D. E., O'Leary, M. R., & Donovan, D. M. (1975). Social skills acquisition and psychosocial development of alcoholics: A review. *Addictive Behaviors, 1,* 111–120.

Pattison, E. M. (1985). The selection of treatment modalities for the alcoholic patient. In J. H. Mendelson & N. K. Mello (Eds.), *The diagnosis and treatment of alcoholism* (pp. 189–294). New York: McGraw-Hill.

Pavlov, I. P. (1927). *Conditioned reflexes* (G. V. Anrep, Trans.). Oxford: Oxford University Press.

Perry, C., Kullen, J., Slinkard, L., & McAlister, A. (1980). Peer teaching and smoking prevention among junior high school students. *Adolescence, 58,* 277–281.

Puig-Antich, J., Orvaschel, H., Tabrizi, M., & Chambers, W. (1980). *The schedule for affective disorders and schizophrenia for school-age children—epidemiologic version (K-SADS-E)* (3rd ed.). New York: New York State Psychiatric Institute and Yale University School of Medicine.

Rachal, J. V., Guess, L. L., Hubbard, R. L., Maisto, S. A., Cavanaugh, E. R., Waddell, R., & Benrud, C. H. (1980). *Vol. I. Adolescent drinking behavior—The extent and nature of adolescent alcohol and drug use: The 1974 and 1978 national sample studies.* Final report to the National Institute on Alcohol Abuse and Alcoholism (Contract No. ADM 281-76-0019). Research Triangle Park, NC: Research Triangle Foundation.

Reuger, D. R., & Liberman, R. P. (1984). Behavioral family therapy for delinquent and substance-abusing adolescents. *Journal of Drug Issues, 14*(2), 403–418.

Rist, F., & Watzl, H. (1983). Self assessment of relapse risk and assertiveness in relation to treatment outcome of female alcoholics. *Addictive Behaviors, 8,* 121–127.

Rounsaville, B. J. (1987). An evaluation of the DSM-III substance-use disorders. In G. L. Tischler (Ed.), *Diagnosis and classification in psychiatry* (pp. 175–194). Cambridge: Cambridge University Press.

Rounsaville, B. J., Spitzer, R. L., & Williams, J. B. W. (1986). Proposed changes in DSM-III substance use disorders: Description and rationale. *American Journal of Psychiatry, 143,* 463–468.

Rounsaville, B. J., Kosten, T. R., Weissman, M. M., & Kleber, H. D. (1986). Prognostic significance of psychiatric disorders in treated opiate addicts. *Archives of General Psychiatry, 43,* 739–745.

Sanchez-Craig, M. (1984). *A therapist manual for secondary prevention of alcohol problems.* Toronto: Addiction Research Foundation.

Schuckit, M. A., Irwin, M., Howard, T., & Smith, T. (1988). A structured diagnostic interview for identification of primary alcoholism: A preliminary examination. *Journal of Studies on Alcohol, 49,* 93–99.

Selzer, M. L. (1971). The Michigan Alcoholism Screening Test: The quest for a new diagnostic instrument. *American Journal of Psychiatry, 127,* 1653–1658.

Siegel, S. (1973). Evidence from rats that morphine tolerance is a learned response. *Journal of Comprehensive and Physiological Psychology, 89,* 498–506.

Simpson, D. D., Savage, L. J., & Sells, S. B. (1978). Evaluation of drug abuse treatments based on first year follow-up (NIDA Monograph No. ADM 78-701). Washington, DC: U.S. Government Printing Office.

Skinner, H. A. (1982). The Drug Abuse Screening Test. *Addictive Behaviors, 7,* 363–371.

Skinner, H. A., & Goldberg, A. E. (1986). Evidence for a drug dependence syndrome among narcotic users. *British Journal of Psychiatry, 81,* 479–484.

Sobell, L. C., Sobell, M. B., & Nirenberg, T. D. (1982). Differential treatment planning for alcohol abusers. In E. M. Pattison & E. Kaufman (Eds.), *Encyclopedia handbook of alcoholism* (pp. 173–203). New York: Gardner Press.

Sobell, L. C., Sobell, M. B., & Nirenberg, T. D. (1988). Behavioral assessment and treatment planning with alcohol and drug abusers: A review with an emphasis on clinical application. *Clinical Psychology Review, 8,* 19–54.

Tarter, R. E. (1990). Evaluation and treatment of adolescent substance abuse: A decision tree method. *American Journal of Drug and Alcohol Abuse, 16*, 1–46.

Tucker, J. A., Vuchinich, R. G., & Sobell, M. B. (1981). Alcohol consumption as a self-handicapping strategy. *Journal of Abnormal Psychology, 90*, 220–230.

Vingilis, E., & Smart, R. G. (1981). Physical dependence on alcohol in youth. In Y. Israel, F. B. Glaser, & H. Kalant, R. E. Popham, W. Schmidt, & R. G. Smart (Eds.), *Research advances in alcohol and drug problems* (Vol. 6, pp. 197–215). New York: Plenum Press.

Watson, D. W., & Maisto, S. (1983). A review of the effectiveness of assertiveness training in the treatment of alcohol abusers. *Behavioral Psychotherapy, 11*, 36–49.

Wechsler, H. (1979). Patterns of alcohol consumption among the young: High school, college and general population studies. In H. T. Blane & M. E. Chafetz (Eds.), *Youth, alcohol, and social policy* (pp. 173–192). New York: Plenum Press.

White, H. R. (1987). Longitudinal stability and dimensional structure of problem drinking in adolescence. *Journal of Studies on Alcohol, 48*, 541–550.

Wikler, A. (1965). Conditioning factors in opiate addiction and relapse. In D. M. Wilner, & G. C. Kassabaum (Eds.), *Narcotics* (pp. 85–100). New York: McGraw-Hill.

Wilson, G. T. (1982). Alcohol and anxiety: Recent evidence on the tension reduction theory of alcohol use and abuse. In K. R. Blankstein & J. Polivy (Eds.), *Self-control and self-modification of emotional behavior* (pp. 91–122). New York: Plenum Press.

Wilson, G. T. (1987). Cognitive processes in addiction. *British Journal of Addiction, 82*, 343–353.

Wolfson, K. P., & Erbaugh, S. E. (1984). Adolescent responses to the MacAndrew Alcoholism Scale. *Journal of Consulting and Clinical Psychology, 52*, 625–630.

Yankofsky, L., Wilson, G. T., Adler, J., Hay, W., & Vrana, S. (1986). The effect of alcohol on self-evaluation, awareness of negative interpersonal feedback and perceptions of control and power. *Journal of Studies on Alcohol, 47*, 26–37.

12

Anorexia and Bulimia Nervosa

DONALD A. WILLIAMSON, C. J. DAVIS, AND
ERICH G. DUCHMANN

INTRODUCTION

It has been our experience that most cases of anorexia nervosa will require inpatient treatment. Hospitalization of the anorexic patient is usually required to accomplish refeeding and weight gain because very few cases will gain weight in outpatient treatment. Bulimia nervosa, on the other hand, can often be treated on an outpatient basis. We find that only about 30% of bulimics referred for treatment will ultimately require hospitalization. Most bulimics are of approximately normal weight and are eating at least one meal per day. Therefore, resistance to eating is usually not as extreme in cases of bulimia nervosa and the need to gain substantial amounts of weight occurs infrequently. Usually, only very severe cases of bulimia nervosa require inpatient treatment. These cases usually binge and purge one or more times every day, and they have very little control over these behaviors. Also, most individuals with severe bulimia are depressed (Williamson, Prather, Upton, Davis, Ruggiero, & Van Buren, 1987) or have personality disorders or other psychiatric problems (Johnson, Corrigan, & Mayo, 1987). When the eating disorder is complicated by other severe psychopathology, hospitaliza-

DONALD A. WILLIAMSON, C. J. DAVIS, AND ERICH G. DUCHMANN • Department of Psychology, Louisiana State University, Baton Rouge, Louisiana 70803-5501.
Inpatient Behavior Therapy for Children and Adolescents, edited by Vincent B. Van Hasselt and David J. Kolko. Plenum Press, New York, 1992.

tion is often required. For both eating disorders, our treatment philosophy is that the primary goal of inpatient treatment is to prepare the patient for intensive outpatient therapy.

The sections which follow describe the procedures that are used for treating adolescents and older children who are diagnosed with anorexia or bulimia nervosa. Assessment and treatment methods that will be presented are derived from cognitive-behavioral formulations of eating disorders (Williamson, Davis, Duchmann, McKenzie, & Watkins, 1990). From this perspective, very intensive, focused treatment can be provided in a hospital setting. This type of treatment is often relatively brief (2 to 8 weeks) and is designed to manage problems that cannot be modified on an outpatient basis.

CLINICAL DESCRIPTIONS

Anorexia Nervosa

Anorexia nervosa is generally conceptualized as the "self-starvation syndrome." This conceptualization is accurate in that most anorexic patients use fasting or starvation as one type of extreme method for losing weight or maintaining thinness. Most clinical researchers agree that the central feature of anorexia nervosa is an intense fear of "fatness" (Williamson *et al.*, 1990). Fatness in this context refers to actually being overweight as well as feeling "fat," which is often conceptualized as a form of body image disturbance. The anorexic patient, fearing fatness, is thus highly motivated to lose weight and maintain a very thin body size. To accomplish this, the person must either avoid eating (i.e., engage in starvation) or engage in purgative behavior (self-induced vomiting) whenever eating occurs. Surveys of anorexic eating habits have found that approximately 50% engage in purgative habits.

The DSM-III-R criteria (American Psychiatric Association, 1987) for a diagnosis of anorexia nervosa are summarized in Table 1. A central

Table 1. Summary of Diagnostic Criteria for Anorexia Nervosa

1. Refusal to maintain normal body weight or failure to gain weight during adolescence.
2. Intense fear of gaining weight.
3. Body image disturbance, for example, feeling fat when emaciated.
4. Absence of three consecutive menstrual cycles.

diagnostic feature of anorexia nervosa is severe weight loss and refusal to maintain a weight level that even approximates normality.

Starvation and extreme weight control methods (e.g., purging) are motivated by an intense fear of weight gain and body image disturbances. The final diagnostic criterion, amenorrhea for three menstrual cycles, has been questioned as an essential characteristic since it is generally considered to result from severe weight loss.

Bulimia Nervosa

Bulimia nervosa is a syndrome with the essential features of uncontrollable binge eating and the use of extreme methods for controlling weight. The most common strategies for controlling weight are self-induced vomiting, laxative abuse, diuretic abuse, and extremely restrictive eating. These behaviors are motivated by fear of weight gain and body image disturbances similar to those described for anorexia nervosa (Williamson, Davis, Goreczny, & Blouin, 1989). Most bulimic patients are approximately normal in weight, though a minority are obese and some are significantly underweight. When evaluating cases where binge eating is a central behavioral problem, it is important to distinguish the syndrome of bulimia nervosa from compulsive binge eating without purging and intense fear of weight gain (Williamson, Kelley, Cavell, & Prather, 1987).

The syndrome of bulimia nervosa has been defined by the American Psychiatric Association (1987) by the diagnostic criteria summarized in Table 2. Using these guidelines, uncontrollable binge eating, purgative behavior, and overconcern with body shape and weight are the central features of bulimia nervosa. The fourth criterion (i.e., at least two binge eating episodes per week) can be considered a measure of severity. It should be noted that some patients present with the symptoms of both anorexia nervosa and bulimia nervosa and that others alternate between the two syndromes over their history.

Table 2. Summary of Diagnostic Criteria for Bulimia Nervosa

1. Compulsive binge eating.
2. Lack of control of eating binges.
3. Use of extreme methods for controlling weight, for example, self-induced vomiting, laxative abuse, diuretic abuse, restrictive dieting, or vigorous exercise.
4. At least two binge-eating episodes per week for at least 3 months.
5. Obsessive overconcern with body shape, body weight, and body size.

BEHAVIORAL AND PSYCHIATRIC ASSESSMENT

Assessment of severe cases of anorexia and bulimia nervosa must be comprehensive. The following sections describe the methods of assessment which we have found to be essential for proper behavioral treatment. In addition to these methods, each case should also undergo a thorough medical examination and dietary consultation.

Clinical Interview

In assessing eating disorder symptoms of children and adolescents, interviews with both the identified patient and his or her family should be conducted. These interviews should attempt to obtain a description of the patient's eating habits, including incidence and severity of binge eating, purgative behaviors (via vomiting, laxatives, diuretics, appetite suppressants, excessive exercise), and restrictive eating patterns. A thorough behavioral analysis of each problem behavior should be conducted. Both environmental events and emotional reactions should be investigated as potential antecedents and consequences which may be maintaining the behavior. For example, bulimic cases may report that binging and purging frequently occur while the individual is alone and during periods of negative affect. Binging may temporarily reduce negative affect, but only if the binge can be followed by purging. When with family members, or when there has been a "good day" at school (a good grade on a test, no peer problems), the individual may report a lower probability of binging and purging. The interview should also identify foods which are avoided because they are "fattening." In bulimia nervosa, these "forbidden foods" (Ruggiero, Williamson, Davis, Schlundt, & Carey, 1988) will usually be consumed only if they can be safely purged. Identification of these forbidden foods is essential for implementing exposure with response prevention treatment.

Several structured interviews for eating disorders have been developed. Palmer, Christie, Cordle, Davies, and Kendrick (1987) constructed an interview format which has been recommended and used for the purpose of diagnosis. Eating behaviors, attitudes, and other symptomatology (e.g., depression, anxiety, obsessions, psychosis) are evaluated. Interrater reliability for most of the 35 items, using five raters, was reported to be high. Cooper and Fairburn (1987) have also presented a structured interview format, which assesses eating patterns over the last 4 weeks. Only current eating behaviors are evaluated, without assessment of historical factors and topography of the eating over time. This method was constructed as a measure of treatment outcome, not as a method for diagnosing eating disorders or providing a behavioral analysis of eating behaviors.

The interview is an integral component of the assessment procedure. We have found that a structured interview which assesses all facets of anorexia and bulimia nervosa is essential for case formulation and treatment planning. We recommend that data derived from the interview can be integrated with other behavioral assessment data to provide objective measurement of the complex of problem behaviors.

Self-Report Inventories

There are many questionnaires which evaluate various symptoms of anorexia nervosa and bulimia nervosa. Four self-report inventories have been fully developed and are widely used. They are the Eating Attitudes Test (EAT) (Garner & Garfinkel, 1979), the Bulimia Test (BULIT) (M. C. Smith & Thelen, 1984), the Eating Questionnaire—Revised (EQ—R) (Williamson, Davis, Goreczny, Bennett, & Watkins, 1989), and the Eating Disorder Inventory (EDI) (Garner & Olmstead, 1984).

The EAT is a 40-item self-rating scale that was developed for evaluating the symptoms of anorexia nervosa. A total score of 30 or more is often used as a cut-off score for anorexia nervosa. The EAT has been reported to be reliable with both clinical and normal subjects.

The BULIT is a 36-item questionnaire which was designed to evaluate the symptoms of bulimia. M. C. Smith and Thelen (1984) reported test–retest reliability of the BULIT to be high; support for concurrent validity, using the correlation of BULIT scores with group membership (bulimics vs. normals) was also satisfactory. More recent research has shown the BULIT to be correlated with frequency of binging and purging, as measured via self-monitoring (Williamson, Goreczny, & Duchmann, 1987).

The EQ—R is a test which, like the BULIT, measures the symptoms of bulimia. It was designed as a brief symptom checklist (only 15 items) and has been found to be highly correlated with the BULIT. Test–retest reliability of the EQ—R has been found to be satisfactory, and internal consistency was found to be quite high.

The EDI is a 64-item test which was constructed as an expansion of the EAT. The EDI samples a diversity of symptoms associated with anorexia and bulimia nervosa. Eight scales are derived from the EDI: (1) drive for thinness, (2) bulimia, (3) body dissatisfaction, (4) ineffectiveness, (5) perfectionism, (6) interpersonal distrust, (7) interoceptive awareness, and (8) maturity fears. Internal consistency of each scale was found to be high, though the scales are intercorrelated. Strong support was found for the convergent and discriminant validity of each subscale, using a variety of measures.

Each of these self-report inventories measures some of the characteristics of anorexia or bulimia nervosa. However, none of these instruments was developed for differential diagnosis and all of them were constructed prior to changes in the American Psychiatric Association's diagnostic criteria in 1987. For these reasons, all of the current self-report inventories must be used as global measures of the psychopathology of eating disorders and cannot be used in place of a comprehensive behavioral assessment.

Body Image Assessment

There is general agreement that body image disturbances play an integral role in the etiology and maintenance of anorexia and bulimia nervosa. There are a number of techniques which have been developed to assess body image distortion. For a thorough discussion of these methods, the reader is referred to Cash and Brown (1987).

Body-part size estimation techniques assess the patient's estimation of the size of specific body regions (Askevold, 1975; Reitman & Cleveland, 1964; Ruff & Barrios, 1986; Slade & Russell, 1973). Results of studies using these techniques have produced mixed results; some investigations have found that anorexics and bulimics overestimate (or distort) body image, and others have not.

Distorting image techniques require the subject to manipulate a visual image of themselves (e.g., using a camera lens) to measure the degree to which their perception of body size matches their actual body size. Studies using this methodology have consistently found that bulimic patients overestimate actual body size (Freeman, Thomas, Solyom, & Miles, 1983; Freeman, Thomas, Solyom, & Koopman, 1985), whereas mixed results have been found in anorexic patients (Freeman *et al.*, 1983; Freeman *et al.*, 1985; Garfinkel, Moldofsky, & Garner, 1979; Touyz, Beaumont, Collins, McCabe, & Jupp, 1984).

Williamson, Davis, Goreczny, *et al.* (1989) have developed a simple procedure for assessing body image disturbances called the Body Image Assessment (BIA). This procedure requires subjects to select body size silhouettes which match their perception of current and ideal body sizes. The BIA has been normed and has been found to be reliable and valid in a series of investigations with bulimia nervosa (Davis, Williamson, Goreczny, & Bennett, 1989; Williamson, Davis, Goreczny, & Blouin, 1989; Williamson, Kelley, Davis, Ruggiero, & Blouin, 1985).

Self-Monitoring

Self-monitoring procedures for anorexia and bulimia nervosa generally require recording (1) the type and amount of food eaten, (2) whether the person considers the eating episode to be a binge, (3) the occurrence of purging, and (4) the environmental and emotional correlates of eating behavior (Williamson, Kelley, *et al.*, 1987). Recent studies of self-monitoring strategies have supported the reliability and validity of these approaches (Williamson, Goreczny, & Duchmann, 1987). Also, most behavioral treatment outcome studies have used self-monitoring data as one index of treatment outcome.

Behavioral Observation

Direct observation of eating behavior can be very useful in the diagnosis and assessment of eating disorders. In an inpatient setting, the most unobtrusive method of evaluating eating behavior is to utilize nursing staff to record (1) food choices, (2) amounts eaten, and (3) the occurrence of purgative behavior and exercise following meals. These data can be invaluable for diagnosing anorexia or bulimia nervosa in patients who deny these problems in interviews and on questionnaires. Also, careful evaluation of the caloric content of foods eaten and types of food eaten (e.g., forbidden foods) can be very helpful in evaluating progress in treatment. When treating anorexia nervosa, it is essential to carefully document daily caloric intake so that changes in weight can be evaluated within the context of objective information related to calories consumed.

Assessment of Family Problems

In a recent review of the literature regarding typical family problems of patients with eating disorders, Kog and Vandereycken (1985) noted several recurring characteristics. Patients with anorexia and bulimia nervosa tended to come from families of higher social class, and their mothers had a tendency to be overweight. Serious physical illness, depression, and paternal alcoholism were commonly observed in the parents of these patients. Marital discord was common in families of eating disordered patients as well. The patient's eating disorder may be a way to divert attention from the problems within the marriage, which may have implications for the level of tension at home as the patient improves with his or her eating disorder. As the family becomes involved with the adolescent's treatment, these problems need to be addressed in family therapy.

In assessing the family of an eating disordered patient, it is often necessary to assess the family's knowledge of eating disorders. Often, the family will believe that the patient has a great deal of control of the disorder, and is acting out or using the eating disorder to control the family, particularly the parents. Educational intervention will often alleviate the anger that the family may have toward the patient. The interview with the family also may yield an accurate assessment of the patient's eating behavior at home (e.g., restrictive eating, food disappearing repetitively) and whether the patient spends a lot of time in the bathroom immediately following a meal.

The Family Environment Scale (FES) (R. H. Moos & Moos, 1980) is often employed to ascertain patients' perceptions of the psychosocial characteristics of their families. The FES, comprised of 10 subscales, measures three underlying domains, including Relationship, Personal Growth, and System Maintenance Dimensions. Several studies which have used the FES with eating disordered patients and their families indicate that low cohesion, expressiveness, and level of independence are often reported (Humphrey, 1986; Strober & Humphrey, 1987).

Assessment of the family, via interview and questionnaire, is integral in the assessment and treatment of the eating disordered patient, especially when the patient is a child or adolescent. Reports of family members may yield important information about the patient's eating behavior, which the patient has denied or minimized. Also, behavioral analysis of the family's response to eating problems should assist in determining whether intensive family therapy should be included as one component of the treatment plan.

Assessment of Secondary Psychopathology

It is well established that anorexia and bulimia nervosa are often accompanied by a variety of other problems (Williamson *et al.*, 1990). Common secondary problems are: depression, conduct disorders, and substance abuse. In severe cases, this secondary psychopathology may negatively impact upon the treatment of problems directly related to eating. (For a more complete review of behavioral assessment techniques related to these problems, the reader should refer to Chapters 4, 8, and 11, in this volume.)

BEHAVIORAL TREATMENT STRATEGIES

Behavioral treatment approaches for anorexia and bulimia nervosa have been developed using both adolescents and young adults as clinical subjects. At present, there are no data suggesting that these interventions are differentially effective for adolescents and young adults. Therefore, no distinctions will be made based on ages of samples used in the various investigations. Also, most treatment studies of bulimia nervosa use outpatient samples. These same treatment techniques are used for treating inpatient bulimics. Therefore, these outpatient studies will be reviewed so that the reader may appreciate the substantial treatment literature which has been developed in support of behavioral treatments for bulimia nervosa. In the sections that follow, specific behavioral and psychopharmacological techniques will be described. Each technique has been developed for the treatment of a specific behavioral component of anorexia and bulimia nervosa (e.g., eating habits, purgative habits, or cognitive errors).

Meal Planning and Behavioral Contracting

Most cases of anorexia and bulimia nervosa have very distorted ideas and beliefs related to dietary habits. Thus, it is important to include basic nutritional counseling in the treatment of these eating disorders (Andersen, Morse, & Santmyer, 1985).

An efficient approach to nutritional counseling is to have patients attend a group in which information regarding basic nutrition is presented. Inclusion of both a therapist specializing in eating disorders and a dietician is recommended to address the wide variety of questions that may be associated with eating for these patients. Following nutritional education, it is important for the patients to have guidance in applying the information they have learned and in developing proper eating skills. Structured meal planning can be used to teach the selection of properly balanced meals with appropriate caloric quantities. The use of a dietary exchange system rather than calories can be less fearful for eating disordered patients and can promote good nutrition as well.

Many of the poor dietary practices exhibited by these patients result from the avoidance of feared or forbidden foods. These are foods which are associated with weight gain, such as high-caloric sweets and high-fat foods. Some patients may find it very difficult incorporating such foods into their meal planning. For these cases, a hierarchy of forbidden foods (from least to most feared or forbidden) can be used in conjunction with behavioral contracting for graduated exposure to foods that are feared.

Exposure with Response Prevention

Exposure with response prevention was developed by J. C. Rosen and Leitenberg (1982) to reduce the purgative behavior of bulimia nervosa. They conceptualized the binge–purge cycle of bulimia as similar to obsessive compulsive disorder in that purging has the effect of "undoing" the effects of binging (i.e., it prevents weight gain). Thus, purgative habits are negatively reinforced by reducing the bulimic's fear of weight gain. Purgative behavior also produces elimination of energy (food) and results in increased hunger which increases the likelihood of further binging. In this manner, a vicious cycle of binging and purging is created (Williamson, Kelley, Davis, Ruggiero, & Veitia, 1985).

Exposure with response prevention requires the bulimic to consume binge foods in the presence of a therapist. This may be carried out either individually or in small groups. The therapist then prevents the patient from purging and usually employs cognitive restructuring to counter irrational concerns about current weight and potential weight gain, as well as misconceptions related to food and eating. This technique also allows for a much more direct analysis of the behaviors and thoughts that occur during eating. Quantification of caloric consumption, ratings of urges to binge and purge, ratings of emotional distress, and investigation of problematic thinking styles can all be used to target idiosyncratic problem areas for each patient.

Cognitive Restructuring

Irrational thinking styles are common in individuals with eating disorders. Abnormal attitudes and ideals regarding body size and shape are often the driving force behind these patients' severely restrictive eating patterns. Therefore, most behavioral treatment approaches for anorexia and bulimia nervosa incorporate some form of cognitive restructuring. This form of cognitive therapy involves identifying and directly challenging irrational beliefs concerning weight, body size, and weight control methods (e.g., dieting, starvation, purging). Usually, the patient is trained to monitor these cognitions and to challenge them by using more rational beliefs which are acquired in cognitive therapy. This type of treatment can most easily be administered in small groups (Williamson, Prather, Bennett, Davis, Watkins, & Grenier, 1989).

Temptation Exposure with Response Prevention

Temptation exposure with response prevention (TERP) was first discussed by Johnson *et al.* (1987) and has been described in more detail by Schlundt and Johnson (1990). TERP is a technique which can be used to extinguish the binge response to environmental cues which set the occasion for binging. In addition to the stimulus characteristics of the food during a typical binge, there are a variety of other external and internal stimulus cues that can come to elicit urges to binge (Johnson *et al.*, 1987). The most common of these cues include being alone at home, being in specific places (e.g., in the kitchen, in front of the television set, etc.), and encountering stressful situations (Hawkins & Clement, 1980; Pyle, Mitchell, & Eckert, 1981; Russell, 1979; Schlundt, Johnson, & Jarrell, 1985). Once these cues are identified, the patient can then be exposed to binge cues and be prevented from binging. Theoretically, this type of treatment should gradually reduce the urgency to binge. In order to assess progress in treatment, subjective ratings of the urge to binge may be measured during the exposure session (Johnson *et al.*, 1987).

Body Image Therapy

Disturbance of body image is frequently observed in anorexia and bulimia nervosa. The most common types of body image disturbance have been referred to as *body size distortion* and *body size dissatisfaction*. Williamson, Davis, Goreczny, and Blouin (1989) have also suggested that extreme preference for thinness may also be regarded to be a third component of the body image construct. Standardized treatment approaches for body image distortion have only recently been developed (Butters & Cash, 1988; J. C. Rosen, Saltzberg, & Srebnik, 1989).

Butters and Cash (1988) were the first to develop a cognitive-behavioral treatment program for body image disturbances. The major components of this treatment included presentation of information concerning body image dissatisfaction (e.g., possible causes, effects), imaginal body image desensitization, and instruction in cognitive techniques, such as challenging irrational beliefs, viewing one's body more positively, and relapse prevention strategies. This treatment approach produced significantly greater improvements in negative body image than a waiting list control condition.

J. C. Rosen *et al.* (1989) compared a cognitive-behavioral treatment condition to a minimal treatment condition for negative body image. At posttreatment and at 2-month follow-up, the cognitive-behavioral treatment was found to produce clinically significant improvements in negative body image which were also superior to those of the minimal therapy condition.

Because these two studies focused on only one aspect of eating disorder symptomatology, it was not appropriate to employ clinical subjects. To date, there have been no controlled investigations of body image therapy as exclusive treatments for anorexia and bulimia nervosa.

Family Therapy

Family interaction patterns, such as enmeshment, overprotectiveness, rigidity, lack of conflict resolution, and involvement of the child in parental conflicts have all been suggested to have possible contributions to anorexia nervosa (Minuchin, Rosman, & Baker, 1978; Sargent, Leibman, & Silver, 1985). In bulimia, binging and purging are secretive behaviors and are seldom discussed openly. From this secretiveness, a great deal of mistrust and miscommunication can result (Schwartz, Barrett, & Saba, 1985). Behavioral approaches to family therapy can be used to modify these problem behaviors.

In addition to targeting family interaction styles, education of the family regarding the nature of eating disorders is very important. As a general rule, some basic understanding about the eating disorder is necessary for patients and their families to communicate effectively about the problem. Other behavioral techniques, such as self-monitoring, goal setting, and contingency contracting, also have been used in family intervention (Root, Fallon, & Friedrich, 1986; Schwartz *et al.*, 1985; Vandereycken, 1987). No controlled investigations of behavioral family therapy for eating disorders have been reported, however.

Psychopharmacological Approaches

A variety of pharmacological approaches have been used with both anorexia and bulimia nervosa. In anorexia nervosa, there is little evidence of the efficacy of pharmacotherapy (Rockwell, Ellingwood, Dougherty, & Brodie, 1982). Yet medications are frequently employed in an attempt to promote weight gain and to reduce anxiety related to weight gain. The most commonly prescribed drugs include major tranquilizers, such as chlorpromazine (primarily because of the inactivity and weight gain side-effects it sometimes produces), antianxiety agents (e.g., benzodiazepines), antidepressants, lithium, L-dopa, and cyproheptadine (a children's antihistamine that has been associated with weight gain).

For bulimia, antidepressant medications have been used most frequently. The use of antidepressants was initially based upon a theory that bulimia was a variant of affective disorders. This hypothesis has not been strongly supported (Hinz & Williamson, 1987). However, there is considerable evidence documenting the efficacy of antidepressant pharmacotherapy for reducing binging, purging, and depression in bulimia nervosa (Agras, Dorian, Kirkley, Arnow, & Bachman, 1987; Hughes, Wells, Cunningham, & Ilstrup, 1986; Pope, Hudson, Jonas, & Yurgelin-Todd, 1983; Walsh, Gladis, Roose, Stewart, & Glassman, 1984).

Other drugs also have been used in treating bulimia because of their effects on proposed etiological factors. Examples of these include phenytoin (based on the conceptualization of bulimia as a seizurelike disorder), fenfluramine (used for its effects on serotonin and carbohydrate cravings), and opiod antagonists (used to inhibit eating proposed to be induced by endorphins). To date, however, outcome research with these drugs in bulimia nervosa has been minimal.

BEHAVIORAL TREATMENT OUTCOME RESEARCH

Earlier behavioral interventions for anorexia nervosa typically employed operant techniques to promote rapid weight gain. Generally, these studies were conducted in a hospital environment where eating behavior and/or weight gain could be reinforced using activities and relief from bed rest. These earlier efforts typically utilized single-case experimental designs and generally showed that short-term weight gain could be accomplished using operant methods (see Bemis, 1987). More recently, however, there has been a growing recognition that for long-term improvement in patients with anorexia nervosa, weight change alone is insufficient (Andersen, Hedlom, & Hubbard, 1983; Garfinkel & Garner, 1982). Most behavioral approaches now combine operant techniques for weight gain with other treatment techniques. These techniques are aimed at altering other common anorexic problems, such as irrational beliefs, body image disturbance, anxiety, poor interpersonal skills, and dysfunctional eating behavior (e.g., Garner, 1986; L. W.

Rosen, 1980; G. R. Smith & Medlik, 1983). However, systematic investigations of the effects of disparate treatment approaches on long-term outcome have not been conducted.

The treatment outcome literature pertaining to behavioral interventions for bulimia has focused on either exposure with response prevention (ERP) or a combination of exposure therapy with various forms of cognitive and/or interpersonal skills therapy (i.e., cognitive-behavioral therapy). Most of this research has involved treating bulimics on an outpatient basis.

Overall, the evidence for the efficacy of ERP in the treatment of bulimia nervosa has been positive. Initial investigations (Leitenberg, Gross, Peterson, & Rosen, 1984; J. C. Rosen & Leitenberg, 1982) found 2 of 6 subjects to be abstinent from vomiting at the end of treatment with a third achieving abstinence during follow-up. Vomiting was significantly reduced in two subjects and only one subject failed to evidence improvement. Giles, Young, and Young (1985) treated 34 bulimics with ERP and cognitive restructuring (CR) and achieved a 50% decrease in vomiting in 65% of these patients. Further, long-term follow-up found 63% of the improved patients to be abstinent from vomiting.

A majority of the studies attempting to examine the differential effectiveness of cognitive and behavioral components have not found the two to differ (Garner, Fairburn, & Davis, 1987). However, in comparing a CR treatment condition to that of ERP with CR, Wilson, Kleifield, & Lindholm (1986) found that the bulimia nervosa patients who received the combined treatment (i.e., ERP and CR) also evidenced significantly greater improvements in their eating disorder symptomatology. A recent controlled investigation conducted by Leitenberg, Rosen, Gross, Nudelman, and Vara (1988) indicated that ERP produced equivalent improvements to that of a cognitive therapy condition on most dependent measures, with evidence of slightly greater reductions in vomiting behavior for the ERP condition.

In general, current research suggests that the combination of cognitive and behavior therapy techniques is very effective in reducing eating disorder symptomatology when compared to waiting list control conditions (Lacey, 1983; Lee & Rush, 1986; Wolchik, Weiss, & Katzman, 1986), and as effective or slightly more effective than other forms of therapy to which it has been compared (see Garner *et al.*, 1987).

Only one study of inpatient treatment of bulimia nervosa has been published (Williamson, Prather, Bennett, *et al.*, 1989). This investigation compared inpatient and outpatient cognitive-behavioral therapy in an uncontrolled experiment. It was uncontrolled because subjects were not randomly assigned to treatment conditions. As one might suspect, inpatients were more severely disturbed than outpatients, which obfuscates interpretation of the results. The study found that inpatient treatment resulted in very rapid improvement; however, a tendency to relapse after discharge was noted over a 6-month follow-up. Outpatients, in contrast, steadily improved over the course of 6 months of treatment and follow-up, with resulting levels of improvement commensurate with inpatient treatment at follow-up.

Together, these studies support the use of comprehensive cognitive-behavioral treatment approaches with anorexia and bulimia nervosa. As noted earlier, most anorexics and the more severe cases of bulimia will require inpatient treatment. Available research suggests that this intervention should address (1) weight gain in low-weight patients, (2) improvement of nutritional habits, (3) elimination of purgative habits, (4) modification of irrational beliefs about weight, dieting, and body size, and (5) improvement of other problem areas unique to the patient, such as depression, family dysfunction, or drug/alcohol abuse. Once the patient is discharged from the hospital, a very structured and intense outpatient program should be implemented and gradually faded over the next 6 to 12 months.

SPECIAL PROBLEMS

Denial

Assessment of eating disorders in adolescents is sometimes complicated by the fact that they are often brought to treatment by parents/guardians and not because they recognize a problem. Because the patient is typically placed into treatment under duress, denial of symptomatology during the assessment process often occurs. During assessment, the patient may minimize or negate any report of affective distress regarding weight gain or eating normal amounts of food. School problems (e.g., grades, social interactions, conduct), family problems, or the presence of accompanying psychopathology may be similarly minimized. If self-monitoring is a component of the assessment process, records may be repeatedly "lost" or "forgotten." Self-report inventories may suggest a guarded or "fake good" pattern of responding. Parents may be able to clarify conflicting reports of eating habits, but, in many cases, their observations may be biased.

Direct behavioral observation can be very useful in such cases. By utilizing observation of eating behavior, one can assess amount of food eaten, anxiety to eating, and foods which are avoided. Utilization of these test meals can often give a more accurate appraisal of the patient's true eating habits. It has been our experience that patients with a strong fear of weight gain cannot easily disguise their avoidance of forbidden foods when purging is prevented. Therefore, careful analysis of which foods are selected, which are eaten, and so forth can provide invaluable information when eating problems are denied. A pattern of avoidance of forbidden foods is usually a valid behavioral sign of anorexia and bulimia nervosa and can usually be used to break the patients' denial.

Resistance to Treatment

When the patient begins treatment, fear of eating and weight gain may lead to a great deal of resistance to the treatment process. This may be expressed by the patient through making "low-calorie" food choices, eating only small portions of the meals, and refusing to select and eat certain forbidden foods. Hiding or disposing of foods which are feared is also common. The patient may make consistent and multiple requests to go to the bathroom after eating a meal, or may attempt to "slip away" in hopes of being able to purge. When the anorexic or bulimic who acknowledges few problems of eating is asked to engage in normalized eating, changes in affect are readily apparent. Exaggerated anger regarding "being watched all the time," unit rules, or being "forced" to eat "unreasonable" amounts of food are common.

With continued resistance to eating, several interventions may be utilized. Nutritional supplements have proven to be useful when the patient consistently does not meet his or her prescribed meal plan. For example, if the patient is only consuming 50% of a 1,500-calorie meal plan, 750 calories are provided via nutritional supplements to make up the difference. Response cost for noncompliance/reinforcement of compliance will often facilitate cooperation. A patient may comply with the prescribed treatment to obtain certain privileges (e.g., phone use) or to avoid certain contingencies (e.g., time-out). Increased caloric intake can be shaped over time so that the fear of weight gain can be challenged gradually. To illustrate, the meal plan of an anorexic patient may begin at 1,000 calories; it may then be increased by the dietician 200 calories every 1 to 2 days until a caloric level producing consistent weight gain is achieved. If shaping, nutritional supplements, and reinforcement contingencies fail to produce weight gain, then tube or intravenous feeding must be initiated.

It is advisable to have strict observation of all bulimics and anorexics, especially after eating. If the patient begins to engage in binge-eating or purgative behaviors, closer observation, direct confrontation of the behaviors, or removal of privileges should be used to facilitate compliance with the treatment regimen.

The resistant patient will often attempt to turn staff against one another, or obtain conflicting recommendations in order to delay or neutralize certain interventions. Regular staffings, both formal and informal, direct confrontation of the patient's behavior, and removal of privileges/reinforcement for cooperation can be used to modify this form of staff "splitting." This type of patient typically will test staff with a period of compliance followed by a period of resistance. If staff are aware of this possibility, resistance can be quickly and consistently dealt with and normal behavioral treatment approaches can be utilized efficaciously. Failure to directly challenge these attempted manipulations can appreciably undermine intervention efforts and result in failure or unnecessary lengthening of the treatment process.

CASE HISTORY

Gail was a 14-year-old girl who was referred for treatment by her pediatrician. At the time of referral, she weighed 65 pounds at a height of 4 feet, 11 inches. Using charts plotting normal weights for heights in children and adolescents, Gail was approximately 28% below expected normal weight. She had lost 20 pounds over the past 8 months and medical evaluations were unable to determine a physical basis for the weight loss. Interviews with Gail and her parents revealed that over the past year she had gradually stopped eating. When she was between 10 to 12 years of age, her parents reported that while she was not overweight, she was a little "pudgy." Her mother was obese and constantly dieted. She remembered frequently warning Gail that she must control her eating so that she would not be fat. About a year ago, Gail began to diet and jog. She began to lose weight, which was praised by her parents, especially her mother. In the previous 6 months, she became very preoccupied with her weight and began even more restrictive dieting. When concern was expressed about her thinness and failure to eat, she said that she just was not hungry or did not like the food.

Comprehensive assessment of her eating habits and other problems indicated a classic profile of anorexia nervosa. Gail was, by history, very perfectionistic and achievement oriented. She was closest to her mother, who reinforced her perfectionism. She was very neat, even showing obsessive-compulsive cleaning habits and she was an exceptionally good student.

Gail was hospitalized immediately upon referral. The initial goals of treatment were refeeding and weight gain. Caloric intake was increased from 500 kcal/day to 3,000 kcal/day over the first three weeks of intervention. All meals and snacks were planned in conjunction with a clinical dietician. She ate all meals with other patients diagnosed with eating disorders. A member of the eating disorders treatment team ate with the patients to supervise and observe their eating. All food consumed was recorded and caloric intake was computed on a daily basis. Privileges on the unit were made contingent upon meeting prescribed caloric intake goals. Over the course of 10 weeks, Gail gained 17 pounds (i.e., to 82 pounds).

In addition to the refeeding process, Gail participated in cognitive-behavioral therapy conducted in an individual and group format. She attended school for 3 hours per day (in the hospital) and participated in about 15 hours of family therapy and unit activities per week. Eating disorder therapy totalled about 20 hours per week. This treatment was directed at improving eating habits, reducing fears of weight gain, and modifying cognitive problems (e.g., body image disturbances and irrational beliefs concerning weight gain).

After 10 weeks of hospitalization, Gail was discharged to intensive outpatient therapy. She attended group therapy for eating disorder problems four times per week during the first month. These groups continued the treatment initiated in the hospital. Over the next 6 months, the frequency of group therapy was reduced to bimonthly. During this period, she gained a few more pounds and weighed 87 pounds at the time of discharge. She has been followed for several years and her progress has been maintained. At last contact she weighed 105 pounds at a height of 5 feet, 3 inches. She expressed only modest concern about her body size. Further, Gail was still a good student and was becoming a very good tennis player. She seldom jogged anymore.

PROCESS MODEL OF TREATMENT

Our experience has shown that most cases of anorexia nervosa and severe cases of bulimia nervosa will require inpatient treatment followed by intensive outpatient therapy. The process model of treatment shown in Figure 1 summarizes how this behavioral treatment can be administered. We have found that the first step of treatment is careful-assessment which leads to diagnosis, case formulation, and a treatment plan. Resistance to treatment and/or denial should be addressed at this time. In some cases, resolution of these problems may require one or more weeks of inpatient treatment.

The next four steps of treatment involve directly modifying eating and purgative habits. We have found that during the initial period of

	Step 1 Pretreatment	Steps 2–5 Behavior therapy	Steps 6 and 7 Cognitive therapy	Step 8 Family therapy
Targets of treatment	1. Diagnosis 2. Case formulation 3. Modify denial and resistance	1. Purgative habits 2. Restrictive eating 3. Binge eating 4. Eating 3 meals/day 5. Normalization of weight 6. Eat forbidden foods	1. Irrational beliefs 2. Body image disturbances	1. Communication 2. Conflict 3. Sabotage
Treatment interventions	Behavioral assessment and family consultation	1. Meal planning 2. Behavioral contracting 3. Exposure with response prevention 4. Temptation exposure with response prevention	1. Cognitive therapy 2. Body image therapy	Family therapy

Figure 1. A process model for behavioral treatment of anorexia and bulimia nervosa.

treatment, behavior change is much easier to attain than is cognitive change. The first goals of treatment should be to eliminate purgative habits and/or restrictive eating. We choose to modify these behaviors first because they directly contribute to weight loss, which is potentially dangerous, and are the most obvious behavioral manifestations of fears of fatness. In cases where binge eating is a severe problem, TERP may be initiated to weaken urges to binge. For bulimic patients, the next goals of treatment are eating three meals per day and reaching a normalization of weight. For persons diagnosed with anorexia nervosa, caloric intake must be increased to produce steady weight gain of 1 to 2 pounds per week. Some bulimic patients may be placed on a 1,200 to 1,400 calorie/day meal plan to allow a *very gradual* weight loss. Once the patient is capable of consistently eating the prescribed meal plan without purging, forbidden foods should be systematically introduced into the meal plan. Forbidden foods can be introduced using an anxiety hierarchy such that the least feared foods are eaten first, followed by foods which produce more anxiety. This process is best administered within the framework of exposure with response prevention and under the supervision of a trained therapist.

As a function of eating larger amounts and types of foods without purging, the anorexic and bulimic patient must directly face fears of fatness. Thus, the process of exposure to feared foods with prevention of purgative habits and restrictive eating arouses the patient's fears and irrational beliefs concerning weight, dieting, and so forth. The behavioral treatment methods, therefore, set the stage for more direct cognitive therapy for these irrational beliefs. For this reason, there is considerable overlap between administration of behavioral and cognitive components of therapy. Challenging these irrational beliefs is the first step of cognitive therapy and is a process which must be continued into outpatient therapy. Body image disturbances are usually most prominent after several weeks of inpatient treatment (i.e., after weight gain has begun and forbidden foods are being consumed on a regular basis). Body image therapy must begin in earnest at this time and continue into outpatient therapy. Similarly, family therapy can begin during hospitalization, but must be continued as outpatient therapy proceeds.

Finally, the patient should be discharged to intensive long-term outpatient behavior therapy. At a minimum, this outpatient treatment should include exposure therapy, meal planning, behavioral contracting, cognitive therapy, and body image therapy. Initially, the patient must be seen from two to four times per week. Some cases may require discharge to partial hospitalization before formal outpatient care can proceed. Over the course of 6 to 12 months, the frequency of outpatient contact may be reduced to once per week or less. Many cases may require some therapeutic contact for several more years.

SUMMARY

Inpatient treatment of anorexia and bulimia nervosa, using behavioral treatment strategies, is now beyond the nascent stage. This chapter summarized the basic assessment and treatment approaches which have been developed. Although many of these strategies were developed using outpatient populations, we have found that they can easily be applied to inpatients as well. In the final section, a process model of treatment was presented to provide a framework for the integration of inpatient and outpatient treatment using cognitive-behavioral techniques.

REFERENCES

Agras, W. S., Dorian, B., Kirkley, B. G., Arnow, B., & Bachman, J. (1987). Imipramine in the treatment of bulimia: A double blind control study. *International Journal of Eating Disorders, 6,* 29–38.

American Psychiatric Association. (1987). *Diagnostic and statistical manual of mental disorders* (3rd ed., rev.). Washington, DC: Author.

Andersen, A. E., Hedblom, J. E., & Hubbard, F. A. (1983). A multidisciplinary team treatment for patients with anorexia nervosa and their families. *International Journal of Eating Disorders, 2,* 181–192.

Anderson, A. E., Morse, C. L., & Santmyer, K. S. (1985). Inpatient treatment for anorexia nervosa. In D. M. Garner & P. E. Garfinkel (Eds.), *Handbook of psychotherapy for anorexia nervosa and bulimia* (pp. 311–343). New York: Guilford Press.

Askevold, F. (1975). Measuring body image: Preliminary report on a new method. *Psychotherapy and Psychosomatics, 26,* 71–77.

Bemis, K. M. (1987). The present status of operant conditioning for the treatment of anorexia nervosa. *Behavior Modification, 11,* 432–463.

Butters, J. W., & Cash, T. F. (1987). Cognitive-behavioral treatment of women's body-image satisfaction: A controlled outcome study. *Journal of Consulting and Clinical Psychology, 55,* 889–897.

Cash, T. F., & Brown, T. A. (1987). Body image in anorexia nervosa and bulimia nervosa: A review of the literature. *Behavior Modification, 11,* 487–521.

Cooper, Z., & Fairburn, C. G. (1987). The Eating Disorder Examination: A semi-structured interview for the assessment of the specific psychopathology of eating disorders. *International Journal of Eating Disorders, 6,* 1–8.

Davis, C. J., Williamson, D. A., Goreczny, A. J., & Bennett, S. M. (1989). Body image disturbances and bulimia nervosa: An empirical analysis of recent revisions of DSM-III. *Journal of Psychopathology and Behavioral Assessment, 11,* 61–69.

Freeman, R. J., Thomas, C. D., Solyom, L., & Miles, J. E. (1983). Body image disturbances in anorexia nervosa: A reexamination and a new technique. In P. L. Darby, P. E. Garfinkel, D. M. Garner, & D. V. Coscina (Eds.), *Anorexia nervosa: Recent developments in research* (pp. 117–127). New York: Alan R. Liss.

Freeman, R. J., Thomas, C. D., Solyom, L., & Koopman, R. F. (1985). Clinical and personality correlates of body size overestimation in anorexia nervosa and bulimia nervosa. *International Journal of Eating Disorders, 4,* 439–456.

Garfinkel, P. E., & Garner, D. M. (1982). *Anorexia nervosa: A multidimensional perspective.* New York: Brunner/Mazel.

Garfinkel, P. E., Moldofsky, H., & Garner, D. M. (1979). The stability of perpetual disturbance in anorexia nervosa. *Psychological Medicine, 9,* 703–708.

Garner, D. M. (1986). Cognitive therapy for anorexia nervosa. In K. D. Brownell & J. P. Foreyt (Eds.), *Handbook of eating disorders* (pp. 301–327). New York: Basic Books.

Garner, D. M., & Garfinkel, P. E. (1979). The Eating Attitudes Test: An index of the symptoms of anorexia nervosa. *Psychological Medicine, 9,* 273–279.

Garner, D. M., & Olmsted, M. P. (1984). *Manual for Eating Attitudes Test (EDI).* Odessa, FL: Psychological Assessment Resources.

Garner, D. M., Fairburn, C. G., & Davis, R. (1987). Cognitive-behavioral treatment of bulimia nervosa: A critical appraisal. *Behavior Modification, 11,* 398–431.

Giles, T. R., Young, R. R., & Young, D. E. (1985). Case studies and clinical replication series: Behavioral treatment of severe bulimia. *Behavior Therapy, 16,* 393–405.

Hawkins, R. C., & Clement, P. F. (1980). Development and contrast validation of a self-report measure of binge eating tendencies. *Addictive Behaviors, 5,* 219–226.

Hinz, L. D., & Williamson, D. A. (1987). Bulimia and depression: A review of the affective variant hypothesis. *Psychological Bulletin, 102,* 150–158.

Hughes, P. L., Wells, L. A., Cunningham, C. J., & Ilstrup, D. M. (1986). Treating bulimia with desipramine: A placebo-controlled double-blind study. *Archives of General Psychiatry, 43,* 182–186.

Humphrey, L. L. (1986). Family relations in bulimic-anorexic and non-distressed families. *International Journal of Eating Disorders, 5,* 223–232.

Johnson. W. G., Corrigan, S. A., & Mayo, L. L. (1987). Innovative treatment approaches to bulimia nervosa. *Behavior Modification, 11,* 373–388.

Kog, E., & Vandereycken, W. (1985). Family characteristics of anorexia nervosa and bulimia nervosa: A review of the research literature. *Clinical Psychology Review, 5,* 159–180.

Lacey, J. H. (1983). Bulimia nervosa, binge eating and psychogenic vomiting: A controlled treatment study and long-term outcome. *British Medical Journal, 286,* 1609–1613.

Lee, N. F., & Rush, A. J. (1986). Cognitive-behavioral group therapy for bulimia. *International Journal of Eating Disorders, 5,* 599–615.

Leitenberg, H., Gross, J., Peterson, J., & Rosen, J. C. (1984). Analysis of an anxiety model and the process of change during exposure plus response prevention treatment of bulimia nervosa. *Behavior Therapy, 15,* 3–20.

Leitenberg, H., Rosen, J. C., Gross, J., Nudelman, S., & Vara, L. S. (1988). Exposure plus response prevention treatment of bulimia nervosa. *Journal of Consulting and Clinical Psychology, 56,* 535–541.

Minuchin, S., Rosman, B., & Baker, L. (1978). *Psychosomatic families: Anorexia nervosa in context.* Cambridge: Harvard University Press.

Moos, R. H., & Moos, B. S. (1980). *Family environment scale.* Palo Alto: Consulting Psychologist Press.

Palmer, R., Christie, M., Cordle, C., Davies, D., & Kendrick, J. (1987). The Clinical Eating

Disorder Rating Instrument (CEDRI): A preliminary description. *International Journal of Eating Disorders, 6,* 9–16.
Pope, H. G., Hudson, J. L., Jonas, J. M., & Yurgelin-Todd, D. (1983). Treatment of bulimia with imipramine: A double-blind placebo-controlled trial. *American Journal of Psychiatry, 14,* 554–558.
Pyle, R. L., Mitchell, J. E., & Eckert, E. D. (1981). Bulimia: A report of 34 cases. *Journal of Clinical Psychiatry, 92,* 60–64.
Reitman, E. E., & Cleveland, S. E. (1964). Changes in body image following sensory deprivation in schizophrenia and control groups. *Journal of Abnormal and Social Psychology, 68,* 168–176.
Rockwell, W. J. K., Ellingwood, E. H., Dougherty, G. G., & Brodie, H. K. H. (1982). Anorexia nervosa: Review of current treatment practices. *Southern Medical Journal, 75,* 1101–1107.
Root, M. P. P., Fallon, P., & Friedrich, W. N. (1986). *Bulimia: A systems approach to treatment.* New York: W. W. Norton.
Rosen, J. C., & Leitenberg, H. (1982). Bulimia nervosa: Treatment with exposure and response prevention. *Behavior Therapy, 13,* 117–124.
Rosen, J. C., Saltzberg, E., & Srebnik, D. (1989). Cognitive behavior therapy for negative body image. *Behavior Therapy, 20,* 393–404.
Rosen, L. W. (1980). Modification of secretive or ritualized eating behavior in anorexia nervosa. *Journal of Behavior Therapy and Experimental Psychiatry, 11,* 101–104.
Ruff, G. A., & Barrios, B. A. (1986). Realistic assessment of body image. *Behavioral Assessment, 8,* 237–251.
Ruggiero, L., Williamson, D. A., Davis, C. J., Schlundt, D. G., & Carey, M. P. (1988). Forbidden food survey: Measure of bulimic's anticipated emotional reactions to specific foods. *Addictive Behaviors, 13,* 267–274.
Russell, G. F. M. (1979). Bulimia nervosa: An ominous variant of anorexia nervosa. *Psychological Medicine, 9,* 429–498.
Sargent, J., Leibman, R., & Silver, M. (1985). Family therapy for anorexia nervosa. In D. M. Garner & P. E. Garfinkel (Eds.), *Handbook of psychotherapy for anorexia nervosa and bulimia* (pp. 257–279). New York: Guilford Press.
Schlundt, D. G., & Johnson, W. G. (1990). *Assessment and treatment of anorexia and bulimia nervosa.* Needham Heights, MA: Allyn & Bacon.
Schlundt, D. G., Johnson, W. G., & Jarrell, M. P. (1985). A naturalistic functional analysis of eating behavior in bulimia and obesity. *Advances in Behaviour Research and Therapy, 7,* 149–162.
Schwartz, R. C., Barrett, M. J., & Saba, G. (1985). Family therapy for bulimia. In D. M. Garner & P. E. Garfinkel (Eds.), *Handbook of psychotherapy for anorexia nervosa and bulimia* (pp. 257–279). New York: Guilford Press.
Slade, P. D., & Russell, G. F. M. (1973). Awareness of body dimensions in anorexia nervosa: Cross-sectional and longitudinal studies. *Psychological Medicine, 3,* 188–199.
Smith, G. R., & Medlik, L. (1983). Modification of binge eating in anorexia nervosa: A single case report. *Behavioral Psychotherapy, 11,* 249–256.
Smith, M. C., & Thelen, M. H. (1984). Development and validation of a test for bulimia. *Journal of Consulting and Clinical Psychology, 52,* 863–872.
Strober, M., & Humphrey, L. L. (1987). Familiar contributions to the etiology and course of anorexia nervosa and bulimia. *Journal of Consulting and Clinical Psychology, 55,* 654–659.
Touyz, S. W., Beaumont, P. J. V., Collins, J. K., McCabe, M., & Jupp, J. (1984). Body shape perception and its disturbance in anorexia nervosa. *British Journal of Psychiatry, 144,* 167–171.

Vandereycken, W. (1987). The constructive family approach to eating disorders: Critical remarks of the use of family therapy in anorexia and bulimia nervosa. *International Journal of Eating Disorders, 6,* 455–467.

Walsh, B. T., Gladis, M., Roose, S. P., Stewart, J. H., & Glassman, A. H. (1984). A controlled trial of phenelzine in bulimia. *Psychopharmacology Bulletin, 23,* 49–51.

Williamson, D. A., Kelley, M. L., Davis, C. J., Ruggiero, L., & Blouin, D. C. (1985). Psychopathology of eating disorders: A controlled comparison of bulimic, obese, and normal subjects. *Journal of Consulting and Clinical Psychology, 53,* 161–166.

Williamson, D. A., Kelley, M. L., Davis, C. J., Ruggiero, L., & Veitia, M. C. (1985). The psychophysiology of bulimia. *Advances in Behaviour Research and Therapy, 7,* 163–172.

Williamson, D. A., Goreczny, A. J., & Duchmann, E. G. (1987). Behavioral and psychophysiological assessment of bulimia. *Annals of Behavioral Medicine, 9,* 8–11.

Williamson, D. A., Kelley, M. L., Cavell, T. A., & Prather, R. C. (1987). Eating and eliminating disorders. In C. L. Frame & J. L. Matson (Eds.), *Handbook of assessment in childhood psychopathology: Applied issues in differential diagnosis and treatment evaluation* (pp. 461–487). New York: Plenum Press.

Williamson, D. A., Prather, R. C., Upton, L., Davis, C. J., Ruggiero, L., & Van Buren, D. (1987). Severity of bulimia: Relationship with depression and other psychopathology. *International Journal of Eating Disorders, 6,* 39–47.

Williamson, D. A., Davis, C. J., Goreczny, A. J., Bennett, S. M., & Watkins, P. C. (1989). The Eating Questionnaire—Revised: A new symptom checklist for bulimia. In P. A. Keller (Ed.), *Innovations in clinical practice: A sourcebook* (pp. 321–326). Sarasota, FL: Professional Resource Exchange.

Williamson, D. A., Davis, C. J., Goreczny, T. A., & Blouin, D. C. (1989). Body image disturbances and bulimia nervosa: Influences of actual body size. *Journal of Abnormal Psychology, 98,* 97–99.

Williamson, D. A., Prather, R. C., Bennett, S. M., Davis, C. J., Watkins, P. C., & Grenier, C. (1989). Uncontrolled evaluation of inpatient and outpatient cognitive-behavior therapy for bulimia nervosa. *Behavior Modification, 13,* 340–360.

Williamson, D. A., Davis, C. J., Duchmann, E. G., McKenzie, S. M., & Watkins, P. C. (1990). *Assessment of eating disorders.* New York: Pergamon Press.

Wilson, G. T., Rossiter, E., Kleifield, E. I., & Lindholm, L. (1986). Cognitive-behavioral treatment of bulimia nervosa: A controlled evaluation. *Behaviour Research and Therapy, 24,* 277–288.

Wolchik, S. A., Weiss, L., & Katzman, M. A. (1986). An empirically validated, short-term psychoeducational group treatment program for bulimia. *International Journal of Eating Disorders, 5,* 21–34.

IV
Special Topics

13

Child Abuse

CHRIS BRADEN AND VINCENT B. VAN HASSELT

INTRODUCTION

Child abuse is a complex problem involving society, the community, and the family. In our social system, children historically have been viewed as the property of their parents, who have the right to punish their children as they see fit (Kempe, Silverman, Steele, Droegemueller, & Silver, 1962). This perspective changed in 1962, when Kempe coined the term "the battered child syndrome" (Kempe & Helfer, 1972). From 1963 to 1968, all states passed laws which required reporting, investigating, and protecting children who were abused (Radbill, 1968). In 1974, the National Child Abuse Prevention and Treatment Act was passed. However, it is only in the past few years that the seriousness and scope of the problem have been fully realized. Indeed, data from more recent nationwide surveys have underscored the magnitude of the problem. For example, there are indications that between 10 and 16 children out of every 1,000 in the United States are abused and/or neglected annually (National Center on Child Abuse and Neglect, 1988). And reports of incidents have risen dramatically across most states.

CHRIS BRADEN • Department of Psychiatry and Human Behavior, University of California, Irvine Medical Center, Orange, California 92668. VINCENT B. VAN HASSELT • Center for Psychological Studies, Nova University, Fort Lauderdale, Florida 33314.

Inpatient Behavior Therapy for Children and Adolescents, edited by Vincent B. Van Hasselt and David J. Kolko. Plenum Press, New York, 1992.

The majority (86.8%) of child abuse is committed by either parents or parent substitutes, and more often by a maternal than a paternal figure (Gil, 1970). However, when there is a male residing in the home, the abusive adult is slightly more likely to be male than female. In only 5% of cases are both parents found to be abusive (B. Justice & Justice, 1975). Also, abusive families have been found to rate high on indices of social readjustment and transition, with excessive changes in family relationships, employment, financial status, and multiple moves (B. Justice & Justice, 1975). Such events promote continual life crises, allowing little opportunity to adapt and creating a state of chronic exhaustion in families.

Interestingly, abusing parents are rarely characterized by major mental illness. Only 2% of abusing parents are psychotic (Lascari, 1972) and about 10% of abusing parents have been described as exhibiting evidence of severe personality disorder (Filippi, 1979). However, abusing parents have evinced certain personality characteristics, such as poor self-image, extreme dependency needs, and social isolation with minimal support from the extended family or extrafamilial contacts.

Further, a personal history of being a victim of abuse, single-parent status, unemployment, and substance abuse by parents are factors that predict abuse by adults. Several characteristics of children also have been implicated in child abuse and neglect. Some of these include: hyperactivity, noncompliance, prematurity, whiny or "colicky" children, and multiple-handicapping conditions (see Ammerman, Cassisi, Hersen, & Van Hasselt, 1986; Ammerman, Van Hasselt, & Hersen, 1988).

Stresses common to abusing families are a high rate of unemployment (especially among fathers) (Light, 1973), frequent moves (85% of abusing parents moved within the last year) (B. Justice & Justice, 1975), financial difficulties (Solomon, 1973), and lack of education (B. Justice & Justice, 1975).

With regard to etiology, most behavioral formulations of child maltreatment consider the problem as multifactorial and complex. According to Ammerman (1990), "there are multiple pathways to maltreatment that combine and interact in nonlinear ways. No single causative factor has emerged" (p. 249). Lutzker (1984) articulated a particularly comprehensive "ecobehavioral" perspective on child abuse and neglect. From this viewpoint, the difficulties in families that precipitate maltreatment involve multifaceted issues, such as poverty, anger, stress control deficits, poor parenting practices, skill deficiencies in children, inadequate home safety, lack of cleanliness, inadequate nutrition, and health risk factors. Consequently, successful behavioral intervention requires a simultaneous focus on these disparate issues.

The purpose of this chapter is to present behavioral strategies that are relevant to assessment and treatment in inpatient settings of abused children. Most behavioral research in this area has been conducted in laboratory or outpatient therapy counseling contexts. However, the problem of child maltreatment has become increasingly relevant in acute treatment centers. Indeed, there are indications that a disproportionately high number of inpatient child and adolescent admissions have a history of some form of maltreatment. For example, Ammerman *et al.* (1988) found evidence of abuse in nearly 40% of psychiatrically hospitalized multihandicapped children. Similarly, Van Hasselt, Ammerman, Glancy, and Bukstein (1991) reported that approximately 60% of inpatient adolescent substance abusers had been subjected to some form of child maltreatment at some point in their lives. These data suggest the need for attention to this problem as a major element of acute care.

After a section on medical evaluation, we will present relevant information on behavioral assessment methods used in cases of child maltreatment. Then, the primary behavioral intervention approaches that have been developed and implemented by behavioral researchers over the past decade will be briefly reviewed. This will be followed by case descriptions illustrating the utilization of behavioral treatment of child abuse in an inpatient setting. Finally, suggestions for directions that future work in this area might take are offered.

ASSESSMENT

Medical Assessment

Physicians, mental health professionals, teachers, nurses, and other professionals working with children must now, by law, be alert to cases of child abuse. Any unexplained injury is cause for suspicion of physical abuse. When the possible explanation that has been offered cannot likely account for the injury, physical abuse also should be considered. When parents delay in obtaining medical attention for an injury, physical abuse should be suspected.

Bruises characteristic of physical abuse include grab marks of finger and thumb prints on a child's arms, choke marks on a child's neck, slap marks, lash marks from beatings, loop marks from cord or rope, strap marks, belt buckle marks, human bite marks, and bruising of the frontal dental ridge, upper lip, and frenulum from forceful feeding. Burns characteristic of physical abuse include cigarette burns and heating appliance burns with their distinctive shapes, dunking burns which include buttocks and possibly thighs and waist but spare hands and feet of the child, and burns from forced immersion of extremities. The latter are characterized by extension of the burns above the wrist or ankle of the child. Traumatic hair loss from yanking of the child's hair is indicated by damaged hairs broken off at different lengths and a normal-appearing scalp, or by bruising or a hematoma in the area of yanking. Retinal hemorrhages without a fracture or bruise of the scalp indicate abuse by forceful shaking of the child.

Subdural hematomas are often fatal or result in serious deficits. Subdural hematomas may result from a blow to the head that causes bruising or swelling of the scalp and a skull fracture. However, subdural hematomas may also result from forceful shaking of the child, with no skull fracture or bruising or swelling of the scalp. Often, grab mark bruises are evident on the arms, shoulders, or thorax. Retinal hemorrhages are almost always evident upon examination. Infants frequently are brought in with seizures, coma, and increased intracranial pressure.

Intra-abdominal trauma, most commonly a ruptured spleen or liver, is another common cause of fatality in abused children. These children are often brought in with repeated vomiting, a distended abdomen, tenderness, or shock. Usually, there are no bruises because of the flexibility of the abdominal wall.

Xray findings of numerous fractures at various stages of healing are evidence of physical abuse. Single metaphyseal chip fractures are also indicative of physical abuse. In children under 5 years of age, the fracture frequently is no longer evident on physical examination within a week following the trauma. Thus, Xrays of the skull, thorax, and long bones should be taken in all children under 5 years who are suspected of being abuse victims. If these show fractures, then Xrays of the pelvis and spine are also needed. In children older than 5 years, fractures are evident on physical examination by findings of bone tenderness, bruising and swelling, limitation of range of motion, and lack of spontaneous motion. If the Xrays are negative following a positive physical exam, they should be repeated in 2 weeks when calcification may confirm the presence of a healing fracture. Bone injuries occur in 10% to 20% of children who are physically abused.

If the parents relate a history of the child's bruising easily, then the child should be evaluated for a bleeding disorder. Bone changes in scurvy and syphilis are symmetrical as opposed to asymmetrical findings from physical abuse. Pathologic fractures in children do not involve the metaphysis as do fractures secondary to abuse.

Behavioral Assessment

Assessing child abuse and neglect is not possible with the standardized devices that are used in intelligence testing or in personality assessment and diagnosis. There are certain environmental variables (e.g., poverty) and adult and child characteristics that predict these problems. Also, direct observation of parent–child interactions, conditions of safety and cleanliness, and the amount of community/social support all warrant attention (Lutzker, 1984; Wahler, 1980). Further, substance abuse by parents, a history of being a victim of abuse, single-parent status, and unemployment are additional factors that predict abuse by adults (see Ammerman & Hersen, 1990). As mentioned, several characteristics of children also appear to predict child abuse and neglect, including multiple-handicapping conditions, whiny or colicky children, hyperactivity, noncompliance, and prematurity (see Ammerman *et al.*, 1986). It has been observed that two behavioral extremes often suggest that a child has been maltreated: (1) extreme social withdrawal or (2) extreme attachment and dependence on nonfamilial adults.

Self-report. A number of self-report and interview strategies have been employed. For example, Hally *et al.* (1980) designed the Childhood Level of Living Scale as a method of scaling critical elements of child care and neglect. This measure focuses on parents of children 4 to 7 years of age. It contains 99 items which encompass nine factors: four of these factors are descriptive of emotional/cognitive (psychological) care, and five are descriptive of physical care.

Milner (1986) developed the Child Abuse Potential Inventory (CAPI) to detect at-risk status of children. The CAPI includes three validity scales (Lie, Random Responding, Inconsistency) and an Abuse Potential scale. This instrument has been employed primarily as a screening tool, although psychometric properties (e.g., convergent and predictive validity, reliability) have been established (Kaufman & Walker, 1986; Milner, 1986).

To obtain reliable parental reports of child maltreatment, Ammerman *et al.* (1988) constructed the Child Abuse and Neglect Interview Schedule (CANIS). This semistructured interview is employed to determine the presence of maltreatment behaviors (e.g., corporal punishment) and factors associated with abuse, such as history of maltreatment. Although originally developed for families of disabled children, this 45-minute interview can be utilized with families of nondisabled children as well.

Indices of anger and arousal levels also have been used in recent child abuse research. Most notable is the Novaco Anger Control Scale (NACS) (Novaco, 1975) that can be administered to ascertain anger control problems that parents may be experiencing. The NACS contains brief descriptions of situations involving provocation (e.g., "You are talking to someone and they do not answer you") in which the respondent endorses the degree of anger he or she would experience if that event should occur. A five-point scale of arousal level is used for scoring each of the items comprising this instrument. Similarly, the MacMillan-Olson-Hansen Anger Control Scale (MOHAC) was specifically designed to evaluate anger experienced by maltreating parents in response to child misbehaviors (MacMillan, Olson, & Hansen, 1988a). The MOHAC asks parents to rate 50 child-related situations (e.g., throws food, refuses to go to bed) as problematic or nonproblematic. Each item is also rated as to the degree of anger evoked in each situation via a 5-point scale. The utility of this measure in determining treatment outcome for anger control interventions has been demonstrated (MacMillan *et al.*, 1988a).

Twentyman, Plotkin, Dodge, and Rohrbeck (1981) developed the Parent Opinion Questionnaire (POQ) to provide a measure of the appropriateness of parental expectations of a wide range of child behaviors. This 80-item measure yields a total score and six subscales: self-care, leaving children alone, proper behavior and feelings, punishment, family responsibility and care of siblings, and help and affection to parents. The POQ has been shown to discriminate between abusive and neglectful mothers from control mothers (Azar, Robinson, Hekimian, & Twentyman, 1984) and abusive from control mothers with abusive partners (Azar & Rohrbeck, 1986).

Another assessment focus of behavioral clinicians and researchers is problem-solving skills in abusive families. To examine ability in this area, Wasik, Bryant, and Fishbein (1980) (cited in Azar *et al.* 1984) developed the Parent Problem-Solving Instrument (PPSI). The PPSI contains 10 "childbearing problem situations" and follows a means–end problem-solving approach. Responses on this device are scored on the following dimensions: number of items on which relevant solutions are provided, total number of means given, number of items on which multiple means are given, number of means on which elaboration occurred, and total number of content categories that were employed. The

PPSI has been found to differentiate groups of abusive/neglectful mothers from normal mothers (Azar *et al.*, 1984).

Problem-solving skill also has been examined using the Parental Problem-Solving Measure (PPSM) (Hansen, Pallotta, Tishelman, Conaway, & MacMillan, 1989). The PPSM classifies problem situations into five domains: (1) anger and stress control, (2) interpersonal problems, (3) child behavior and management, (4) financial, and (5) child-care resources. Responses to this 25-item instrument are rated for number and effectiveness of solutions generated.

Direct Observation. In a more direct observational approach to assessment of child abuse and child management, MacMillan *et al.* (1988a) developed the Home Simulation Assessment. This strategy utilizes an adult actor to present deviant child behavior and assesses the parent's child management skills in realistic problem situations. The assessment entails providing the parent with 10 tasks (e.g., dry the dishes) and asking him or her to do his or her best at prompting the actor to complete the tasks. The actor displays deviant scripted responses to each of four types of control or parental discipline efforts, including prediscipline warnings, instructions, initiation of time-out, and maintenance of time-out. Actors' behaviors are under the control of a clinician who observes the interaction behind a one-way mirror and listens with a bug-in-the-ear. To ascertain parental skill, the percentage of parent's correct instructions and responses to the disparate deviant and compliant actor behaviors are calculated.

The High-Deviance Home Simulation Assessment (HDHSA) (MacMillan, Olson, & Hansen, 1988b) is an adaptation of the aforementioned approach which focused on relatively low-demand situations. Used to examine anger and stress responses to child behaviors, the HDHSA introduces higher levels of child demand and deviance by means of an additional child actor and increased rates of deviant actor responses. Responses to child deviance in the 10 tasks used with the earlier measure are coded. In addition, parent ratings of stress, anger, and anxiety are obtained.

TREATMENT

The major behavioral intervention strategies for child-abusing families have included parent training and behavior management, stress reduction, and multiple-component treatments. Most illustrative of the former approach is the systematic program of research conducted by David Wolfe and his colleagues (e.g., Wolfe, 1987; Wolfe & Sandler, 1981; Wolfe, Sandler, & Kaufman, 1981; Wolfe *et al.*, 1982) at the University of Western Ontario over the past decade. In an early single-case study, Wolfe *et al.* (1982) employed the "bug-in-the-ear" device to give feedback in parent training sessions to a mother with a history of aversive behaviors toward her three children. During parent–child interactions, the mother was provided with prompts and feedback in order to diminish rates of hostile verbal statements and physical gestures. As part of this procedure, the mother was trained (via instructions, prompting, and feedback) to increase her frequency of positive parenting behaviors (hugs, praise, pats). Results indicated a substantial reduction in negative parent behaviors and increased positive responses with training. In addition, gains were maintained in clinic and home settings at a 2-month follow-up evaluation.

Wolfe and Sandler (1981) expanded on the previous effort by training three abusive mothers in parent effectiveness strategies and contingency contracting. In the parent training component, readings on child management techniques and instructions in problem-solving approaches were provided. Contingency contracting involved the delivery of reinforcers to parents contingent on the application of certain child management programs (e.g., token reinforcement). Results revealed that the combined interventions led to sharp reductions in maladaptive parent–child interactions. Gains were still evident at a 1-year follow-up.

In an examination of the utility of a group treatment format, Wolfe *et al.* (1981) used a tripartite behavioral intervention consisting of (1) child management training—problem-solving and modeling of appropriate child management approaches; (2) stress management and anger control training—deep muscle relaxation, reinforcing self-statements; and (3) developmental education—films and readings in human development and child management. Training and behavior rehearsal in the home setting also was carried out. This combined approach was effective in improving parenting skills as assessed by direct observations in the home and by parental and caseworker reports. Especially noteworthy was the finding that no episodes of child abuse occurred among treated families over a 1-year follow-up period.

Egan (1983) examined the differential effectiveness of the behavioral strategies employed by Wolfe *et al.* (1981). In this investigation, stress management, child management training, and waiting list control conditions were compared. Application to abusive parents resulted in improved parental feelings for those receiving stress management while those involved in child management training developed enhanced parenting skills.

John Lutzker and his colleagues (e.g., Lutzker, 1990; Lutzker & Van Hasselt, in press; Lutzker, Frame, & Rice, 1982; Lutzker, Wesch, & Rice, 1984) have been the major proponents of "ecobehavioral" approaches to the remediation of child abuse and neglect. From this perspective, child maltreatment is viewed as a multifaceted problem requiring multifaceted and comprehensive behavioral assessment and intervention. A major emphasis is on the implementation of treatment procedures directly in the setting where problems are occurring (in the home, community, day care, or foster home sites). However, a number of the targeted problem areas and remedial procedures have potential value in the child inpatient setting as well.

Illustrative is a report by Campbell, O'Brien, Bickett, and Lutzker (1983) who used relaxation training to reduce migraine headaches in a mother who was concerned that she might kill her noncompliant 4-year-old daughter if she did not obtain relief and assistance. After headache frequency decreased, parent training was initiated and led to increased child compliance. Marital counseling was then provided which improved marital satisfaction.

In another study, Dachman, Halasz, Bickett, and Lutzker (1984) trained a neglectful mother of a 4-year-old boy to use descriptive praise and discrete, simple commands during structured, unstructured, and academic sessions with her son. Observational data revealed that as praise and appropriate commands by the mother increased, child compliance also improved. Further, maternal criticisms of the child, which occurred at high rates during baseline, decreased to near zero levels following treatment.

Affective parent–child interactions were assessed in two abusive families in an investigation by Lutzker, Megson, Webb, and Dachman (1985). Here, parents who lacked affect when dealing with their children were taught a variety of interactive skills (e.g., voice intonation, passive touch, talking with their children at their eye level) to remediate this deficit. Affect training for parents resulted in increased positive child behaviors and high rates of compliance. Interestingly, findings indicated improvement not only in skills parents were taught with "target" children, but with those children's siblings with whom parents had not been trained. Lutzker, Touchette, and Campbell (1988) contended that affect training is more natural and perhaps more effective in the long-run than more traditional behavior management strategies.

John Fantuzzo and his associates at the University of Pennsylvania conducted three investigations that attempted to determine the efficacy of behavioral interventions for abused children. Each of the studies targeted economically disadvantaged preschoolers with serious social dysfunction. The treatment strategies employed in this series of studies were adapted from peer-mediated methods developed by Strain and his colleagues to increase rates of social interactions of socially isolated preschoolers (e.g., Odom & Strain, 1984).

In the first of these investigations, Fantuzzo, Stovall, Schachtel, Goins, and Hall (1987) examined the impact and generalization of a peer-mediated intervention with four preschool children with a history of neglect. As in previous peer-mediated approaches, two maltreated children with high-baseline rates of appropriate social behavior were trained to initiate positive play activities with withdrawn children during free-play periods. Results of a reversal design indicated that targeted children showed significant increases in prosocial interactions for the withdrawn children as a function of the behavioral intervention.

The second effort (Fantuzzo *et al.*, 1988) compared peer and adult social initiation strategies across multiple areas of functioning. Thirty-six maltreated children (victims of neglect) were randomly assigned to peer-treatment, adult-treatment, or control conditions. As in the first investigations, high functioning maltreated peers were trained to initiate prosocial interactions during play periods. The adult-treatment condition was similar except that an adult initiated play activities with maltreated children. Results indicated that children in the peer-treatment condition displayed significantly increased rates of positive social behavior. Children with adult interventionists exhibited a significant decrease in social behavior after treatment. Standardized tests and measures of developmental level, however, revealed that all subjects improved on these indices over the course of the study.

In the third investigation, Davis and Fantuzzo (1989) replicated the findings of the second study by exposing withdrawn, neglected and withdrawn, and nonneglected preschool children to comparable peer- and adult-mediated interventions. In addition, the efficacy of these interventions was examined with physically abused preschoolers who were overly aggressive. Direct observational data were obtained on social behavior of two withdrawn, nonmaltreated subjects; two withddrawn, neglected subjects;and three aggressive, abused subjects. A particularly innovative feature of this report was the collection of data on a nonwithdrawn, nonmaltreated subject during baseline to serve as a comparison for purposes of social validity analysis.

In this alternating treatment design, a play session with a peer confederate was alternated with a play session with an adult confederate. In baseline and follow-up periods, confederates responded positively to play initiations of subjects but made no initiations themselves. Davis and Fantuzzo (1989) reported the following pattern of results: (1) withdrawn, nonmaltreated children displayed equal levels of interaction with peer and adult initiators; (2) withdrawn, neglected children demonstrated a clear preference for interaction with peers over adults; (3) peer initiations led to increased rates of reciprocal play behavior; however, adult initiations resulted in brief positive responses and no social initiations; and (4) the aggressive, abused children responded differentially to the peer and adult initiator and, overall, did not respond favorably to the initiation intervention.

Case History

Sam was an 11-year-old boy who had been living with his mother, Cynthia, and Pete, her boyfriend, in a two-bedroom apartment in a large metropolitan area. Both Sam and Cynthia described Sam's depression as beginning 2 years prior and gradually escalating to the point that during the past year, Sam had attempted suicide on several occasions. Specifically, Sam had tried to drown himself by tying a pool chair to his leg and jumping into the deep water. However, upon experiencing the discomfort of not being able to breathe, he eventually released himself. Frequently, Sam would hold his breath, thinking this would cause his death. The day prior to his admission to the child psychiatry inpatient unit, Sam attempted to suffocate himself by tying a trash bag over his head; however, he panicked when he could not breathe and tore a hole in the bag.

Sam complained of feeling very lonely and of having few friends, which he attributed to his obesity. Sam had gained 50 pounds over a 2-month period so that at a height of 5 feet 1 inch, he weighed 184 pounds. At the same time, Sam related that food no longer tasted good, although his thoughts were often preoccupied with food. Sam had lost his interest in usual childhood activities and had become even more isolated and withdrawn from both children and adults. He would frequently react to any frustration by becoming physically aggressive toward himself with suicide attempts or by hitting his head with wooden spoons and pans, screaming that he wanted to die. At other times, aggression (hitting and kicking) was directed toward his mother. Sam had frequent crying spells and related feelings of hopelessness. Often, he spoke of not wanting to grow up and of hating his life. In school, Sam complained that nobody liked him. His teachers were frustrated, being unable to motivate Sam to turn in any work, thus receiving D's and F's, even though Sam appeared to know the material. He often "tuned out" his teachers during much of the school day. Since kindergarten, Sam had been socially immature and withdrawn from his peers, but for the past 2 years he had become even more isolated and restricted his play to solitary activities.

Cynthia's pregnancy with Sam was planned and she delivered at term but with forceps. Cynthia breast-fed Sam until he was 6 months old when, on her doctor's advice, she "starved him into taking the bottle" because of "bad breast milk." At 8 months, Sam's feeding was again changed to a soybean formula. Sam was a colicky, sickly infant with frequent diarrhea. Cynthia described him as an overly active child with frequent temper tantrums. Cynthia and John, Sam's father, had frequent disagreements on how to raise and manage their son. When Sam was 6 months old, Cynthia's younger teenage brother and sister moved in with them, but were incorrigible and did not get along with John, adding further stress to the family situation. Cynthia's siblings were later placed in group homes. When Sam was 3 years old, Cynthia began considering divorce; when Sam was 4 years old, Cynthia and John separated. Sam had very little contact with his father after the separation.

Cynthia and Sam then moved to live with Cynthia's father. Together Cynthia and her father ran a small business. When Sam was 5 years old, he was repeated sexually abused by a friend of his cousin. When Sam was 8 years old, Cynthia moved to Arizona with Paul, her live-in boyfriend of 4 years, to begin another business. This venture soon failed, and the relationship was overwhelmed due to the financial stress. When Sam was 9, Cynthia and Paul began couples therapy. It was during this time that Sam's depression began. Within 6 months, Cynthia left Paul, who had been a father to Sam for 5 years, and she and Sam moved again. Cynthia then became involved with Pete, another live-in boyfriend, and there was considerable conflict in this relationship. Pete and Sam did not get along and Pete physically abused Sam, hitting him on the arms and legs and leaving characteristic hand print and belt buckle bruises. Pete and Cynthia argued frequently and Pete had recently destroyed their television during one of his angry rages. Approximately 1 month preceding Sam's hospitalization, Pete attempted to rape Cynthia in front of Sam. Cynthia was in the process of separating from Pete at the time of Sam's hospital admission. Cynthia had at times sought therapy for her own depression.

Cynthia first took Sam to an outpatient Child Guidance Clinic during the peak of her conflicts with Paul, to whom Sam was quite attached. Sam was seen in weekly individual therapy and biweekly group therapy until the time of his hospitalization. At the Child Guidance Clinic, the physical abuse by Pete was reported to local Child Protection Services.

At the onset of his inpatient admission, Sam presented as an obese, sloppily dressed, and very depressed, soft-spoken boy. His affect was both constricted and restricted. Psychomotor retardation was evident. Sam depicted himself as a passive, helpless victim, who was harassed by others. He was preoccupied with fears of rejection and abandonment by his mother.

With staff, Sam, although very needy, was often noncompliant in response to their requests and directions, but did respond to positive reinforcement in the form of attention. Initially, Sam was very withdrawn and isolative with other children. He was very easily frustrated and would respond either by further withdrawal or by provoking and controlling peers. Sam would also threaten and strike out aggressively at his peers, alienating the other children. However, Sam would then blame his peers' rejection of himself on his being overweight. Sam had great difficulty expressing his feelings directly and frequently changed the focus to food.

The unit schoolteacher also noted Sam's low frustration tolerance. Although he completed his assignments in response to positive reinforcement, his work generally was sloppy. A sixth grader, Sam scored at the twelfth-grade reading level on the Woodcock Johnson test, but he was unable to read beyond the sixth-grade level in the actual classroom. Throughout his schooling, Sam had difficulties in math and attended a resource classroom for this subject as well as private tutoring. Sam scored in the fourth-grade level in math on the Woodcock Johnson.

Both Sam and his mother were involved in family therapy twice a week with the unit social worker. Cynthia, who described herself as depressed and shy, was advised to again resume her own individual therapy which had been helpful in the past. Throughout the hospitalization Sam was also involved 3–4 times a week in psychodynamic psychotherapy with a child psychiatry fellow. A multiple-component behavioral intervention was developed to target the various deficits identified in Sam during the evaluation phase of his admission. First, as mentioned above, Sam had a number of deficiencies falling under the rubric of social skills. Specifically, he was passive, withdrawn, isolative, and displayed difficulty in making new friends and in initiating or maintaining conversations. In addition, it was apparent that he had considerable difficulty expressing positive or negative feelings. Therefore, part of his treatment regimen involved participation in a daily social skills group on the unit. The focus of the unit was on the development of interpersonal skills requisite to adequate socialization. Targeted skills included: friendship making, conversational skills, positive assertion (expressing praise and appreciation), negative assertion (standing up for one's rights, denying unreasonable requests, adapting refusal behaviors in high-risk situations), identifying the feelings and emotions of others (i.e., role-taking and social perception skills), and being socially reinforcing toward others.

Second, to increase compliance with unit rules and to decrease aggression toward peers, Sam participated in the unit-wide level system. This traditional token economy program consisted of the administration of generalized conditioned reinforcers (stars and points) that were redeemable for special reinforces (e.g., toys, treats) or activities (e.g., outings, playing games with staff) at the end of each day. In addition, Sam and his mother participated in the unit's behaviorally oriented, weekly parent training group. The purpose of this intervention was to provide parents with the child management skills needed to control their children's misbehavior. Topics covered were: positive reinforcement strategies, punishment and time-out, extinction/ignoring, contingency management, behavioral contracting, and problem-solving skills. Parent training consisted of four 2-hour evening sessions each week over the course of the inpatient stay. In each session, some time was spent in having parents practice their newly acquired skills and techniques with the child under the supervision of the group leader.

Further, in an effort to reduce his weight, Sam and his mother met with the unit nutritionist who provided dietary suggestions and menus to facilitate better and restricted eating habits. Also, Sam was provided with a self-monitoring form on which to record food intake. He was reinforced (stars applied to daily totals) for adhering to his diet and accurately monitoring his food intake. Sam also participated in ongoing educational and occupation therapy programs that were administered to all children on the unit.

Initially, Sam was on suicide precautions; and although his suicidal thoughts greatly subsided in response to the intensive therapies, his other depressive symptoms responded only minimally during the initial 3 weeks of hospitalization. Therefore, a trial of desipramine was instituted and gradually titrated up to 150 mg. Sam tolerated the antidepressant well, and his EKGs remained normal with each increment in dosage.

From the fourth week onward, Sam made steady improvement and was more energetic and involved in his therapies. His treatment team noted a gradual lifting of his depression and a brightening of his affect. Sam's interactions with the teacher and other children on the unit improved, and his work reflected his enhanced self-esteem; he readily completed assignments. In occupational therapy, Sam began to show enthusiasm for his projects and required less assistance. His organization and frustration tolerance also improved. On the unit, Sam's social skills and play skills matured to age level. Concurrently, his aggression and provoking of his peers greatly subsided. Sam also lost 12 pounds during his admission. Food became less of a focus as did his weight, and Sam was able to begin to accept greater responsibility for his own behavior.

After 9 weeks of hospitalization, Sam and his mother had progressed to the point that continued intensive outpatient therapy with the Child Guidance Clinic was recommended. In addition to the individual and group therapies Sam had received, continuation of the behavioral program and the antidepressant was recommended. Cynthia was also advised to continue her own individual therapy as well as participate in family therapy and parent training with Sam at the Child Guidance Clinic.

SUMMARY AND CONCLUSIONS

Epidemiologic and survey research over the past several years has provided a convergence of empirical evidence attesting to the alarmingly high magnitude of child maltreatment. Such findings have served as the impetus for accelerated clinical and investigative efforts in the area. Behavioral researchers, in particular, have directed increased attention to the problems of child abuse and neglect. In this chapter, we reviewed a number of behavioral assessment and treatment strategies that have been utilized in recent approaches to the problem. Assessment strategies have included a variety of self-report and structured interview techniques, and, more recently, direct observational methods.

A wide range of behavioral treatment procedures also have been developed and implemented, including parent training, contingency contracting, stress management, relaxation training, anger control training, and peer-mediated interventions. Preliminary data regarding the effectiveness of these approaches generally have been positive. Unfortunately, there is a modicum of information concerning the application of such intervention methods in inpatient settings. To date most of the work in this area has been carried out in the laboratory or in outpatient settings. The case study that we described here, however, illustrated the potential heuristic value of utilizing such methods in the psychiatric inpatient setting. In light of the growing awareness and prevalence of maltreatment in children who present in psychiatric hospitals (Ammerman *et al.*, 1988; Van Hasselt *et al.*, 1991), there is an urgent need for services directed specifically to this problem.

REFERENCES

Ammerman, R. T. (1990). Etiological models of child maltreatment. *Behavior Modification, 14*, 230–254.

Ammerman, R. T., & Hersen, M. (Eds.). (1990). *Children at risk: An evaluation of factors contributing to child abuse and neglect*. New York: Plenum Press.

Ammerman, R. T., Cassisi, J. E., Hersen, M., & Van Hasselt, V. B. (1986). Consequences of physical abuse and neglect in children. *Clinical Psychology Review, 6*, 291–310.

Ammerman, R. T., Van Hasselt, V. B., & Hersen, M. (1988). Maltreatment of handicapped children: A critical review. *Journal of Family Violence, 3*, 53–73.

Azar, S. T., & Rohrbeck, C. A. (1986). Child abuse and unrealistic expectations: Further validation of the parent opinion questionnaire. *Journal of Consulting and Clinical Psychology, 54*, 867–868.

Azar, S. T., Robinson, D. R., Hekimian, E., & Twentyman, C. T. (1984). Unrealistic expectations and problem-solving ability in maltreating and comparison mothers. *Journal of Consulting and Clinical Psychology, 52*, 687–691.

Burns, R. (1973). as quoted in V. J. Fontant, *Somewhere a Child is Crying*, New York, Macmillan, 1973.

Campbell, R. V., O'Brien, S., Bickett, A., & Lutzker, J. R. (1983). In-home parent-training, treatment of migraine headaches, and marital counseling as an ecobehavioral approach to prevent child abuse. *Journal of Behavior Therapy and Experimental Psychiatry, 14,* 147–154.

Dachman, R. S., Halasz, M. M., Bickett, A. D., & Lutzker, J. R. (1984). A home-based ecobehavioral parent-training and generalization package with a neglectful mother. *Education and Treatment of Children, 7,* 183–202.

Davis, S., & Fantuzzo, J. W. (1989). The effects of adult and peer social initiations on social behavior of withdrawn and aggressive maltreated preschool children. *Journal of Family Violence, 4,* 227–248.

Egan, K. (1983). Stress management and child management with abusive parents. *Journal of Clinical Child Psychology, 12,* 292–299.

Fantuzzo, J. W., Stovall, A., Schachtel, D., Goins, C., & Hall, R. (1987). The effects of peer social initiations on the social behavior of withdrawn maltreated preschool children. *Journal of Behavior Therapy and Experimental Psychiatry, 18,* 357–363.

Fantuzzo, J. W., Jurecic, L., Stovall, A., Hightower, A. D., Goins, C., & Schachtel, D. (1988). Effects of adult and peer social initiations on the social behavior of withdrawn, maltreated preschool children. *Journal of Consulting and Clinical Psychology, 56,* 34–39.

Filippi, R. K. (1979). Child abuse. In B. N. Irving & S. A. Lawrence (Eds.), *Basic handbook of child psychiatry,* Vol. IV, pp. 364–374. New York: Basic Books.

Gil, D. G. (1970). *Violence against children.* Cambridge: Harvard University Press.

Hally, C., Polansky, N. F., & Polansky, N. A. (1980). *Child neglect: Mobilizing services* (DHHS Publication No. OHDS 80-30257). Washington, DC: U.S. Government Printing Office.

Hansen, D. J., Pallotta, G. M., Tishelman, A. C., Conaway, L. P., & MacMillan, V. M. (1989). Parental problem-solving skills and child behavior problems: A comparison of physically abusive, neglectful, clinic, and community families. *Journal of Family Violence, 4,* 353–368.

Justice, B., & Justice, R. (1975). *The abusing family.* New York: Human Sciences Press.

Kaufman, K. L., & Walker, C. E. (1986). Review of the Child Abuse Potential Inventory. In J. D. Keyser & R. C. Sweetland (eds.), *Test critiques* (Vol. 6, pp. 55–64). Kansas City, MO: Westport.

Kempe, C. H., & Helfer, R. E. (Eds.). (1972). *Helping the battered child and his family.* Philadelphia: Lippincott.

Kempe, C. H., Silverman, E. N., Steele, B. E., Droegemueller, W., & Silver, H. K. (1962). The battered-child syndrome. *Journal of the American Medical Association, 181,* 105–112.

Lascari, A. (1972). The abused child. *Journal of Iowa Medical Society, 62,* 229–232.

Light, R.J. (1973). Abused and neglected children in America: A study of alternative policies. *Harvard Educational Review, 143,* 559.

Lutzker, J. R. (1984). Project 12-Ways: Treating child abuse and neglect from an ecobehavioral perspective. In R. F. Dangel and R. A. P. Polster (Eds.). *Parent training: Foundations of research and practice* (pp. 260–291). New York: Guilford Press.

Lutzker, J. R. (1990). Behavioral treatment of child neglect. *Behavior Modification, 14,* 301–315.

Lutzker, J. R., Frame, R. E., & Rice, J. M. (1982). Project 12-Ways: An ecobehavioral approach to the treatment and prevention of child abuse and neglect. *Education and Treatment of Children, 5,* 141–155.

Lutzker, J. R., Wesch, D., & Rice, J. M. (1984). A review of Project 12-Ways: An ecobehavioral approach to the treatment and prevention of child abuse and neglect. *Advances in Behaviour Research and Therapy, 6,* 63–73.

Lutzker, J. R., Megson, D. A., Webb, M. E., & Dachman, R. S. (1985). Validating and training adult-child interaction skills to professionals and to parents indicted for child abuse and neglect. *Journal of Child and Adolescent Psychotherapy, 2,* 91–104.

Lutzker, J. R. Touchette, P. E., & Campbell, R. V. (1988). Parental positive reinforcement might make a difference: A rejoinder to Forehand. *Child and Family Behavior Therapy, 10,* 25–33.

MacMillan, V. N., Olson, R. L., & Hansen, D. J. (1988a, November). *Low and high stress analogue assessment of parent training/stress minimization package with physically abusive parents.* Paper presented at the meeting of the Association for the Advancement of Behavior Therapy, New York.

MacMillan, V. N., Olson, R. L., & Hansen, D. J. (1988b, November). *The development of an anger inventory for use with maltreating parents.* Paper presented at the meeting for the Association for the Advancement of Behavior Therapy, New York.

Milner, J. S. (1986). *The Child Abuse Potential Inventory: Manual* (2nd ed.). Webster, NC: Psytec.

National Center on Child Abuse and Neglect. (1988). *Study of national incidence and prevalence of child abuse and neglect: 1988* (Contract No. 105-85-1701). Washington, DC: U.S. Department of Health and Human Services.

Novaco, R. W. (1975). *Anger control: The development and evaluation of an experimental treatment.* Lexington, MA: Lexington Books.

Odom, S. L., & Strain, P. S. (1984). Peer-mediated approaches to promoting children's social interactions: A review. *American Journal of Orthopsychiatry, 54,* 545–557.

Radbill, S. X. (1968). A history of child abuse and infanticide. In R. E. Helfer & C. H. Kempe (Eds.), *The battered child.* Chicago: University of Chicago Press.

Solomon, T. (1973) History and demography of child abuse. *Pediatrics, 51,* 775.

Twentyman, C. T., Plotkin, R., Dodge, D., & Rohrbeck, C. A. (1981, November). *Inappropriate expectations of parents who maltreat their children: Initial descriptive survey and cross-validation.* Paper presented at the Association for the Advancement of Behavior Therapy Convention, Toronto.

Van Hasselt, V. B., Ammerman, R. T., Glancy, L. J., & Bukstein, O. G. (1991). *Maltreatment in psychiatrically hospitalized dually diagnosed adolescent substance abusers.* Unpublished manuscript, University of Pittsburgh School of Medicine.

Wahler, R. G. (1980). The insular mother: Her problems in parent-child treatment. *Journal of Applied Behavior Analysis, 13,* 207–219.

Wolfe, D. (1987). Child abuse. In R. T. Ammerman & M. Hersen (Eds.), *Treatment of Family Violence.* New York: Wiley.

Wolfe, D., & Sandler, J. (1981). Training abusive parents in effective child management. *Behavior Modification, 5,* 320–335.

Wolfe, D., Sandler, J., & Kaufman, K. (1981). A competency-based parent training program for child abuser. *Journal of Consulting and Clinical Psychology, 49,* 633–640.

Zalba, S. (1971). Battered children. *Trans-Action, 8,* 61.

14

Academic and Educational Aspects

LINDA L. LOAR

INTRODUCTION

Until the 1960s, there was little acknowledgment of the educational rights of children and adolescents with social and emotional problems to an appropriate academic program. Before this time, students with such problems were systematically excluded from educational programs and were denied the right to procedural due process. Eventually, student's rights were established in several important legal decisions. In 1967, the *In re* Gault case was heard before the U.S. Supreme Court and the rights of minors to due process procedure, which is guaranteed by the Fourteenth Amendment, were acknowledged. In 1968, Hewett introduced strategies for teaching school-aged children with social and emotional problems. In 1970, publications from the Joint Commission on Mental Health of Children reported the need to reorganize the mental health treatment offered to children with a major emphasis on the area of prevention (Kessler, 1988). In 1975, with the passage of the Education for All Handicapped Children Act (Public Law 94-142), all students who were labeled *emotionally disturbed* were guaranteed a free, appropriate, and public education and all related services.

LINDA L. LOAR • Association for Children and Adults with Learning Disabilities, 4900 Girard Road, Pittsburgh, Pennsylvania 15227.

Inpatient Behavior Therapy for Children and Adolescents, edited by Vincent B. Van Hasselt and David J. Kolko. Plenum Press, New York, 1992.

The regulations of Public Law 94-142 define the category known as *seriously emotionally disturbed* (SED) as:

> 1) An inability to learn which cannot be explained by intellectual, sensory, or health factors; 2) an inability to build or maintain satisfactory interpersonal relationships with peers and teachers; 3) inappropriate types of behavior or feelings under normal circumstances; 4) a general pervasive mood of unhappiness or depression; or 5) a tendency to develop physical symptoms or fears associated with personal or school problems. (34 Code of Federal Regulations 121.a.5(8))

This regulation also noted that the student exhibits these characteristics "over a long period of time and to a marked degree which adversely affects educational performance (34 Code of Federal Regulations 121.95(8))." It also noted that the term *seriously emotionally disturbed* did not include children who were socially maladjusted unless they were also classified as seriously emotionally disturbed.

The purpose of this definition of seriously emotionally disturbed was to assist in determining a student's eligibility for special education programs and services (Turnbull, 1986). Unfortunately, however, students labeled *socially maladjusted* were excluded from the definition and, thus, were often denied educational services. In 1984, Congress requested the Secretary of Education to evaluate the need for changes in the category and definition of seriously emotionally disturbed children and the effects that this change would have on the identification and delivery of services to students with emotional and social problems (Turnbull, 1986). In 1985, at the Midwest Symposium of Leadership in Behavior Disorders, educators debated the merits of including socially maladjusted children and adolescents into the definition of handicapped. The educators in favor of inclusion reported that the group labeled socially maladjusted was already included in the services for handicapped students in two thirds of the states and that the definition only needed to be expanded to represent the students already served. The educators against the inclusion noted that the students labeled socially maladjusted demanded assistance from many social agencies and that the educational system would fail with this population because of the unavailability of a meaningful definition, limited skills in offering services, and insufficient funds (Benson, Edwards, Rosell, & White, 1986).

Although educators and researchers continued to discuss the definition of students to be served in the category of seriously emotionally disturbed children, others have attempted to evaluate existing special education programs for students in this classification. Kauffman *et al.*

(1985) reported that the development of appropriate services for this group was hampered by a lack of descriptive evidence of successful programs. In a rare study completed by Grosenick, George, and George (1988), 97% of 192 programs for emotionally/behaviorally disturbed students were noted to have a definition of the populations they served. However, only 37% had descriptions of instructional methods, 33% had evaluation procedures, and 11% noted any involvement of community agencies in their program.

As reported in this brief synopsis of the educational opportunities and rights afforded to youth who are labeled as socially and emotionally disturbed, progress has been achieved since 1960 in refining the definition of the children who are eligible for special education services and the programs offered to these students. In a parallel development, clinicians in child and adolescent psychiatry have refined the behavioral criteria of childhood disorders in an attempt to avoid personal interpretation in the diagnosis of aberrant behaviors (Kessler, 1988). The process of interviewing children and adolescents has become standardized and measures, such as the Interview Schedule for Children (Kovacs, 1985), Kiddie-SADS (Chambers, Puig-Antich, & Tabrizi, 1978), and the Child Behavior Checklist (Achenbach & Edelbrock, 1983), are used extensively to assist clinicians in the diagnosis of disorders in youths. Treatments available to children and families have broadened to include behavioral therapy, social skills training, and cognitive therapy in addition to the more traditional models of play therapy, individual therapy, and family therapies. Another treatment often recommended to serve the needs of these students is special education. When recommended, this treatment should address all the needs of the student and should involve the parents, the educational system, and the mental health program in the community.

The term *special education* reflects the provision of specially designed instruction at no cost to parents or guardians in order to meet the unique needs of a handicapped child. This right to instruction includes teaching that is offered in hospitals and institutions (34 Code of Federal Regulations 300.14). The educational services offered to children and adolescents in inpatient psychiatric settings provide a unique challenge to educators and all members of the treatment team in that they represent educational efforts conducted in a very restrictive setting. The rights of students to a free and appropriate public education in a medical setting demands an interpretation of the Education for All Handicapped Children Act of 1975 in light of available information on social, medical, and psychiatric issues usually unavailable to educators in the public and private school setting.

EDUCATIONAL SETTING

The educational program for children and adolescents with social and emotional disorders in an inpatient setting is unique in that necessary services are available within the hospital setting. In this educational setting, the emphasis is not only on the programming within the hospital setting but also on the coordination of the educational and mental health needs of the student beyond hospitalization.

The inpatient setting increases the responsibilities of the educator who must assume the role of classroom teacher, treatment team member, school liaison, and child advocate. The educator must have a working knowledge of the rights of exceptional students and the present practice of the local educational agency (LEA) and state educational agency (SEA). In addition, the educator must develop the ability to diagnose both the learning and behavioral abilities and disabilities of the student, and then interpret and communicate the student's needs to the treatment team, parents, and home school personnel.

The educator must establish a classroom setting that will facilitate the collection of information vital to the diagnosis, treatment, and dispositional planning for the student. As a treatment team member, the educator must expand his or her usual view of the student to include social, medical, and psychiatric information. The members of the treatment team will often ask the educator to respond to and analyze all information presented on the student. The role of the school liaison with the LEA is the focal point for continuation of educational treatment after hospitalization. From the day of admission, the inclusion of personnel from the student's LEA is necessary to ensure consideration of all treatment needs and the appropriate educational placement in the least restrictive environment. While the student is hospitalized, the educator will assume the role of child advocate. This includes helping the parents or guardians to understand the educational needs of the students and the procedure for ensuring that the LEA safeguards the educational rights of their child.

A child or adolescent is hospitalized because he or she has, by observed or reported behaviors, presented the need for a placement in a restrictive setting. The goal of the hospitalization is to observe and diagnose the student, initiate treatment, and prepare for continued treatment through the family, school, and mental health agency. This chapter will include information on the educational and academic program that should be provided to protect the educational rights of students and ensure the necessary treatment for the student.

EDUCATIONAL PROGRAM

The educators in an inpatient setting should be professionals who are trained in special education with experience in curriculum and behavioral management. The educators must expand their role beyond classroom teaching while operating a classroom that maintains a high standard for behavioral and academic performance by the students.

The role of classroom teacher will be the role most familiar to the educator in an inpatient setting, and the classroom will be an important area for collecting information on and observing the behaviors of the student that is necessary for appropriate placement. The academic planning for the student will be determined by the previous educational placement and/or the age of the student. For clients previously placed in specialized settings for multiply disabled students, the teacher may continue the educational programming with an emphasis on functional living skills. Planning for elementary age students will focus on academic skills appropriate to the grade level, whereas teachers of high school students may request textbooks and lesson plans from the home school to ensure that academic requirements for graduation are fulfilled. For older students who have failed to complete graduation requirements, the educational focus may be on academic skills necessary for the completion of the graduation equivalency diploma.

The types of educational materials used in the classroom will be determined by the developmental level of the students and the length of the hospital stay. Although it is common for classroom teachers to order specific textbooks or reading series for the students, in an inpatient setting it is rarely practical to equip the classroom with this type of material. With students who are developmentally delayed, materials geared toward the instruction of daily living skills would be appropriate for the continued practice and generalization of the Individual Educational Program (IEP) objectives. For students in the elementary and middle schools, consumable workbooks, duplicating materials, computers, and subject-specific software will be cost-efficient and useful in continuing the practice of skills. At this level, it is important to purchase materials for group lessons because this type of instruction allows the students to practice skills necessary for appropriate participation in large-group instruction. At the high school level, as mentioned above, students usually use their own textbooks with lessons planned by the home school teacher. The use of computers in these classrooms will be of assistance for practice of particular skills and for enhancing computer literacy.

Across all settings, the educator must set realistic expectations and goals in light of the length of hospitalization. The IEP for each client should include realistic goals established through assessments and information from the previous educational placement. The IEP should be included in the total treatment plan for the student to ensure compliance to the regulation of parental involvement.

Educational assessments administered to the student may be formal and informal. The formal assessments, including intelligence and achievement testing, should be administered under optional conditions. Accordingly, if a student is being withdrawn from medication or a behavioral and/or medication treatment is to be initiated, the testing should be scheduled for a time and condition which may help in providing the most accurate results. Through liaison with the LEA, the educator will be aware of the achievement tests used most frequently in determining educational placements and will be responsible for recommending the appropriate tests. The psychologist will be responsible for interpreting the tests, completing a written report, and making educational recommendations. The educator may assist the psychologist in making the recommendations by inviting the psychologist to observe the student in the classroom and participate in the educational and treatment teams.

The behavioral management program used in the classroom may be prescribed by the management system of the inpatient setting on which the classrooms operate or may be at the discretion of the educators. If the classroom expectations are included in the general behavioral program, the educators must have a thorough knowledge of all expectations and consequences and must devise a procedure for enacting the consequences immediately after the student exhibits or performs the behavior. The classroom teacher must also communicate daily to the other staff members any consequences which may influence the student's privileges in the living area of the inpatient setting. If the management system of the classroom is unique to the classroom, the educator must establish expectations and consequences which are similar to behavioral expectations in the classrooms of public and private schools.

The classroom expectations should be stated in simple phrases and in a language the students can understand. These expectations should include goals in the areas of completion of academic assignments, appropriate peer and adult interacting, and self-evaluation of the student's behavior. The expectations will need to be reviewed and frequently role-modeled by the teacher. Students should be involved in the role-plays of appropriate behaviors because this will help the teacher assess the student's present ability to perform the behavior. The establishment of these expectations is actually the first phase of the management system of the classroom. Often, the educator must take the next step, instructing the student, following the same steps as academic instruction, in the development of appropriate classroom behaviors. The expectations and consequences, targeting both positive and negative behavior, should be consistent across all classrooms in the inpatient setting and, as with the use of the unit-wide behavioral programming, information as to a student's success should be communicated to all members of the staff.

In both academic and behavioral areas, the teacher will be requested to maintain anecdotal records and/or complete checklists and observation forms on the student's performance. The requested measures will be vital in assessing the effectiveness of the setting and management program, in decreasing problem behaviors, and in promoting positive behaviors. In addition, the response of the students for specialized therapies, such as social skills training, cognitive therapy, and individual therapy, should be documented in order to assess the appropriateness of the treatment. The effect of medication treatment for attention deficits, hyperactivity, seizure disorders, and symptoms of psychosis can be documented through the use of behavioral checklists which are designed for the assessment of these targeted behaviors.

The classroom is a valuable environment for collecting information on the academic and behavioral strengths and weaknesses of the student. The classroom is a setting to which the student will return upon discharge, and all information on the successful behavioral treatment of the student will be of assistance to the receiving school in continuing the treatment initiated in the inpatient setting.

THE TREATMENT TEAM

The treatment team is a group of professionals, chosen or assigned, who are given the responsibility of diagnosing the student, initiating treatment, and preparing the dispositional plan for the client. The teacher represents the educational needs of the student on the treatment team and makes treatment recommendations regarding the dispositional needs of the student. The information presented by the educator will be in three areas: educational history, behaviors exhibited by the student in the classroom, and dispositional plans.

The information on the educational history of the student should include the following: (1) all prior schools the student has attended; (2) any changes in types of service offered; (3) test scores; (4) parental involvement; (5) present academic and behavioral performance; and (6) appropriateness of present placement (see School History Form, Appendix 1). This information should be presented in the correct chronology and in written form that is available to all treatment team members. This school history is especially important to the members of the team as it may be the most reliable source of information available on the child.

The teacher must also report on the academic and behavioral performance of the student while participating in the classroom in the inpatient setting. The teacher must combine information on educational problems obtained from the home school, as well as the problems presented by the parents upon admission. The teacher must assess the strengths and weaknesses of the student as reported by the entire educational staff. The teacher must report on the frequency of the behavior, antecedent events, and both effective and ineffective consequences. In addition, all information from formal checklists and observation forms should be incorporated into the report to the treatment team. The teacher should report all updates on dispositional planning at the treatment team meeting (see Treatment Team Report, Appendix 2). The educator must record the student's progress on the unit, in individual therapy sessions, in group therapy, with medication therapy, and in family sessions, and then inform the other members of the educational team of all changes/updates on the treatment plan.

The treatment team meeting also provides a forum for the educator to inform all members of the treatment team of the educational rights of students and the federal, state, and local regulations regarding the due process procedures. The team may recommend placements that appear to match the present needs of the student, even though this placement may be a violation of the regulations of the least restrictive environment for the student. For example, if a student had participated in regular education before hospitalization and the treatment team members are recommending a change to a full-time special education program, the educator would have to review the cascade of services available for the student and determine if a resource room or part-time program would be more appropriate, balancing the student's right to specialized educational programming and placement in the least restrictive environment. The educator, through knowledge of the educational rights of the students and active participation on the treatment team, will assist all members of the team in becoming informed of the procedure for appropriate educational placements.

As a member of this team, the educator will also be informed of procedures, policies, and statutes of mental health/mental retardation agencies, outpatient clinics, and child protective services. These agencies will be responsible, in conjunction with the home school, for continuation of treatment and protection of the student. The educator should participate in all meetings with these agencies in order to provide a cohesive plan for dispositional treatment.

The treatment team is responsible for analyzing and adapting the treatment plan for the student and is the center for information exchange. The academic and educational needs of the students will be discussed and decided by all members of the team and within the parameters of the rights and services available to the student.

SCHOOL LIAISON

The inpatient hospital is a service unfamiliar to most educators in the community. It is imperative for the educator in the psychiatric hospital to initiate and maintain contact with the personnel of the student's LEA in order to facilitate appropriate educational dispositional planning. By involving the home school personnel in the treatment plan from the day of admission, these professionals will be able to have a complete and unique understanding of the student's educational needs.

The LEA and/or home school should be notified by letter and/or phone of the admission of the student to the inpatient setting. The staff of the inpatient school must address and be knowledgeable of the attendance policies of the system and establish a policy within the inpatient setting for monitoring the status of the student. Some inpatient settings operate a certified academic school within the setting whereas others may offer homebound instruction or a school operated by the local education agency. Each type of program may involve slight variations of the procedures, but all programs will need to maintain liaison with the LEA to protect the student's status in the educational program (see Educational Liaison Form, Appendix 3). In addition to attendance, the LEA should be notified of the proposed length of the hospitalization, programs offered by the hospital, and dates of the meetings to discuss the treatment for the student and the recommended dispositional plan. Each interaction with the LEA personnel should be recorded to ensure accountability by all personnel and agencies involved in the treatment of the student. Other professionals may be involved in the student's present educational program and it may be necessary to initiate several calls in order to collect all necessary information vital to the treatment of the student. The Educational Liaison Form should be maintained on each student in the program.

The School History Form will be completed by the classroom teacher with facts obtained from the personnel of the LEA. In addition to the historical information, the teacher will need information of the current performances of the student. The teacher will be able to obtain the required information from the principle, teacher, counselor and/or special education director. This information includes the following: type of programming, related services, mainstreaming, academic and behavioral strengths and weaknesses, successful academic and behavioral interventions, attendance, suspensions, and medication treatment. The type of programming may be regular education, regular education with remedial service, special education (full-time, part-time, resource, and itinerant), or special education with related services (speech/language services, occupational/physical therapy, adaptive physical education and/or counseling). The teacher should also request information on the number of students and adults in the classroom and if the program is self-contained or departmentalized. If the student is in special education, the teacher should request information on the date of placement, reason for placement, all related services offered and progress in these services, classes in which the student is mainstreamed, and progress in these classes.

A major part of the discussion with home school personnel should focus on the academic and behavioral strengths and weaknesses and successful behavioral interventions. The teachers should request specific and descriptive information on all problems listed by the home school personnel. For example, if the home school personnel report that the student never does her work, the teacher will need to ask the following questions: "Is the student distractible?" "Does the student become frustrated easily?" "Does the student have academic difficulties?" The gathering of this specific information will provide a foundation for building the educational treatment plan for the student. The teacher should also request information on attendance of the students and any suspensions which have been imposed during the student's school career. The teacher should request the reason for the suspension, length of the suspension, and effectiveness of this consequence (see Home School Information Form, Appendix 4). If the student has had medication treatment for specific behaviors, the teacher should inquire about the name of the medication, length of the treatment, and any changes observed while the student was on medication. It is important to note any communication regarding the medication treatment with the parents and mental health agency and/or treating physicians (see Medication Treatment Form, Appendix 5). By maintaining contact with the home school personnel, the educator will be informed of all possible placements and related services available to the student.

The LEA may request formal documentation and recommendations from the personnel of the inpatient setting. These documents often include educational reports, the psychological report and recommendations, the psychiatric report including diagnoses, treatment, and recommendations, medical reports, speech and language evaluations, and plans for continued treatment upon discharge. All requested reports and recommendations should be sent to the LEA before discharge or presented to the personnel at the dispositional meeting. Although the educational placement of the student may be a priority for the personnel of the inpatient setting, the LEA personnel have many students in need of services. The processing of all requested documentation should be completed in a timely manner.

The liaison with the home school personnel is the link between the local education personnel and the staff of the inpatient setting in regard to the initiation and continuity of educational treatment for the student. Information received from the home school personnel is vital to assist the treatment team in recommending the most appropriate and least restrictive placement for the student.

CHILD ADVOCACY

The inpatient setting is unique in that the parents/guardians of the student will be accessible to the educational staff through appointed meetings with the staff and visits to their child. The presence of the parents/guardians provides an opportunity to inform them of the educational rights of the student in the school system and available supports for them after the student is discharged from the inpatient setting. As noted previously, the treatment team members have the responsibility of gathering a complete medical, social, psychiatric, and educational history of the student. This information will be shared with the parents/guardians through the treatment plan and their meetings with members of the treatment team. The teacher may meet with the family to gather information on the student's educational performance or may receive the information from the social worker assigned to the student. This information will assist the teacher in two ways. First, the information will aid in the interpretation of the educational history and home school performances as reported by the home school personnel. Second, the information reported by the family will assist the members of the treatment team in understanding the parents' knowledge of the rights of the student in the school system.

The education staff members may arrange meetings with the parents through the social worker at a time when there are no competing issues in need of discussion. The teacher should review the student's academic skills that were observed by the educational team and the student's test results (both intelligence and achievement) and then interpret this information for the parents/guardians. The psychologist may be included in this meeting if the test results are complicated or have direct implications on the placement recommendations. The teacher should address the behaviors exhibited by the student in the classroom and explain the ramifications of these behaviors on school performance. If the treatment team members have recommended a change in placement, the justification and procedure to establish the change should be discussed in detail. The teacher should provide written information for the parents/guardians regarding the procedure for placement. In addition to the formal information exchanged, the teacher should provide the parents with the names and phone numbers of the LEA personnel so that the parents/guardians can become involved in the placement change.

The teachers may expand their parental contact beyond the meeting regarding the change of placement by arranging an additional session to inform the parents of the educational rights of the student with regard to appropriate placement, least restrictive environments, mainstreaming, related services, suspensions, and expulsions. The teacher may provide the parents/guardians with names and phone numbers of educational advocacy services to assist them after hospitalization.

The teacher, in the role of school liaison, provides the recommendations for educational placement upon discharge. Follow-up arrangements with the home school personnel and parents/guardians should be a definite part of all dispositional planning. This follow-up arrangement will benefit all members of the dispositional planning team in that it will assist the teacher in evaluating the appropriateness of the recommended placement, assist the home school personnel in assessing their follow-up on all treatment recommendations, and guarantee the parents/guardians support in monitoring the student's progress in the educational program.

SUMMARY

The educational and academic needs of children and adolescents in an inpatient setting present a unique challenge to all members of the treatment team. Through contact with vital information sources—the student, the personnel of the LEA, the parents/guardians, and the inpatient staff—the educator begins to form an ecological view of the needs of the student. The classroom provides an environment for collecting information on the academic and behavioral performance of the student. The treatment team incorporates educational information into a comprehensive treatment plan. Home school personnel provide information on the availability of educational placements and, through their involvement in the hospitalization, become a vital link to treatment continuity. The parents/guardians, through education provided by the treatment team, are made aware of the advocacy necessary to safeguard the educational rights of the student. Each one of these areas is important in and of itself, but educational programming is only complete when all personnel and agencies cooperate in providing the best treatment for each individual student.

APPENDIX 1

School History Form

Academic History

Name: Glenn	Age: 9
Age, Level, and School	Tests/Results/Placement
4, Preschool, Head Start	None
5, Kindergarten, Scott Elementary	Low average on Readiness Test
6, 1st grade, Scott Elementary	Group IQ Testing: 92
7, 1st grade (repeated) Scott Elementary	Referred for formal testing for poor academic performance. WISC-R v. 92, p. 91, fs. 91; WRAT Rd. 1.1, Sp. 1.2, Math 1.6. Referred for reading services.

8, 2nd grade, Scott Elementary	Continued with remedial services. WRAT Rd. 1.13, Sp. 1.3, Math 2.5. Behavior problems reported by teacher and parents.
9, 3rd grade, Scott Elementary	Remedial services were increased. Behavior problems have escalated. Temper tantrums 1 time/day. Several suspensions from school; school social worker referred child to the hospital.

Parent Involvement

Parents have always been involved in the student's education. They are concerned about his academic and behavioral problems and have followed suggestions by school personnel. They were reluctant to hospitalize their son but agreed when the child's behavior escalated.

Appropriateness of Present Placement

Home school personnel are suggesting a placement in a program for children with emotional problems.

APPENDIX 2

Treatment Team Report

Background

Name: ______ Age: __ Grade: __ Educational placement: ____________

Problem List

Home/school	Parents	Hospital
	Problem 1: Inattentiveness	
Fails to complete tasks	Never follows directions	Needs structured environment to remain on tasks; usually on-task 5–7 minutes
Daydreams	Off in a world of his own	Verbal positive reinforcement is motivating to him
Rarely completes homework		Needs directions repeated many times

	Problem 2: Easily Frustrated	
Gives up easily on all assignments	Gets upset while doing his homework	Works well if task is on the "practice" level; new tasks must be introduced slowly with constant support and praise; when this is followed, frustration lessens
	Problem 3: Stealing	
Students report that he frequently takes things and when confronted, says he was just borrowing them	No reported incidents	No reported incidents
	Problem 4: Temper Tantrums	
Able to follow rules of the classroom; needs supervision during recess especially during competitive games	Few friends in the community because he often becomes angry when he does not get his way	Initially tested limits; with introduction, reminders of rules and consequences; he is able to earn all points each day
	Treatment Progress	
Group Therapy	Social Skills Training	Family Sessions
More attentive to group discussion	Using skills, developed friendship with peer	Mild improvement in compliance to instructions

APPENDIX 3

Educational Liaison Form

Background Information

Student's name: ______________________ Age: ______________________

Address: ______________________

Parent/guardian: ______________________

School: ______________________ Grade/program ______________________

Address: ______________________

Principal: ______________________ Phone: ______________________

Teacher: ______________________ Phone: ______________________

Counselor/master teacher: ______________________ Phone: ______________________

Special education director: ______________________ Phone: ______________________

Release of information signed: ____________ Date: ____________
Notification of admission: ____________
Personnel: ____________ Date: ____________
Attendance at meetings: ____________
Personnel: ____________
Date: ____________
Personnel: ____________
Date: ____________
Personnel: ____________
Date: ____________
Dispositional meeting: ____________
Personnel: ____________ Date: ____________

Dispositional Responsibilities

Home/school district	*Inpatient personnel*
____________	____________
____________	____________
____________	____________

Records sent: ____________
Personnel: ____________ Date: ____________

APPENDIX 4

Home School Information Form

Name: ____________ Age: ____________
If regular education: *Programming*
Regular full-time: _____
Regular remedial reading: _____ periods/week: _____
remedial math: _____ periods/week: _____
Self-contained: ____________ Departmentalized: ____________
Adult/student ratio: _____
Number of teachers working with the student: _____
If special education (list periods/day or percentage of the day):
Full-time: ____________ Resource: ____________
Part-time: ____________ Itinerant: ____________
Classification: ____________
Date of placement: ____________
Reason for placement: ____________
____
____
____
Related services provided: ____________
____
____

Is the student mainstreamed? ______
If yes, list mainstream classes: ______

Behavior/academic progress in mainstream: ______

Peer interactions: ______
Adult interactions: ______

Academic functioning (list present levels)

Reading: ______	Science: ______
English: ______	Social Studies: ______
Spelling: ______	______

Behavior functions

Strengths	Weaknesses
______	______
______	______
______	______
______	______

Major behavior problems: ______

Successful behavioral interventions: ______

Attendance: ______
Suspensions: ______

APPENDIX 5

Medication Treatment Form

Medication: ______
Dates of treatment: ______
Length of treatment: ______
Observed/reported response to treatment: ______

Is medication administered at school? ______
Is the student compliant to medication scheduled? ______
Personnel responsible for liaison with mental health agency/treatment physician: ______
Frequency of communication: ______

REFERENCES

Achenbach, T. M., & Edelbrock, C. (1983). *Manual for the Child Behavior Checklist and Revised Child Behavior Profile.* Burlington, VT: University Associates in Psychiatry.

Benson, D., Edwards, L., Rosell, J., & White, M. (1986). Inclusion of socially maladjusted children and youth in the legal definition of the behaviorally disordered population: A debate. *Behavioral Disorder, 9,* 11–17.

Chambers, W., Puig-Antich, J., & Tabrizi, M. A. (1978). *The ongoing development of the Kiddie-SADS* (Schedule for Affective Disorders and Schizophrenia for School Aged Children). Paper presented at the annual meeting of the American Academy of Child Psychiatry, San Diego, California.

Education of All Handicapped Children Act of 1975 and Federal Regulations. Public Law 94-142; 20 U.S.C. §§ 1401–1461.

Grosenick, J. K., George, M. L., & George, M. P. (1988). The availability of program descriptions among programs for seriously emotionally disturbed students. *Behavioral Disorders, 13,* 108–115.

Hewett, E. F. (1968). *The emotionally disturbed child in the classroom: A developmental strategy for educating children with maladaptive behavior.* Boston: Allyn & Bacon.

In re Gault, 387 U.S. 1 (1967).

Joint Commission on Mental Health of Children. (1970). *Crisis in child mental health: Challenge for the 1970's.* New York: Harper & Row.

Kauffman, J. M., Beirne-Smith, M., Eichberg, C. G., Hart-Hester, S., McCullough, L., & Williams, R. (1985). Guidelines for describing programs for behaviorally disordered children and youth. *Journal of Special Education, 9,* 11–17.

Kessler, J. W. (1988). *Psychopathology of childhood.* Englewood Cliffs, NJ: Prentice Hall.

Kovacs, M. (1985). The Interview Schedule for Children. *Psychopharmacology Bulletin, 21,* 991–994.

Turnbull, H. R. (1986). *Free appropriate public education: The law and children with disabilities.* Denver: Love Publishing.

15

Social and Family Work

JACK FUNDANISH

INTRODUCTION

The Joint Commission on Accreditation of Healthcare Organizations (1988) has outlined five standards for inpatient social work services in their *Accreditation Manual for Hospitals*. These standards, accompanied by 25 required characteristics, emphasize the need for readily available social work services to patients and their families, including significant others, that encompass crisis intervention, assessment, treatment, and discharge planning. These services are to be provided by a sufficient number of qualified social work personnel who are responsible to an administrative or medical designee, and are to be implemented in collaboration with appropriate clinical and administrative representatives. Guided by written policies and procedures, the services should be adequately documented in patients' medical records with an emphasis on the need for regular communication among all care providers. These policies and procedures are supposed to be reviewed regularly and, if necessary, revised, and are subject to the hospital's quality assurance programs which provide a systematic process for monitoring and evaluation, as well as a mechanism for problem resolution.

It is clear that a wide range of social work and family services can be

---

JACK FUNDANISH • Attention and Conduct Evaluation Service, Western Psychiatric Institute and Clinic, 3811 O'Hara Street, Pittsburgh, Pennsylvania 15213.

Inpatient Behavior Therapy for Children and Adolescents, edited by Vincent B. Van Hasselt and David J. Kolko. Plenum Press, New York, 1992.

included within these broad parameters. This chapter is not intended to be an exhaustive review of social work methods, nor will it detail all appropriate or necessary social work interventions and treatment with children, adolescents, and their families based upon specific psychosomatic disorders or psychiatric conditions. However, it will examine the changing role of the inpatient social worker and the evolving family and social work issues impacting upon service provision within the context of a child and adolescent psychiatric inpatient setting that is not impervious to volatile economic, political, and social forces.

Overview of Services and Functions

The rapid increase in child psychiatric inpatient services seen in the 1970s continues today and is accompanied by increased specialization as well as economic forces dictating shorter term hospitalizations. Jemerin and Philips (1988) discussed the transformation of child psychiatric units in hospitals from treatment settings similar in concept to traditional residential care into a "modality with specific capabilities and goals not duplicated elsewhere in the service spectrum" (p. 397). Where social workers once had several months to engage families in working alliances and a variety of therapeutic strategies, they now have several weeks or less to assess the family system and implement treatment planning. Interventions are brief and the phases of treatment—engagement, assessment, education, and therapeutic efforts—are, by necessity, blended to accommodate time constraints. Social workers are forced to place increasing emphasis on crisis intervention strategies, short-term problem resolution (often related to issues surrounding the hospitalization itself), and related efforts which focus on stabilizing the family for continued treatment once the child is discharged. Dispositional planning begins even prior to admission. This transformation requires inpatient social workers to function less as therapeutic agents and more as therapeutic liaisons with families and outpatient resources. Unfortunately, this practice coincides with social forces and economic factors that have resulted in overburdened outpatient clinics, greatly diminished residential resources for children, and hastily conceived in-home family services such as have appeared within the past few years. Jemerin and Philips (1988) briefly described and discussed the advent of a "revolving door" for child inpatient hospitalization that is due to the increasingly fragmented community care now provided to children. In this light, inpatient evaluation is too costly a resource to be used as a dispositional catalyst for a system designed to protect the welfare of children that is now floundering because of political and economic forces far removed from family crises. The social services slogan of the 1980s has been "Do More with Less." The slogan for the 1990s may well need to be "Accept Less No More." Inpatient social workers are beginning to feel increasing pressure to advocate for more adequate service provision across the social service spectrum.

Social workers in a child and adolescent inpatient setting are in a unique and challenging position. Their involvement with the child and the family begins prior to hospitalization with intake, screening, orientation, and admission, and proceeds through evaluation, treatment, discharge, and follow-up. Generally, this involvement entails further contact with other systems usually comprised of the patient's extended family, significant others, and community agencies or resources that interface on various, and often disorganized, levels. As indicated by Woolston (1989), "the most pressing current concern for inpatient child psychiatry is the challenge to utilize the enormous mass of information gathered during a child's hospitalization in an expeditious, effective manner" (p. 20). Social workers lead the effort to meet this challenge by functioning as liaisons between these complex systems and the inpatient treatment team of psychiatrists, psychologists, nurses, educators, child care workers, and a host of ancillary professionals. Concomitantly, they are viewed by these systems as a member of this team and, as such, are also responsive to its needs and demands. Therefore, the tasks of focusing and disseminating the flow of information while remaining sensitive to the needs of these sometimes competing systems present an enormous challenge to social workers who must maintain a delicate balance between being a family advocate and a team player.

This role duality need not present a major conflict for the social worker who is functioning in an inpatient setting that focuses on enhancing family integrity and that accepts the premise that viable treatment plans and realistic goals can only be developed and implemented with ongoing family awareness, support, and cooperation. More importantly, what are the overall goals of hospitalization now and what will they be in the coming years? Nurcombe (1989) listed five aims of brief hospitalization which envelop the concept of stabilization and proposed that the purpose of hospitalization is to "stabilize those problems that prevent the child from being treated safely outside the hospital" (p. 27). Engaging family systems and outpatient resources in a working alliance that focuses on continuity of care and realistic planning is the initial task of the social worker and begins at intake (see Appendix).

INTAKE

The first contact with the family or other related systems primarily occurs via a telephone inquiry. These calls originate from a variety of professionals (physicians, therapists, educators, caseworkers, etc.) and occasionally from a concerned family member. Because a large majority of children requiring hospitalization have had at least one prior treatment experience, the contact is usually made by someone who is familiar with the child and the family and who can provide information to determine the necessity and/or expediency of hospitalization.

A successful treatment outcome is based on the attainment of realistic treatment goals that are shared by the family, hospital staff, and other significant outpatient and community resources. The conceptualization of these goals begins with the statement of presenting problems: (1) What does the referral source hope hospitalization will accomplish? (2) Is the family aware of this referral? (3) To what extent is the family involved in the decision to hospitalize the child? and (4) What are the family's expectations in light of the child's prior treatment history and outcome? It is important that these and other issues be explored in order to assess the need for an inpatient evaluation and delineate mutually acceptable goals for hospitalization. At any time during the intake process, the social worker should be prepared to suggest treatment options for those who do not appear to require hospitalization, emergency referrals for those in need of immediate attention, and alternatives for children who fail to meet inclusion criteria, including inadequate financial coverage. A working knowledge of outpatient resources is essential.

Once the intake information sheet is completed, and financial issues are addressed to assure adequate insurance coverage, the information is presented to the admissions review committee. This committee is comprised of a representative from each professional discipline who is prepared to discuss the appropriateness of the referral and the urgency of need.

The decision to hospitalize a child often involves consideration of the following: (1) severity of symptomatology and relative family dysfunction; (2) a review of outpatient resources thus far utilized and their impact on child and family functioning; (3) the degree of risk posed to the child with the continuation of current circumstances; and (4) the resources that might be called upon as a deterrent to hospitalization. In recent years, shrinking community resources for children and expanding inpatient waiting lists have required increased scrutiny. If admission is warranted, the committee formulates provisional goals for hospitalization that will be refined throughout the initial assessment period. The process continues by contacting members of the family to confirm the referral and elicit their concerns and views of the child's current problems which may differ from those of the referral source. Family members are also asked to state their goals for hospitalization. At this time, permission is requested to contact current care providers (if these should differ from the referral source) in order to enlist their support and cooperation which is vital to the continuity of family care. A preadmission screening appointment is then scheduled and immediate questions and issues are addressed. Beginning with this interaction, the intake social worker should assess the strengths and motivations of family members as well as their potential for active involvement throughout hospitalization.

It is also useful to send to the family a copy of a parent manual that provides a comprehensive program description and an overview of policies and procedures which impact most directly on the child and the family (e.g., the child's daily schedule, visitation privileges). This helps the family prepare for the screening appointment and provides a basis for constructive use of this time.

The screening appointment with the social worker is attended by a minimum of the child and one parent (or guardian) and is an important first step toward engaging the family in a working relationship. It is helpful if either the family's outpatient therapist or the referral source can attend this meeting so as to enlist support and ongoing involvement in the child's hospitalization and to begin dispositional planning as to which target resources are to be contacted prior to discharge. Families and outpatient clinicians are usually quite cooperative with requests in light of their desire for an inpatient evaluation. Parents, children, and others in attendance are provided ample time to ask questions and are given honest answers that convey a realistic view of hospitalization. Information, support, and reassurance are the underpinnings of this initial personal contact that should be combined with an accurate overview of the demands of the admission day and of the overall hospitalization experience.

Formal assessment of the family begins at this point in the intake process by obtaining a brief genogram that will be expanded upon during the admission process. McGoldrick and Gerson (1985) elaborated on this method of assessment and its many uses and benefits with families. For example, they suggested that several areas of exploration can be made more easily available, such as the assessment of the family's attitudes toward treatment through a discussion of current and past treatment experiences that highlights the efforts the family found useful or ineffective. The child is encouraged to be involved in this discussion but is not necessarily the focus. Family issues of importance are often explored through questioning that is centered on significant others' attitudes about an impending hospitalization. Relationship patterns may begin to emerge as details are gathered regarding those family members who may, or may not, be supportive of a decision to hospitalize the child. Information releases are signed to access pertinent records from all other sources involved, especially public welfare agencies and community mental health centers. A tour of the facility is given, and "preemptive" information is shared regarding predictable problem areas following admission (e.g., homesickness issues, loss of clothing items). Predicting the likelihood of common minor problems prior to admission appears to minimize any ensuing disruption and hostility should they eventually occur. Finally, provisional treatment goals as outlined by the admissions review committee are discussed and agreed upon, and the family is encouraged to contact the social worker with any further questions, concerns, or problems pertaining to hospitalization while awaiting the admission date.

ADMISSION

Many of the steps taken during the preadmission process are designed to decrease the family's anxiety regarding hospitalization of the child, increase their awareness of realistic treatment outcomes, and lessen the trauma of the actual physical separation on admission day. However, if the treatment team is ill-prepared and admission procedures appear disorganized and hurried, any progress made in this direction can easily be lost. Therefore, social workers are responsible for sharing intake information with the treatment team and discussing pertinent issues that may impact upon the family at admission. All members of the team are encouraged to review screening information and meet, if only briefly, prior to the family's arrival to coordinate the task that lies ahead. Efforts are made to reduce the amount of repetition that inevitably occurs by having the family meet initially with the entire team. At this time, more detailed information is obtained and family members are often easily engaged in this "mapping" of their history. An informal schedule is then presented to the family to prepare them for individual interviews to follow with a rationale provided for each. Eventually, the child is weaned from the family by a staff nurse who begins the orientation process on the unit with assurances that the child and family will be given adequate time to say goodbye.

The most sensitive aspect of the admission process is often the presentation of necessary legal and release forms which require parents' signatures and which may symbolize the loss of control over their child, if only temporarily. It is important for social workers to be familiar with the legal aspects of admissions, including patient and family rights and responsibilities, and be prepared to answer any questions that arise. Families with strong ambivalence toward hospitalization often need to be reassured that the admission is voluntary, and should be informed of their rights regarding discharge against medical advice. Many families may feel pressured by schools or community resources to accept hospitalization and may deny the severity of the child's problems. The crisis of hospitalization often serves as the family's Achilles' heel and forces the family to realize the possibility that a child may suffer from a more serious illness that requires lengthy treatment and the involvement of other institutions and treating professionals. Social workers can assist the family to accept this type of "loss" and promote the acquisition of greater coping skills. Family members can then be supported with information that will instill a sense of hope and be reminded that hospitalization, which is both necessary and helpful, will require their continued close involvement with the child and the treatment team.

The social worker, who may have the most frequent contact with the family during hospitalization, is often the last person on the team to meet with them. All "final" concerns are then addressed, and an appointment is made to meet again at the earliest possible date to continue the ongoing assessment. The social worker facilitates the separation between family and child and provides necessary support. In some cases, separation is not the major issue. In chronically dysfunctional families and/or families that have experienced multiple hospitalizations of their children, the task of the social worker is to motivate the family to return for continuing assessment and eventual treatment planning which may ultimately include a change in placement for the child.

Finally, the entire treatment team assembles to review the admission, compare notes, and discuss pertinent issues. Initial target problems are outlined and discussion is elicited regarding the perceived needs of the child and family that require further exploration. The strengths and weaknesses of the family system are postulated and the more obvious subsystems are identified while family patterns of interaction are reviewed. Social workers play an important role in helping the team remain family-focused and view the child in the context of his or her natural environment which counteracts the tendency of staff to over-identify with the child. This role is maintained throughout the hospitalization, but, if abandoned, can lead to a schism among hospital staff which is counterproductive for the child and the family.

MANAGING RESISTANCE

In simple terms, hospitalization can be viewed as a therapeutic time-out for families, children, and outpatient resources that are feeling the strain of frustration at the lack of progress or deterioration in functioning commonly associated with the decision to admit the child for evaluation. Relief is often one of the primary feelings expressed by all systems following the admission. However, several minor issues may arise once the child is the patient and the anticipatory anxiety of hospitalization dissipates.

Resistance to involvement in the therapeutic aspects of hospitalization is perhaps the most common major issue social workers face from families and outpatient resources. This resistance takes many forms and may be related to feelings of anger and frustration over the seeming futility of outpatient services, and resentment the family and outpatient clinician may feel at having to look to the hospital for help. There is a tendency to emotionally decompress and to view the inpatient evaluation as the solution to the problem. Consequently, families may fail to keep appointments with the social worker, whereas outpatient clinicians may be slow to provide additional information on treatment history. The child becomes the problem to be fixed and eventually is to be returned to the family to live happily ever after. Outpatient clinicians look to inpatient social workers to perform the same function with families. Efforts to obtain in-depth family and social history and to scrutinize prior treatment interventions vital to the assessment process are often perceived critically and may meet with defensive maneuvering or passive noncompliance. Later efforts to share information regarding successful behavioral treatment interventions may also be undermined and accepted as working only within the structural confines of the hospital. Family relationships with unit staff may also suffer, and the child may be precipitously discharged if feelings of anger, guilt, and a sense of failure are not addressed and directed more appropriately. This type of resistance may be inadvertently perpetuated by inpatient social workers and staff who implicitly accept the omniscient role bestowed upon the hospital. Early and tactful confrontation of these negative views is essential but can only be achieved when social workers support both the family's involvement and the vital role of outpatient resources in the treatment planning process. Liaison work with both systems is the most labor intensive aspect of hospitalization.

LIAISON WORK WITH FAMILIES

Families are encouraged to meet with the social worker a minimum of one time each week during the child's hospitalization to provide pertinent information, complete standardized assessments for the treatment team, and establish a sense of trust that their decision to hospitalize the child was in the family's best interests. Upon completion of the team's formal evaluation and subsequent diagnostic review conference (approximately 2 to 3 weeks after admission), the family is informed of the diagnoses given to the child and the recommendations made by the treatment team as well as the approximate time it will take to complete the inpatient phase of treatment. Parent education regarding diagnoses and psychopharmacological interventions are best addressed by medical staff, though the treatment team can be called upon for support in family meetings. A specific family plan is then developed which clarifies expectations and corroborates clinical recommendations that may include family therapy, parent management training, or a referral for treatment of a serious psychiatric disturbance in one or both parents, such as alcoholism or drug addiction. The actual physical separation that occurs between child and family through hospitalization can be a prime motivator for parents to examine such treatment-resistant issues, which they fear may result in out-of-home placement of the child. Parents are often more susceptible to learning and practicing new ways of managing the child's behavior. Education regarding behavioral management techniques that are used within the hospital and that are tailored for use within the home may be important when dealing with families who use harsh punishment, and may be an effective means to help the child generalize gains made during hospitalization. These techniques are easily modeled by staff and are accessible to families formally and informally, that is, during visitation. Initially, families can be quite reactive when staff exerts control over a child's negative behaviors that were unmanageable prior to admission. This emotional reactivity can be directed into parent management training presented to a single family or to multiple family groups which provide the added benefit of support from other parents and extended family members who may share in caretaking responsibilities. Creative use of videotaping and the use of electronic devices that make it possible to give instruction or suggestions to parents without the social worker's physical presence can enhance family relationships by increasing interactional skills. Usually, such "high-tech" therapeutic activities are well received by parents and children and can be stimulating for all those involved. Parents often report that with growing respect for basic child management techniques comes newfound respect for themselves and their children. This positive view of treatment may be easily transferred to outpatient resources.

In severely dysfunctional families, it may be necessary to share a recommendation of out-of-home placement for the child and perhaps raise such sensitive issues as physical or sexual abuse. Also, in cases where it seems likely that the child will require more structure than the family could reasonably provide upon discharge, work may begin to prepare the family for this placement. As a result, it is necessary for social workers to be aware of child welfare laws and procedures regarding dependency issues as well as the hierarchy of available placements which will address the child's and the family's specific needs. In the case of residential placement, social workers will need to have confidence in this recommendation in order to adequately manage the family's increased anxiety and fear, and to convey the rationale for such a plan. It is helpful for social workers to visit placement sites and collect concrete information on these resources for presentation to families.

More recently, brief treatment models of family therapy have been developed and are being embraced by inpatient social workers who are eager to enhance their clinical repertoire and effective work with families. Alexander and Parson's (1982) functional family therapy model is an example of a brief intervention that shows promise in helping families with difficult interactional problems. In child-focused or enmeshed families, the admission of the "problem child" usually results in an escalation of tension between parents and/or other family members. By tracking this anxiety and tension, the social worker can highlight the alliances most vulnerable in the family system and can provide the appropriate interventions via marital therapy or family treatment. Hospitalization of the identified patient may also exacerbate such underlying illnesses as depression and severe anxiety problems in remaining family members which can also be more easily identified and addressed by the social worker.

Some families have become long-accustomed to dysfunctional ways of interacting and are only able to be reactive. Parents in these families may not be able to identify any remaining strengths in the child or in themselves. The social worker can play a vital role in restoring family structure by first acknowledging these feelings and then strategically identifying strengths through reframing techniques and redirecting their energies in more positive ways through the assignment of tasks (Haley, 1973). These tasks are designed to reduce reactivity and provide family members with a greater sense of control over their actions, which can help redefine appropriate family boundaries and create a healthier equilibrium in the system. In selecting such interventions, social workers must understand their long-term effectiveness and availability to the family upon discharge. Inpatient social workers are in a position of strength and have an array of techniques and interventions that can be tailored to the family's personal style and/or mode of presentation. A captive audience is usually at hand, as well as an entire team of inpatient and outpatient supports. Cooperative efforts with these supports and a willingness to persist in the face of resistance are the key ingredients in inpatient family and social work. Again, any efforts to enhance parent and family functioning during brief hospitalization will be most effective when shared with outpatient therapists who have remained actively involved with the family during the child's hospitalization.

LIAISON WITH OUTPATIENT RESOURCES

Shafii, McCue, Ice, and Schwab (1979) have contended the "recognition that inpatient care of children is only one small phase of the therapeutic process" and have called for the "integration of outpatient and inpatient resources to provide continuity of care rather than the traditional division" (p. 429). Community mental health centers that were struggling to survive during the 1980s have placed increasing pressure on their clinicians to raise productivity while doing little to stimulate professional growth. Many, if not all, consultation and education monies have dried up and salaries have not kept pace with the private sector. Outpatient staffing patterns rely heavily on the attraction of novice social workers who are eager for experience yet lack opportunities for the acquisition of skills necessary for the treatment of chronically or severely dysfunctional families. These clinicians are therefore receptive to efforts made to include them in the child's and the family's experience of hospitalization. As a high percentage of children are referred for evaluation by these clinicians and will return to their care upon discharge, it would seem logical that a more concerted effort should be mounted to provide hospital-based consultation and education programs for community-based resources.

It is unlikely that moves to integrate inpatient and outpatient services will occur rapidly because of economic and political factors which regulate service delivery and its geographical boundaries. Inpatient social workers who are concerned with continuity of care issues must then take the lead in directing increased attention toward cooperative efforts with outpatient resources.

Notification of outpatient clinicians regarding the child's admission should be made on the day of admission if not sooner. Usually, an invitation is extended to meet with the clinician to discuss treatment issues. The clinician is then expected to remain as actively involved as possible with the child and the family to promote the preservation of their clinical relationship. Time constraints are often an obstacle not easily overcome, yet active support of this end usually results in workable accommodations. At a minimum, inpatient social workers and their outpatient counterparts should agree on regular weekly telephone contact to update and review inpatient efforts and formulate dispositional plans. Outpatient clinicians are encouraged to attend the diagnostic review conference, and care is taken to be sensitive to scheduling needs. With prior permission from families, written information regarding specific behavioral interventions can be mailed to outpatient clinicians as well as formal written evaluations and summaries.

When more than one community resource is actively involved with a hospitalized child, a dispositional conference can be arranged prior to discharge to coordinate services, refine dispositional planning, and review the course of hospitalization. This is an excellent time to discuss options available to the family if behavioral and treatment goals are unrealized, or if gains made during hospitalization are not generalized upon discharge. Child case managers who are charged with monitoring service delivery to children and families who are active within the public mental health sector can be invaluable resources toward this end. The entire treatment team's attendance at this meeting is helpful and creates a climate supportive of continued work with families.

DISCHARGE

Families and children rarely report feelings of being fully prepared at the time of discharge despite discussion of dispositional planning throughout the hospitalization. Children are somewhat fearful about leaving the hospital and parents are mistrustful that the gains made will be maintained. Regression in functioning is common, and staff must be alert to, and accepting of, this phenomenon. Social workers should be supportive to families during the confusion surrounding discharge and should encourage children to use skills that were acquired during hospitalization. Children should be assured that mixed feelings of fear, excitement, sadness, happiness, and even anger are normal reactions to anticipated discharge, and should be reminded of the outpatient supports and dispositional plan in place for them.

Inpatient social workers may share the family's concern regarding the consolidation and maintenance of treatment gains and may also question the impact of the services provided. Inpatient staff and members of the treatment team may be reactive to the child's likely regression prior to discharge and convey a sense of doubt to the social worker about the degree of change in the family system or the adequacy of the dispositional plan. Social workers must continually guard against accepting too much responsibility for family change. Therefore, it is also important for the treatment team to meet prior to the child's discharge in order to internally process the course of hospitalization and resolve any conflicts which may have risen. If too little attention is paid to the reactivity surrounding discharge issues, the morale of the entire team may suffer and affect the quality of future service provision.

SUMMARY AND CONCLUSIONS

Even with the aforementioned constraints of increasingly briefer hospitalizations, inpatient social workers remain in an enviable therapeutic position with families. The child's hospitalization provides powerful treatment leverage to elicit the involvement of nuclear and extended family members, as well as significant supportive members who might otherwise resist such involvement. This experience can supply a wealth of family information and insights regarding current and past family functioning. Formal, and even informal, opportunities should be created to observe, assess, and monitor family interactions, and to clarify and confront family issues that are likely to remain undisclosed or ambiguous throughout a course of outpatient treatment.

Inpatient social and family work is entering a period of virtual redefinition as it approaches a new decade. As the implications of briefer hospital stays are felt and the awareness of constraints in service provision increases, social workers will have to struggle with the transition from therapeutic agent to therapeutic liaison. This transformation will require an acceptance of the need to advocate for improved service delivery to children and families across the mental health service spectrum. This task will demand the enlistment of all related disciplines concerned with the enhancement of family integrity and the future needs of children.

There are many reasons to be hopeful in light of advances that are being made in the field of child psychiatry. Changing social, political, and economic forces are moving inpatient social work beyond the confines of the hospital and into the communities that provide long-term direct service to children and families. Inpatient social workers are poised at the forefront of these advances and will play a leading role in their dissemination toward the evolution of more effective service delivery.

APPENDIX

Intake Information Form

Child's Name: ________ Date of Call: _____/_____/_____
Age: ___ Admission Date: _____/_____/_____
Date of Birth: __________ Team: __________
Parents/Guardians: ____________________
Address: ____________________

____

____

Phones: Work ( ) __________ Home ( ) __________
Insurance Company: __________ Phone: ( ) __________
Insurance Information Number: _______ _______ _______
Financial Clearance: Yes ____ No ____
Referral source:
Agency: ____________________
Name: ____________________
Address: ____________________
Phone: ( ) ____________________
Relationship to Family: ____________________
Child's Current Placement: ____________________
Mental Health Catchment Area: ____________________
Child Case Manager: ____________________
Phone: ( ) __________
Current Treatment:
Agency: ____________________
Therapist/Physician: ____________________

Phone: ( ) ____________________
Past Treatment:
Agency: ____________________
Therapist/Physician: ____________________
Phone: ( ) ____________________
Comments: ____________________

____

____

Child Welfare Involvement: Yes ____ No ____
Caseworker: ____________________
Phone: ( ) ____________________
Legal Involvement: Yes ____ No ____
Worker: ____________________
Phone: ( ) ____________________
Diagnoses: ____________________

____

____

Presenting Problems (includes dates of onset, duration, and severity):

____

____

____

____

____

____

____

Medical Problems: ____________________

____

____

Current Medications: ____________________

____

____

Recent Medication Changes: ____________________

____

History of Suicidal Ideation: Yes ____ No ____
Describe: ____________________

____

Homicidal Ideation: Yes ____ No ____
Describe: ____________________

____

Stressors: ____________________

____

____

____

Family Issues/Relationships: ______________________________

____

____

____

History of Physical Abuse: Yes ____ No ____
Alleged Perpetrator: ______________________________
History of Sexual Abuse: Yes ____ No ____
Alleged Perpetrator: ______________________________
Legal Status or Interventions due to Physical or Sexual Abuse: ____________

____

____

School Information: ______________ Grade: ____________
Name/District: ______________ Failed: ____________
Type of Class: ______________________________
Teacher/Principal: ______________________________
Phone: ( ) ______________________________
Academic Problems: ______________________________
Behavioral Problems: ______________________________

____

____

Goals of Hospitalization:

____

____

____

____

Comments/Special Circumstances:

____

____

____

____

Admissions Review Committee Meeting: Date: ____/____/____
Admission Warranted: Yes ____ No ____
If Yes: Urgent ____ Preferential ____ Routine ____
If No: Referrals Made ______________________________

____

Provisional Goals of Hospitalization: ______________________________

____

____

____

Signature of Medical Director: ______________________________

Notes Regarding Contacts prior to Admission: ______________________________

____

____

____

____

____

____

____

REFERENCES

Alexander, J., & Parsons, B. (1982). *Functional family therapy.* Monterey, CA: Brooks/Cole.

Haley, J. (1973). *Uncommon therapy.* New York: W. W. Norton.

Jemerin, J. M., & Philips, I. (1988). Changes in inpatient child psychiatry: Consequences and recommendations. *Journal of the American Academy of Child and Adolescent Psychiatry, 27,* 397–403.

Joint Commission on Accreditation of Healthcare Organizations. (1988). *Accreditation manual for hospitals.* Chicago, IL: Author.

McGoldrick, M., & Gerson, R. (1985). *Genograms in family assessment.* New York: W. W. Norton.

Nurcombe, B. (1989). Goal directed treatment planning and the principles of brief hospitalization. *Journal of the American Academy of Child and Adolescent Psychiatry, 28,* 26–30.

Shafii, M., McCue, A., Ice, J. F., & Schwab, J. V. (1979). The development of an acute short-term patient child psychiatric setting: A pediatric-psychiatric model. *American Journal of Psychiatry, 136,* 427–429.

Woolston, J. L. (1989). Issues in child and adolescent psychiatric hospitalization. *Journal of the American Academy of Child and Adolescent Psychiatry, 28,* 20.

Author Index

Subject Index

Printed in the United States
201083BV00001BD/6/A

9 780306 440793